Masterful Health & Wellness Coaching

Deepening Your Craft

Michael Arloski, PhD, PCC, NBC-HWC

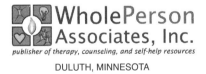

WholePerson Associates, Inc.

publisher of therapy, counseling, and self-help resources

DULUTH, MINNESOTA

Whole Person Associates, Inc.
101 West 2nd Street, Suite 203
Duluth, MN 55802-5004

800-247-6789

books@WholePerson.com
www.WholePerson.com

Masterful Health & Wellness Coaching, Deepening Your Craft

Printed in the United States of America

Editorial Director: Jack Kosmach
Art Director: Joy Dey
Cover Design: Joy Dey
Editor: Peg Johnson

Library of Congress Control Number: 2021934050

ISBN: 978-1-57025-361-4

For Deborah, my love, my friend, my muse.
My dance partner who puts legs under all I do.

Foreword

More than anything with this Foreword, I want to impress upon you how essential Dr. Michael Arloski is to the creation and development, and advancement of the health and wellness coaching profession. I've been his colleague and friend for almost four decades and witnessed how he stands head and shoulders above a field of coaching experts for multiple reasons. Here are the top ten.

1. His humanism is unrivaled.

From the first workshop I took with Dr. Arloski at the National Wellness Institute in early 1990s, I appreciated how he centered his coaching philosophy and practice on the foundational work of pioneers in the humanistic psychology movement, namely, Carl Rogers and Abraham Maslow. This is a branch that revealed how psychotherapy needed a reset from pathologizing to exploring attributes of positive mental health, such as empathy and caring. You'll discover his deep appreciation for that foundation in his opening chapters, where he gives credit to his own teachers.

2. He is an expert in scope of practice.

I can think of no other coaching expert who could write so effectively about how to advance your coaching skills without violating the scope of practice boundaries and thereby falling into the territory of psychotherapy. As both a coach and a counseling psychologist, he knows those grey border areas better than most. No doubt, among the thousands of health and wellness coaches he has trained, many have had moments of thinking, "Oh dear, how did we wind up talking about existential misery or this childhood issue? I've offered empathy and taken a moment, but now what?" We all have lives filled with painful moments or traumatic histories that are pushed into the dark recesses of the human psyche. What can emerge, even in the most upbeat coaching relationship, is a confessional moment that stuns the novice coach.

But don't worry. You'll have a master health and wellness coach, the best one I know of, guiding you through those encounters. Ethical, professional coaches stay within their scope of practice. This book will show you how to respectfully redirect the dialogue and refer to mental health providers or physicians when appropriate.

3. His love of continuous lifelong learning.

Advanced level coaches embody a commitment to improve and learn continually. It is actually a coaching competency, highlighted by both the ICF and NBHWC. Michael demonstrates that commitment in spades. He captures health and wellness coaching trends, further elucidating advanced techniques in a step-by-step fashion. He welcomes input from Jim and Janice Prochaska of the Transtheoretical Model and experts in Motivational Interviewing and then translates the information in a way that ensures readers can understand and apply the tools. These are solidly researched tools and techniques tailored to healthy behavior change.

4. His networking is world-class, and you will benefit from it.

Dr. Arloski is a person who always goes out of his way to help others succeed in their careers. He loves to put people in touch with other people who could help them. As a great networker, he thoroughly enjoys his time traveling with his wife and business partner, the formidably resourceful Deborah Arloski, whether in Brazil, China, or Ireland. I've had the pleasure of sharing a pint with Michael and Deb from London to Stevens Point, and I cherish how he maintains friendships and professional resources. If you're part of the global universe of Arloski-trained coaches, you know what I'm referring to.

5. He is a tireless advocate of widespread placement of health and wellness coaches.

Dr. Arloski has been instrumental in bringing coaches to a variety of settings: insurance plans, disease management companies, self-insured plans, corporate wellness programs, community centers, government agencies, universities, and more. He has championed the inclusion of health and wellness coaches with physical therapy teams, occupational health, diabetes management and prevention, and weight management programs. He has taught countless providers to be more "coach-like" in their managerial communications and interpersonal exchanges. He always seems to keep top of mind awareness that nearly 80% of healthcare costs are due to chronic illnesses such as heart disease, stroke, cancer, type 2 diabetes, chronic respiratory conditions, obesity, and arthritis, all of which are preventable.

6. He is the consummate teacher of coaching methodology.

He has innovated the actual teaching of coaching for over 30 years. I have participated in trainings with him and learned directly from him. He has provided a key service to students and participants in every corner of the globe. Here's something I'll readily admit in print, although he probably won't. Many start-up coach training companies have shamelessly copied his work without credit, and while he and Deb have for the most part accepted it as a form of flattery, I'm using this platform to insist that Michael receive the acknowledgement that he was the first and remains the best. His tools and techniques are duplicated everywhere.

7. He walks his talk, as a living example of coaching-in-practice.

Let me share about the man himself, beyond his work, his books, his teaching. He naturally gravitates to the positive unless he senses I need to unload with a fuming rant for a minute. Then he's the empathetic listener and ally, helping me to calm down with a humorous remark that often allows us to laugh at ourselves, at life, at those things we can't control.

8. He knows the concerns of those with health challenges forced to seek a "new normal."

Michael and I used to sit on the National Board for Health and Wellness Coaching (NBHWC), swapping tales about how there were growing legions of folks who, just because they looked good in yoga pants and could make a decent smoothie, were calling themselves health coaches. Hence, we shared the urgency for national standards for education and training and a new national board certification. We each dedicated a decade to that advancement with renowned colleagues from academic and private training firms. At the same time, as those first competencies were mapped out by NBHWC, Michael was a firm advocate for not over-medicalizing the profession or we would lose the initial need and impetus for non-clinical folks who could serve as behavior change experts to stem the rising tide of chronic disease and help others with lifestyle improvement. Health coaches need to know healthy lifestyle information, but they don't need to be medical practitioners.

One of the many places this book really excels and offers something unique from other behavioral coaching guides is in giving you tremendous insight into the mind of someone newly diagnosed with a medical condition that has them stunned, saddened, or in full denial. Dr. Arloski's descriptions within the final chapter are pure gold for this profession. He chips away at the exteriors of bravado, stoicism, or even stunned immobility that beset individuals (and their families) when faced with troubling medical news. As a former cardiac rehabilitation and CCU RN, I am thoroughly impressed with the exquisite detail that prepares lay coaches with just the right amount of information so they can confidently navigate these corridors for clients.

9. He embodies a cross-cultural sensitivity to diverse perspectives.

I've taught coaching on three continents, and I can assure you, people the world over tend to slide into directive, top-down conversations, telling clients what to do. Michael understands this reflex fully, having broad experience in China, the UK, Ireland, South American, and more places than I can keep track of. His teaching is unwavering; it is the commitment to coaching principles while being aware of radically diverse communication styles among various societies. If you've struggled to refrain from expert-speak, rest assured you have plenty of tips to help you overcome it here.

10. He overflows with life experience.

His editor may want to eliminate this bit, but I have to disclose at least one humorous habit of his. Watch out when he says: "...long story, short..." It's not. Settle back, and grant the man his due. He's earned it. He will be channeling a tale that will have relevance for your predicament, and it will most likely end with a lighthearted anecdote about fishing or something I have no clue about.

Finally, it's been said that the purpose of coaching is to change behavior, but as we uncover more about neuroscience, I think the type of masterful coaching that Dr. Michael Arloski imparts in this book involves not just techniques but real-world wisdom that can alter the nature of the mind. You will sense in these pages that he is actually coaching you, not just imparting a lot of great information. He will teach you how to bring out the best through a whole-person approach, which ultimately transforms lives with less anguish and more positivity. Michael Arloski is a masterful guide, and this culmination of his advanced coaching philosophy strikes me as a profound homage to the humanistic psychology that he cut his teeth on many years ago. In fact, I think it is the next evolution of the human potential movement, disguised as a coaching manual. Enjoy the journey to masterful coaching.

—Meg Jordan, PhD, RN, NBC-HWC, ACC

Preface

The awareness that how we live our lives has a tremendous effect upon our health has never been greater. The wellness field has grown from "helping well people be well-er" through health-risk identification and education, to a more mature recognition of how truly behavioral health is. Lifestyle medicine conferences are doubling in size each year. Acknowledgment that health and wellness coaching is a viable and effective way to individualize wellness has arrived.

Wellness coaching has grown exponentially since I began training wellness professionals to be coaches in the late 1990s. Seeing not only its acceptance, but its embrace by so many individuals, corporations, and organizations has given me gratification beyond anything ever hoped for. So many people have benefited by having the assistance of a real ally to finally succeed at lasting lifestyle improvement. Healthcare and wellness professionals now have a methodology and a way of building alliances with people that makes the job of health improvement and personal growth so much easier. All of this gives me the ultimate satisfaction for the part my colleagues and I have played in developing this field.

Over the course of training thousands of coaches at our Real Balance organization I have reviewed thousands of case studies. I have listened to hundreds of recordings of wellness coaches in action. Observing the direct application of our teachings and methodology has provided great insight into the way wellness coaches do their work and awareness of their strengths and where they struggle to be effective. It has not only resulted in continual improvement of our curriculum but has been a great teacher for me about what wellness coaches can benefit from learning. Working with students in our advanced classes and mentoring coaches seeking credentialing through the International Coaching Federation (ICF), and those pursuing their certification through the National Board for Health and Wellness Coaching (NBHWC), I have seen the need for wellness coaches to develop their craft to a higher level. That experience provided much of the impetus for this book.

In 2006 Whole Person Associates published my book, *Wellness*

Coaching for Lasting Lifestyle Change, with an updated version in 2009 and a completely revised and expanded Second Edition in 2014. This groundbreaking book is used as the primary text in many wellness coach training programs and college and university courses. It has had a powerful impact around the globe. It has even been published in Mandarin. In 2009, Whole Person Associates published *Your Journey to a Healthier Life: Paths of Wellness Guided Journal, Vol. I.* I wrote this book primarily to be used by wellness coaching clients in individual or group coaching as a personal workbook/journal through the coaching process. Many coaches have found it a valuable coaching guide for both their clients and themselves. As much as these books covered, there is a need to provide a deeper dive into the advanced topics of coaching such as collusion and self-disclosure. An aid to help coaches truly polish their craft became self-evident.

Adding graduate school years into the mix, I practiced psychotherapy for a total of twenty-seven years. Recognizing that coaching was something different than therapy, in the mid-1990s I sought out training in the emerging field of life coaching through the Coaches Training Institute (CTI). That was 1996, one year after the International Coach Federation (ICF) was formed.

As a psychologist and coach, I am the first to say that being a better coach does not mean attempting to become a faux-therapist. My background positions me to be acutely aware of the distinctions between coaching and therapy and I will elaborate on these later in this book. My point here is to say that as we deepen our way of coaching we remain in the realm of coaching. Being a better coach does not mean adopting the intricate theories or practices of psychotherapists or some self-help experts. In fact, there is great danger in the person who is not a trained mental health professional wading into that water with a client and not knowing how to really swim.

Wellness coaching could be considered part of the profession of life coaching. Yet, there has been recognition that the work of wellness coaching is something that builds on the life coaching foundation but takes it in distinctive directions. Wellness coaches focus on helping people to succeed in changing attitudes, beliefs, and health behavior. They are often focusing upon daily lifestyle behaviors that are quite specific. At other times they find that the key to changing those behaviors for the better are often rooted in concepts like self-efficacy, social isolation versus connectedness, or environmental and cultural factors. Our approach needs to be both holistic and behavioral, acknowledging the whole person in their environment, and grounding our work in our knowledge of behavioral change. It is my intention in this book to contribute to the continued learning needed for building the quality of wellness coaching services to a higher level. The time to take the profession of wellness/health coaching deeper, to enrich the skills and concepts, is now.

Introduction

Health and wellness coaching, though still nascent, is now a recognized and established profession. We are fortunate that so many individuals and organizations have helped this profession to grow. Now seen as an integral part of any comprehensive wellness program, it is a best practice.

As health and wellness coaching has grown, so have the coaches practicing it. To be attracted to this book most likely you are such a person. You want to learn more and to grow as a coach. You want to go beyond the basics of just goal setting and accountability, beyond tracking calories and sit-ups. Students of coaching, such as yourselves, want to become scholars of coaching. You want to develop greater understanding of the process of behavioral change. You want to learn more about wellness and what the entire field of health promotion has discovered about being well. Such wellness coaching scholars want to become skilled craftspeople.

Health and wellness coaching is saving lives. While coaches do work with clients who arrive stating that all they want to do is lose twenty pounds, the majority of wellness coaches today are working with folks with medical conditions where lifestyle improvement is vital. Chronic illnesses such as diabetes, heart disease, cancer, and COPD, often show up as the health challenges coaching clients are facing. Coaches are now beginning to be integrated into the medical treatment teams that help people improve their health and well-being. Coaches also continue to play a vital role in prevention and with helping wellness programs to individualize the delivery of their services.

We have observed that approximately one-quarter to one-third of the students training to be wellness coaches are preparing to develop their own independent business as a coach or add to the coaching work they already do by specializing in wellness coaching. For the vast majority of coaches practicing in the field, the setting varies including corporate employee wellness programs, hospital wellness programs that serve employees and possibly the public, disease management companies, insurance companies, and various clinical settings.

To bring the quality of the profession to a competent and trustworthy level the National Consortium for Credentialing Health and Wellness Coaches was formed and forged a path to national standards and credentialing. This organization, of which I was a founding member, evolved into the National Board for Health and Wellness Coaching (NBHWC.org). I am now a member Emeritus of the National Board.

The terms wellness coach and health coach are often used interchangeably. At times an organization might make a distinction and refer clients who are working on improving their lifestyle as a way to help with the management of their health challenge (chronic illness, disease) to the health coach. In other organizations the very same referral goes to a wellness coach. The NBHWC decided early in its work to eliminate any such distinction since it is often arbitrary or even contradictory. For the purposes of this book we will most often use the term wellness coach.

Like any true profession, the more we learn about wellness coaching the more we discover we need to learn. I'm fond of the quote I learned as an undergraduate about my major, psychology. Freud's contemporary William James would say, "Our knowledge is but a drop and our ignorance a sea."

The work of this book therefore will be to focus on advancing the process of coaching in the health and wellness setting and attaining a greater level of expertise in that process. Honing our craft as wellness coaches is our goal.

This book is composed of three parts. We will begin with the concept that great coaching is really all about transformation. Changing behavior needs to be viewed not through a unitary lens, but in the context of growth and development. We'll look at how this can be done for both the client and for the coach. The second part will focus on "How to Be," that is, our coaching presence, our way of being in the world and with our client, and the powerful effect this has upon the coaching process. Part Three will examine "What to Do" at a more masterful level, a deeper dive into the craft of wellness coaching. Throughout we will be referencing what we can learn from relevant theory and research, but the emphasis will be on application.

Acknowledgments

It may be safe to say that all books are a result of some grand act of pulling together. It is a gathering in, a harvesting, an inclusion of so much of what has come before. What made this book possible was a pulling together of support and knowledge. The support came from loved ones, colleagues, and my publisher. The knowledge came from many sources, primary among them the thousands of students that our company, Real Balance Global Wellness Services, Inc., has trained.

Dr. Meg Jordan is a wellness professional I have known for many years and for whom I have the utmost respect. Her contributions to the field of health and wellness promotion have been invaluable. I'm blessed with her dear friendship and very grateful, indeed, for the Foreword that she provided for this book.

It is with deep and special appreciation that I extend my thanks to Drs. Janice and James Prochaska for their review and editing of my section on the transtheoretical model of behavior change. Also, sincere thanks to Dr. Adam Archega (Loma Linda University, School of Public Health) for his review and editing of my section on motivational interviewing.

Special thanks go to Nancy Gilliam who supplied an actual case study for me to draw upon. Her work exemplified masterful coaching while working with challenging clients.

For me as a writer, nothing accelerates my ability to fashion my work into a coherent whole as contiguous time in retreat from the day to day world. Thanks to Kim and Fred Devore, for the use of their cabin in the heart of the Rockies.

I speak of coaches being allies and I was fortunate to have the best of such in my Whole Person Associates editor, Peg Johnson, and the rest of that company's ownership and staff. The alliance that, of course, has seen me through this project from start to finish, before and beyond, is my wife and colleague Deborah Arloski. Her content knowledge of this same field, her practical wisdom, patient love, and support has been my greatest gift and asset.

Table of Contents

TABLE OF FIGURES

PART ONE
TRANSFORMATION

Chapter 1—Life Transformation

CHAPTER 1

Life Transformation

*The root of "coach" can be traced to a village in Hungary,
Kocs, where carriages were made in the 1500s. Coaches love
metaphors and what is better than this one: A "coach" takes
you from where you are to where you want to go. Perfect.
The client is the one with the reins and it is the coaching
process that facilitates the journey.*

Evoking Transformation

When people change their lives, they change who they are in the
world. To one degree or another we adapt, we grow, we think, we feel,
and we behave differently. Sometimes the shift is so significant that it
is as though we become a different person—we transform. Ideally, we
are like the moth or butterfly breaking free of the chrysalis and spread-
ing our wings. Our old ways of being seem to no longer serve us. For
clients, life shifts to a new normal. This sort of profound change happens from the inside out yet seems to often need a catalyzing agent to
ignite it and fan the spark into a sustainable flame. It may be the hope
that comes from realizing that one finally has a true ally on the quest.
It may come from an effective methodology for change and growth
that provides structure, support, and accountability. Perhaps reversing
an age-old pattern of negativity and problem-focus into a new model
of positivity and possibility allows the tipping point to be reached. It
most likely comes from a combination of factors like these that unite
into success. When we act as that ally in the growth process, how can
we bring out the best in our client? How can we provide that catalytic
spark that begins the transformational process?

Evocation may be the ideal word to describe how we are engaging with our coaching clients when it comes to life transformation. The Merriam-Webster Online Dictionary (merriamwebster.com, n.d.) defines evocation as: the act of bringing something into the mind or memory. Another online dictionary defines evocation as the "Creation anew through the power of memory or imagination." (merriamwebster.com, n.d.) When we transform we do create anew. What emerges are new ways of behaving, new ways of looking at the world, new ways of being.

Merriam-Webster's secondary definition speaks metaphorically with even more power: "the summoning of a spirit." Rather than a misty apparition at a séance, we are instead summoning the spirit of that person, the energetic essence they have that embraces life and makes the most of it. Call it what you will, perhaps "inner chutzpa." It is the part of us that drives self-actualization, reaching to maximize our human potential.

The coach's challenge is how to facilitate the bringing forth of this essential part of our client. Without the context or trappings of a religious setting, the coaching session serves to provide an invitation to change, to growth—an invocation for the spirit to be with us. In coaching we are inviting the person to connect with the part of them that is most in touch with their own values, the part of themselves that represents who they truly are. This is the part of the person we hope will be guiding the coaching process, steering a course that serves them best. Yet our true self has sometimes not seen the light of day for a very long time. A myriad of doubts, conditions, and other reasons may have buried its expression. To allow it to reemerge the connection has to be made and then the feeling of safety will allow it to surface. Guiding that connection (re-connection actually) and providing the facilitative conditions of trust and safety is the coach.

In the foundational book *Co-Active Coaching*, the authors encourage coaches to take a stand for evoking transformation in our clients. They embrace it as one of their *Four Cornerstones of Coaching*. Our client will often be speaking to us about a concrete goal such as smoking cessation, getting more sleep, or losing weight that represents only a part of their life. They may have a perspective that is narrowly focused on their desire for a better outcome for this goal. "But if we follow that leaf to the branch and then travel from the branch to the trunk and the root—there is always a deeper connection possible" (Kimsey-House, 2018). The coach's job is to hold a larger vision for the client, to see how the topic being discussed, or the actions being taken towards a goal, are in fact connected to that person's fulfillment as a complete human being. Coaches must hold sight of what's possible, even when our clients aren't there yet. "And when that connection ignites between today's goal and life's potential, the effect is transformative" (Kimsey-House, 2018). Now our client realizes that they are not trapped by their circumstances. They are suddenly infused with more confidence that the good life is possible. It is truly within their reach even though it might require a stretch.

In the day-to-day work of a wellness coach it is easy to forget that bigger picture. When coaching is referred to as an "intervention," as it is in some settings, it reflects the medical view of working with people in acute care, as though behavioral change is a treatment to be administered to specific maladies. Part of what has allowed wellness coaching to become a valued and integral part of effective health promotion programs is the realization that lifestyle behavioral change in the non-pathological population does not require therapy or treatment. Behaving in ways that may work against our best health are not pathological behaviors to be "treated." This recognition allows professionals who are not licensed mental health professionals or medical personnel to function effectively as wellness coaches and assist people in achieving lifestyle behavioral change.

Coaches working in larger coaching systems deal with a high number of clients each day. Most of these clients are struggling with health challenges and often challenged to get some basic needs met as well. Coaching for maximizing human potential and the words of Abraham Maslow could sound like academic fantasies. Yet, if we look back to what really motivates behavioral change that lasts, we are once again on Maslow's Pyramid, moving around his Hierarchy of Needs. Yes, we definitely meet the client where they are at and coach them to get their survival needs met first, but even as we are doing that, the coach has to envision the whole pyramid. We keep the perspective that yes, when our client finds childcare that allows them to work part-time it is a step, not just for economic survival, but a first step towards that better life that will allow them to be healthy and well.

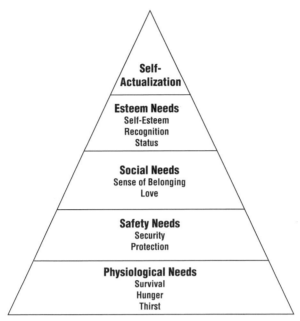

FIGURE 1—MASLOW'S HEIRARCHY OF NEEDS

The Hierarchy of Needs has come under considerable criticism in recent years. We need to loosen our thinking around it and acknowledge new ways to adapt it. It is most important to understand that Maslow's work is about motivation. It does not purport to state that all behavior works in this absolute way. Must we get all of our survival needs met in order to reach out to others and improve our self-regard? Of course not. However, are we *motivated* by survival, gasping for that next breath, as that primal baseline? That is hard to argue. Even Maslow, in his book *Motivation and Personality* (Maslow, 1954), warned us not to get the false impression that a need had to be 100% satisfied before the next need would emerge. All of our needs continuously influence our motivation to varying degrees.

As we consider Maslow's work, let's take in such criticism as that brought forward by Pamela Rutledge (Rutledge, 2011), and acknowledge the greater role that social connection plays while also recognizing that our motivations (as well as our behaviors) are not so ordered into a neat hierarchical triangle. As Rutledge states, "Life is messier than that." While we might not agree that social connection is the singular hub around which all behavior emerges, we should, as she urges us, consider Maslow's pyramid as more of a dynamic interactive circle. The need for "relatedness" discussed in *Self-Determination Theory* (Deci, 2000), and the need for "affiliation" discussed in *Achievement Motivation Theory* (McClelland, 1988), also bring up the importance of our connectedness to the world around us. Bandura's *Social Cognitive Theory* (Bandura, 1977) also shows us how our behavior is an interplay between what we observe in the world around us, how we self-reflect about it, and how we decide to go forward with action.

Regardless of the function of pyramids and circles in our attempts to conceptualize human motivation, we must remember that what has really been the contribution of Maslow and many of the humanistic psychology thinkers is the idea that we are not just locked into a deficit way of functioning. We are here to grow and become all we can be. Our drive to actualize our potential is intrinsic and when we succeed in removing the barriers we naturally actualize more of that potential.

The mindset of the coach can enhance this process of growth and personal development. There is potentially so much more going on in coaching than just increasing or decreasing the frequency of some behavior or behaviors. When a coach operates in a simplistic behavioral fashion there can be immeasurable losses of the "path not taken." If the coach is being true to a wellness mindset, that implies, by definition, operating with a holistic approach. (We will explore the coaching mindset more in Chapter Four.) Successful coaching clients continually report that one thing that allowed them to improve their lives was the belief that their coach showed in them. The coach conveyed that not only was success possible in this world, but that the client themselves could be successful.

What holds wellness coaches back from embracing this transformative approach? Perhaps there are two reasons. First, many coaches, like their clients, aren't aware of what is possible. They may have been trained in a one-dimensional approach that emphasized assessment, goal setting, and accountability. While all three of these are important elements in effective coaching, they are inadequate by themselves. We might ask was the assessment more of a diagnostic evaluation, or was it a client-driven self-exploration that may have integrated external information (such as medical information and inventories)? Was the goal-setting part of a fully integrated Wellness Plan, or just simply goals set as topics came up? Was accountability the only other element present in the coaching process?

Too often wellness coaching is presented as a way to help people with very specific problems, such as weight loss or medical compliance. All efforts are focused on the targeted behavior and the whole process is modeled on either a research process model or a symptom reduction medical model. When coaches are trained in a thorough methodology that is steeped in life coaching principles, holistic, and yet also grounded in behavioral science, and when it follows a positive psychology framework, so much more is possible.

The second reason that many wellness coaches hold themselves back from a more transformative approach may well be the health-risk reduction model that many operate on. Think about it. Health risk-reduction, by definition, only addresses the ground floor of Maslow's Pyramid, survival. Certain behaviors are associated with greater probability of deterioration of one's health through accident, disease, etc. Eliminate these behaviors and the person gains a much greater chance at health. Anytime we succeed in helping a person eliminate a risky behavior it's time to celebrate! The emphysema patient who succeeds at smoking cessation definitely has something to rejoice in.

If, however, we look at what may very well help that same emphysema patient to remain tobacco-free we will probably discover that they need something more. We are stepping up to the next level of Maslow's Pyramid, looking at social connectedness and support, into the dimensions of relatedness and affiliation of which our more recent theorists speak. Does our coaching continue, helping the person solidify their behavioral gains by increasing their connection with other sources of support in their lives beyond the coaching relationship? Can we help them take things further by connecting their accomplishment to that greater vision of living their best life possible? When motivation becomes positive, not just fear-based (avoiding illness), when we strive towards the attraction of a life well-lived, lasting lifestyle, change takes root.

Wellness Is About Personal Growth

As the field of wellness evolved from the work of Halbert Dunn (Dunn, 1959) to that of Don Ardell (Ardell, 1986), John Travis (Travis, 2004), and others, much of their foundational influence was the writings of Abraham Maslow and his contemporaries of the then-called Human Potential Movement. There was a realization that studying how people lived their lives in ways that increased the probability of good health was being overlooked. When we look at the models for wellness that Ardell and Travis in particular postulate, we see how grounded their work is in this humanistic and holistic approach to psychology. Travis's "Iceberg Model Of Health" (Travis, 2004) conveys this, affirming that our state of health is a function of three underlying levels: Lifestyle/Behavioral Level; Cultural/Psychological/Motivational Level; Spiritual/Meaning/Being Realm.

The medical/physiological and the psychological elements of health continue to be recognized as inexorably intertwined. Physiologists constantly bring forth research that continues validating the mind-body connection. Sophisticated neuroscience technology, such as functional MRIs (fMRI), shows us through brain imagery how our very thoughts bring about changes in our physiology. Now the field of lifestyle medicine looks at how improving our lifestyle behavior can be used as a first-line treatment for many illnesses.

> Recent clinical research provides a strong evidential basis for the preferential use of lifestyle interventions as first-line therapy. This research is moving lifestyle from prevention only to include treatment—from an intervention used to prevent disease to an intervention used to treat disease. (Harinath, 2010)

With increased awareness that how the way we live our lives, even the very thoughts we think, have influence on the manifestation of our health, we see that health, whether personal, public, or medical, is much more about behavior and psychology than earlier imagined. When we talk about wellness we are talking about our ways of being and doing that affect health in many ways. When we see this larger picture we realize that while health-risk behavior is certainly one determinate of our health, there is so much more.

So, how can we bring about transformational change in wellness coaching? What will help us to co-create the experience where our clients find themselves saying, "I'm a whole different person now!"

Coaching for Transformation

Maslow often spoke of "self-actualization" versus "self-image actualization." The later being the way we often work on accomplishing an image of who we think we ought to be, that may not actually be congruent with our own true nature. When we express ourselves genuinely, when we achieve our unique measure of success, we do indeed transform our lives. We become who we truly are. The worried mother or father who is holding the family purse strings tight finally has the income to relax and become the generous person they really are. As they see their children thrive and their own self-esteem soar, they do indeed transform, not into someone else, but into their true self.

Our clients often come to wellness coaching hoping that this service will help them to lose weight, stop smoking, manage their stress better, etc. Health risk behaviors are hopefully reduced during the time the coaching takes place. This basic service, if effective, provides the competent, adequate job we hope for.

If we take our services a step further, coaching at a more masterful level so that our clients experience changes in additional areas of their life, even more growth takes place. The wellness coaching client who expected help losing weight would have liked to have improved their time management skills but did not come through the door expecting that to happen. Now they are thrilled that their work/life balance has improved and they actually have time for family, friends, fun, and recreation.

Given the time and opportunity to work more deeply with our client, a holistic and more masterful approach to coaching may yield even greater results. The same client we've been referring to had no idea that the coaching process would help them find more meaning in their life. They discovered, through the insights gained in the coaching conversations and the real-life experiments that they engaged in, that meaning and purpose, or perhaps a greater connectedness with others, nature, and their community, could make such a transformative difference. Such a client is happy to say, "I'm truly a different person!"

Going from "good" to "great" is not just a book title, *From Good to Great* (Collins, 2004). How can we improve the work we do in coaching so that our customer, our client, doesn't just experience a bare minimum service, but experiences coaching delivered by a craftsperson who is an expert at lifestyle behavioral change? Such a coach must possess a combination of skills and mindset that allow growth to occur and be maintained. Taking those skills to a higher level and fostering a mindset that goes beyond "What's wrong, and how can we fix it?" to "What's possible?" is the journey of the coach becoming masterful.

When coaches see their role as agents not just of change, but also of transformation, great things can happen. Evoke transformation!

The Transformation Process

There are many paths available to one who wants to transform their life and accelerate their growth as a whole person. Such a "seeker" could travel on the path of adventure by participating in an Outward Bound trip or traveling to a new country. Life transitions such as launching into a new and rewarding career, a meaningful relationship, even the experience of loss and grief can propel us into profound personal growth. There are infinite possibilities. What wellness coaching offers our seeker is a transformation of their lifestyle, their way of living. When lifestyle improvement happens in a lasting, meaningful, and fulfilling way it can indeed be transformational.

Wellness coaching can help people allow themselves to reconnect with parts of themselves that they are seldom in touch with, or give expression to. When I've asked the client who states that they want to lose 40 lbs., "What will your life be like when you've lost those 40 lbs.?" I hear about feelings and behaviors that they have abandoned, sometimes for years, which they want to reclaim. The person who loved to swim, but won't allow themselves to be seen in public in a bathing suit; the dancer who hasn't danced in years; the light-hearted person who has literally been weighted down by their obesity is yearning to be rediscovered. To "remember" is to reconnect with a part of one's self that has been severed in some way, like a severed member of the body.

Personal transformation is a process of becoming who we truly are and what we are actually capable of. It is giving expression to the qualities that make us special. As our clients cope with life circumstances and operate out of their own belief systems and perceptions of their world, a level of functioning is achieved as best as the person can. An external analysis may reveal that some of their attitudes, beliefs, and behaviors are self-defeating. Pointing these out from the outside brings up mainly shame and defensiveness. As clients engage in some kind of helpful process such as therapy, self-help, coaching, or personal growth through life experiences, they are often able to identify and shift these attitudes, beliefs, and behaviors. As barriers are lifted and change occurs, we see the realization of more of the person's potential and greater expression of their true self. This is in line with basic self-actualization theory.

It is often the challenge of internal and external barriers to change that a coaching ally can help with. Our own belief systems, blind spots (lack of awareness), and self-defeating behaviors may be hard to tackle alone. Our life circumstances may require strategies that are best developed through the mill of conversation and engagement, not just introspection.

> *If you could have done it by yourself,*
> *you probably would have done it by now!*
>
> **— Patrick Williams**

With barriers reduced or eliminated motivation can shift from extrinsic to intrinsic and lasting change can occur more easily. This is where the coach, through the coaching conversation and coaching methodologies, does what no self-help book or computer program can ever do.

— — —

Jay—A Story of Transformation

Three short steps led to the front door of Jay's home. Hand over hand Jay pulled his 305-lb. frame laboriously up each step, tightly gripping the iron handrail. His deteriorating hips screamed with a pain he had become all too familiar with. His muscular dystrophy didn't help either. It was the end of another long day of sitting at the computer, working, making a living, and supporting his loving family. He knew the bigger health challenges he faced, but right now the three short steps were a more than adequate obstacle.

Inside the house, the forty-year-old man dropped into an easy chair and breathed to get his heart rate down. Recently a co-worker had died of a heart attack, and still feeling the exertion of walking across the front lawn and up the simple three short steps, he worried about his chances of remaining around for his family that he loved.

The day before, his appointment with his physician had been what might be described as a consciousness-raising session. Jay experienced a pivotal moment during that doctor's visit. He was diagnosed with a condition called avascular necrosis. The condition was causing pain in his left hip due to the limited blood supply getting to the area. He was in need of a total hip replacement, but the doctor was reluctant to do the surgery because of the complications that often accompany surgery on a person who weighs over 300 lbs. (136 k). He was told that the risk of post-surgical infection was a major concern for a person carrying that much weight. For him to heal and recover well from such a procedure Jay needed to change. He needed an ally to help him do it.

Fortunately, Jay found that ally in a wellness coach/nurse who had become certified as a health and wellness coach. Nancy Gilliam had received both initial and advanced training in wellness coaching. Her work with Jay was captured in a case study (partially presented here) that she wrote for her certification requirements.

At the initial discovery coaching session, Nancy met with Jay and his wife, Dianne.

We spent most of this coaching session gathering information about Jay's current situation. I found that Jay was highly motivated; he said that he had been telling his wife for years that he needed to lose some weight. Just as it was with Jay, it is not unusual for many of us to stall out in the contemplation stage of change. We frequently think that our health can wait until a better time. The fact is, "the better time" is now and every day for the rest of your life. If we wait until the perfect time it will never come.

During this first session we worked through the Wellness Wheel (aka Wheel of Life). The Wellness Wheel is a tool that coaches use to get a snapshot of the areas in life where the client may be dissatisfied. I asked Jay to rate, on a scale of one to ten, how satisfied he was with eight key areas of his life. Through this evaluation process, Jay was able to identify the areas that most needed change. The Wellness Wheel is just one of the many tools that coaches use that allow the client to examine what change needs to occur.

Over the past few years, Jay had noticed that his weight was becoming an issue for him. His knees, hips, and joints continued to cause him pain due to the extra weight that he was carrying. The sports sideline reporting that he loves to do for the radio stations was not as enjoyable because he was in constant pain. Dianne mentioned that Jay was finding it difficult to help with his son's band activities because he "pays for it" the next day. Like many Americans, Jay was starting to experience the burden of carrying too much weight. His weight was not only a threat to his health, but it was starting to affect his family life as well.

When I asked him, "Why now? What is different than all the other times you told your wife you need to lose some weight?" Jay mentioned several things. The first thing he spoke about was that of a co-worker who passed away from a heart attack. Jay said, "He was a big man, kind of like me." We frequently learn from other people's experiences. Other people's journeys can give us a sneak preview of what's likely to occur if we follow that same path. Often, this is just what we need to create the change that we desire in our lives.

The next thing Jay mentioned was that it is very important that he be around to take care of his family. When Jay spoke of a plan he and his wife had been working on to become debt free, I glanced over at Diane to see her reaction. She was looking straight at him through eyes of pride, love, and comfort. I knew that she was going to be a big source of support. Helping relationships are a big part of creating lasting change. The most effective support mixes praise and understanding with encouragement to stick to the work that needs to be done.

The last thing that Jay said was that it was very important that he be able to walk his daughter down the aisle. I could tell by the emotion in his voice that this was something imperative for him. This is where the hip comes in. Walking down that aisle would require two working hips, but at this stage of the game, one was being overtaken by avascular necrosis. Jay looked straight at me and said, "I need to change. I have to change. I need to create a new normal!" Jay's starting weight was 305 with a goal weight of 230.

At the end of the discovery session, I asked Jay if he would be willing to track all of his food and exercise on an easy-to-use app called "Lose It!" I encouraged him not to feel that he had to change anything, but just compare his current diet against what is considered a healthy diet. I also gave him a copy of a healthy eating guide for him to use as a reference. It was important for Jay to have some type of resource in order to make the adjustments he needed to his diet. The goal of this exercise was for Jay to discover for himself the adjustments he could make that would improve his diet and health.

As a coach, I understand the importance of creating small action steps to prevent frustration and the feeling of being overwhelmed. When faced with a health crisis, we often think we need to go from fat, sick, and nearly dead to completely juicing everything we eat. That concept makes for a great documentary, but it is not realistic for the majority of people, and it can leave individuals feeling disappointed and discouraged when they can't stay with the plan. I encouraged Jay to not go on a "diet." Why? Because diets usually fail! I explained to Jay that we would be working together to find his real, authentic diet, one that will naturally promote good health and weight loss.

It only took Jay one day to make a very valuable observation as he compared his diet to what was recommended in Harvard's Healthy Eating Plate. As I was checking my email the next evening I found this message from Jay. "Wow! I am killing myself with sodium." Jay had been looking over his food journal for the day. Food journaling, or tracking, is somewhat like Toto the dog in *The Wizard of Oz*: It pulls back the curtain to reveal what a person may or may not want to see. Jay's calories were well under budget for the day, but he made a very valuable observation. His sodium level was over 7,000 mg, more than triple what it should be.

Frequently, as health care providers, we are tempted to give our clients all the answers. We are tempted to tell them all the things they are doing wrong and how to fix them. That's what we do; after all, we are "health professionals." Health coaching is different in the fact that it allows the client to discover for him or herself the adjustments that need to be made. I never know what will be the shift that turns a client. Sometimes it's the amount of fat or sugar that he or she is consuming. For Jay it was sodium. So instead of me telling him what he should or shouldn't do to improve his health, he was intrinsically motivated to create change for himself.

Jay and I coached for several sessions and developed strategies to bring the sodium down to a level that would be more in line with a healthy diet. His outrage over the amount of sodium he was consuming brought up many discussions about healthy and unhealthy processed meats and processed foods, as well as the amount of sodium in fast foods. Jay started comparing food labels and looking up sodium content prior to eating foods. After a few weeks he cut his sodium back to 1,500 mg per day.

The important thing to know about coaching is that the client gets to choose what is going to best fit his or her needs at that time in the coaching process. Health and lifestyle coaching is a very powerful process because it allows the client to create the change that he or she wants to see in their life. Through health coaching Jay created and took ownership of his own well-life vision. At each session, he created action steps that would bring him closer to his wellness goal. As change occurred, his confidence skyrocketed. Through the process of coaching, Jay increased his self-awareness and self-knowledge about the changes he needed to make.

At the end of 90 days, Jay had lost 43 lbs. In less than four months after our first coaching session, he has lost over 50 lbs. Jay is well on his way back to health!

—Nancy Giliam

— — —

Jay's journey back to health continued with great success. I was fortunate to interview Jay a year later and got his permission to share the rest of his story. He went on to lose over 100 lbs. and make grand reductions in key biometric markers.

Jay's Biometrics—Then
Weight = 315 lbs.
Total Cholesterol 215
HDL = 33
LDL = 114

BP = 108/75

Fasting Blood Glucose = 85

Sodium daily intake = 3,500-4,500 mg

And Now

Weight = 199.5 lbs*

Total Cholesterol 140

HDL = 57

LDL = 62

BP = 105/56

Fasting Blood Glucose = 71

Sodium daily intake = <1,500 mg

Jay was able to have both hips surgically replaced, which improved his quality of life dramatically. As we explored together what had made the wellness coaching so effective he pointed to a number of things, but what stood out was his "Well Life Vision." With the Wellness Mapping 360° Methodology™ we emphasize the need for a positive motivation that pulls the client towards wellness instead of only relying on the negative motivation of avoiding illness and death. After a thorough self-assessment of one's wellness and current state of health, we help the client to create a vision of what living their best life possible would look like. For Jay it was to *"be a rock for my family and participate in life . . . I'm a physically fit 215 lbs. and my health no longer holds me back from my family. I'm physically able to look forward to what the future holds and I'm able to participate in life."*

Jay said that the work his coach, Nancy, did with him simply made sense. He realized that it was the sum of all the little things he was doing every day that made the difference. The way Nancy combined great coaching with key educational guidance pointed him in helpful directions and filled in some gaps, especially in his knowledge and awareness of what he was eating and its effect upon his health. He made healthier choices, abandoned diet soft drinks, and found healthy alternatives. His reduction of sodium drew him away from a lot of packaged foods. Tracking, using his phone-based app, allowed him to avoid self-deception and maintain progress. *"I didn't know where to go. I had so much confusion about what's healthy or not. I was able to find the keys to success that seemed locked away. She (my coach) was able to help me clear out the noise that I would hear . . . and focus."*

Much of Jay's work was with improving his diet and finding the best ways to exercise. He worked with a personal fitness trainer five times a week. However, he attributed a great deal of his success to the accountability that coaching provided. Checking in at each session on the commitments to action that he had made kept him consistent. When he plateaued in the 220-lb. range, Nancy helped him to work with his own frustration and view of his own progress. Together they worked through these internal barriers and set doable five-pound weight loss targets.

As I spoke with Jay, in our post-coaching interview, what came forward was the value of having a true ally, someone he could open up with and process what he was experiencing and feeling through this whole journey. He could share and process his emotions, and deal with his frustrations. Coaching helped him reframe his experience in ways that allowed him to see solutions and gain new perspectives. *"I had a lot of emotional baggage and she helped me unpack it and put it away in the right spots."*

What made my own heart soar was when he told me of his former struggles pulling himself up his three front steps with the handrail, and then said, *"You know what happened today? I jogged up those three steps effortlessly before I realized what I had done! Health Coaching has saved my life! My lifestyle of eating, emotions, spiritual wellbeing, and overall health was in a downward spiral. If left unchecked I would have taken an early exit on life's highway. Now I have the keys to change my life and not just health but overall. I have received my life back."*

Lasting Health Behavior Change

How do people transform their actual health-related behavior? Transformation, by definition, means that the change is lasting, enduring. Yet, we see so many people succeed only at "temporary lifestyle change." When we think even for a moment about it, lifestyle improvement, to be successful, must endure for a lifetime. What do we truly know about how enduring health behavior change is, and how to achieve it?

The theme of the 41st Annual National Wellness Conference was "Spotlight On Sustainability." While we often think about sustainability and our environmental practices, as a wellness coach and psychologist, I immediately thought of sustainable behavioral change. As I prepared for my presentation on this topic, my research revealed that we actually know very little about how effective our efforts actually are at helping people improve their lifestyles in a way that will last.

Maintaining success at lifestyle change is often daunting. Most wellness coaching clients have a history of initiating efforts at losing weight, stopping smoking, managing stress, etc. Many experienced success at making this changes, if only for a while. For many, however, there is a trail of failures at maintaining those new ways of living in the long run. The result is a lowering of self-efficacy and lingering feelings of discouragement.

As I deepened my research quest, I found that other behavioral scientists had been concerned enough about this issue to establish an impressive research consortium to tackle it. The result was a journal article entitled "The science of sustaining health behavior change: The health maintenance consortium" (Ory, 2010). The authors did a thorough research synthesis of articles spanning 2004-2009, amassed resources, and funded 21 projects to look at this issue of lasting change in health behavior. Asking how long can positive gains be sustained without additional long-term support, here is what they concluded:

- In most cases this is unknown because studies only track maintenance for a year or two after the post-intervention phase.

- In the majority of cases, intervention effects on lifestyle behaviors are often strongest in the one or two years closest to active intervention.

- Without additional support, positive effects tend to diminish over time, or treatment differences vanish.

- It's not realistic to expect long-term maintenance based on initial interventions (single-variable research).

- Moderate-intensity behavioral interventions may need to be coupled with more environmental changes to sustain long-term effects.

- In other words people need the support of healthier communities and workplaces, peer groups, etc.

- "Incorporation of physical activity into the *self-concept* emerged as the strongest predictor, with self-efficacy having a major indirect influence confirming it as an important predictor for both behavioral initiation and maintenance" (Ory, 2010).

In summary: The authors conclude "that no single mediator makes a large impact; rather, there is a long and winding road with maintenance achieved through a multitude of modest interrelated meditational pathways from behavioral initiation to maintenance."

There are many reasons for our scarcity of knowledge. One is that much research of this nature is done by universities where graduate students need short-term projects that allow them to finish up and . . . graduate! We may learn more from larger sociological and epidemiological studies such as The Framingham Study (National Heart, Lung, and Blood Institute and Boston University, 2019), the work of The Blue Zones (Buettner, 2012), etc. However, here we are not isolating variables. We can't really say if it was the plant-based diet, the supportive extended family, or the red wine that made the healthy difference. It seems we have to be satisfied with the shotgun approach and put our best bets on culture and environment.

What can we conclude about making positive changes in health and wellness behavior last?

- Changes must be sustainable over a lifetime.

- Intrinsic motivation trumps extrinsic every time.

- Most research looks at single interventions and doesn't track more than one or two years.

- Long-term studies that have been completed show that a combination of environmental support and "internal" shifts sustain lifestyle improvement better. Culture, environment, attitude, and beliefs!

- We must ask how can coaching support shift towards wellness attitudes and beliefs?

The finding that this research consortium could really identify was two-fold: a shift in self-concept and community support. While we should have known how vital community support in all of its forms can be, the idea of focusing more on a transformation of self-concept—the way we see ourselves—is most interesting. This gets at the outcome of truly well-crafted and effective coaching—the client's report that they are "a whole different person now."

Does our coaching and the process of change that our clients engage in engender a new identity for that person? *Now I'm a runner! Now I'm a cyclist! Now I'm an outdoors person—a backpacker, hiker, camper, etc. Now I'm a dancer!*

Much of the work in health and wellness coaching emphasizes the attainment of a list of goals, changes in specific behaviors: reduction of calories, medical compliance, increased physical activity. While all quite legitimate, are we missing what allows these behavioral changes to become locked in place and evolve into healthy habits of a lifetime? Perhaps the overall process of coaching is meant to help our clients build the support they need for the transformation that they seek.

The Five Keys of Coaching for a Lifetime of Wellness

1. Build Self-Efficacy
2. Nurture Visionary and Intrinsic Motivation
3. Focus on the Maintenance Stage (TTM)
4. Co-create Relapse Prevention Strategies
5. Coach for Connectedness

1. Build Self-Efficacy

For the wellness coaching client, self-efficacy is the degree to which they believe that they can affect their health. How much do they believe that all of their lifestyle improvement efforts will bring them the success they seek? How confident are they that they can make these changes and maintain them, especially in the face of temptation? What we often call a lack of motivation is really the appearance of low self-efficacy developed through a history of attempt and failure at lasting lifestyle improvement.

Social psychologist Albert Bandura deeply explored the concept of self-efficacy, which is foundational to wellness coaching. His social cognitive theory (formerly known as social learning theory) shows tremendous congruity between it and the foundational principles of coaching. We will explore how to help clients improve their self-efficacy in Chapter Six.

2. Nurture Visionary and Intrinsic Motivation

Much of our coaching work is around helping people to envision the outcome they want. When we have a clear picture of both where we are (our current state of wellness) and where we want to be (our Well-Life Vision) we can "coach to the gap" between the two and coach around what needs to change to attain that Well Life Vision. Such a positive psychology approach is foundational to coaching and motivates better than simply fear and illness avoidance.

We know that when clients experience intrinsic joy in activities they will be more motivated to engage in them. Look at the work of Jay Kimiecik, *The Intrinsic Exerciser: Discovering the Joy of Exercise* (Kimiecik, 2002), and Daniel Pink's book *Drive: The Surprising Truth About What Motivates Us* (Pink, 2009).

To coach for intrinsic motivation:

- Notice!—Help your clients to focus on the enjoyment, the pleasure that they perceive as they are performing the behavior.

- Inquire!—Ask about the details of their experience. When a client reports about taking a walk, hike, or bike ride outdoors ask about what they saw, what they experienced, what they felt.

- Inquire about Bonus Benefits. Clients sometimes fixate on their goal of weight loss, for example, but what else is happening during their efforts? Are they experiencing more energy? Better sleep? More mental concentration?

- Avoid incentivizing. Incentives tend to decrease intrinsic motivation.

Take a Kai Zen Approach (Maurer, 2014). Coach with your client to set up action steps that are so small that they are very doable and allow continuously successful progress towards their goals.

3. Focus on the Maintenance Stage (TTM)

Of all of the Stages of Change that James Prochaska talks about in the *Transtheoretical Model of Change* (Prochaska, 2016), coaching around the maintenance stage may be the most vital. Here the coach again takes a positive psychology approach and acknowledges and reinforces what is working. As the old saying from coaching goes, "Nothing succeeds like success!" A key in this stage is for the client to see the value in tracking behavior and to do it regularly. Avoiding self-deception is key. Use whatever works for keeping track of new healthier behaviors: calendars, charts, apps, activity monitoring devices, etc. Then the accountability that coaching provides makes the process conscious and deliberate, and increases consistency. Lastly, coaches really prove their worth here as they coach their clients through the barriers and the "push-back" that clients sometimes receive from those they were hoping would provide support.

4. Co-Create Relapse Prevention Strategies

We might say, "Relapse happens! Count on it!" James Prochaska is fond of back-up plans. We all know that life throws us curveballs all the time. Our best-laid plans run up against life realities. This is where coaching can get creative! Coach clients to come up with their own back-up plans for when things don't go as they would like, or when temptation increases. Going to a potluck dinner where the dietary direction of friends tends to be sabotaging of your wellness efforts? Be sure to bring an entrée to share that will satisfy your own needs. Not enough time to do your hour-long exercise routine? Having a quick and simple set of exercises you can do anywhere fills in "better than nothing" and maintains engagement in your program.

Pivotal to this key is self-compassion. There is a real difference between excuse-making and true compassionate understanding. Coach your client to be less self-critical and more forgiving. Help them keep a healthy perspective on their Wellness Plan.

5. Coach for Connectedness

More masterful coaches are coaching for connectedness from day one. The amount of time any client spends in coaching is a brief moment compared to the lifetime they have to live in a new way. In addition to the support of the coach, other sources of support must be encouraged, discovered, or consciously developed. For each step of action we ask "Who or what else can support you in this?" If our client has little support then making the development of such support a deliberate area of focus to work on in coaching is vital. This is where the role of culture, community, workplace, peer groups, family, friends, and relationships becomes a part of coaching that cements lasting lifestyle change.

Living a wellness lifestyle is a lifetime job! Providing the kind of coaching that goes beyond simplistic goal-setting and allows our clients to transform who they are can build the foundation for a lifetime of wellness.

Meaning and Purpose

The purpose of life is to live it, to taste experience to the utmost, to reach out eagerly and without fear for newer and richer experience.

— Eleanor Roosevelt

Personal transformation and growth seems to inevitably connect with achieving a greater sense of meaning and purpose in life. Those in the helping professions have long observed that people who have a sense of meaning and purpose in their lives appear to do better with their lives in general and their health in particular. Research over the last ten years is showing us that our observations were spot on. A clear, if even very simple, sense of one's values, meaning, and purpose is linked with greater longevity, fewer heart attacks and strokes, better diabetes management, better sleep, less depression, less sedentary behavior, less Alzheimer's disease, and even better sex! (Boyle PA, 2010), (Hill, 2014), (Kim, 2013), (Kim ES1, 2015), (Rasmussen, 2013), (Prairie BA, 2011).

As early as 1977 in the first edition of *High Level Wellness* (Ardell, 1986), wellness author Don Ardell included Meaning and Purpose in his model of wellness under the dimension of Self-Responsibility.

*An aim in life can help you obtain the kind of rewards
needed for fulfillment and balance, and is crucial to your
feeling centered and reasonably content with your life.*

— **Don Ardell**

Ardell notes that the famous stress researcher, Hans Seyle "Believes that a goal or purpose in life is fundamental to positive health and well-being." Ardell continued to emphasize meaning and purpose in his 1977 book *14 Days to High Level Wellness* (Ardell, 1977, rev. 1982) by including it as one of his five dimensions of wellness. In 2016 he and wellness psychologist Judd Allen collaborated on a new book on purpose and leadership (Allen, Ardell, 2016) continuing to develop this important theme.

Business leaders, life coaches, and executive coaches have continuously linked Meaning and Purpose with better work and career performance. Kevin Cashman, author of one of the best books ever written on leadership, *Leadership from the Inside Out*, (Cashman, 2017), included "Purpose Mastery" as one of his "Seven Pathways To Mastery of Leadership From Within." He sees it as a way to lead by expressing our gifts to create value.

> Purpose gives meaning and direction to all life. It is the context that frames all of our life experiences into a meaningful whole. If we have it, all the challenging experiences of life serve to forge our identity and character.
>
> Purpose may be the most practical, useful connection to an effective life. It is bigger and deeper than our goals. It is life flowing through us. Purpose releases energy. The higher the purpose, the greater the energy. Purpose also frees us. The more profound the purpose, the greater the sense of freedom. Purpose opens up possibilities.
>
> Purpose is not a goal to be set. It is not something you create. It is something you discover. It calls you.
>
> — **Kevin Cashman**

For Cashman, having purpose allows average-performing individuals and organizations to become highly effective ones. He urges us all to live our lives on purpose.

In recent years there has been more attention given to this topic in the media and in the work of people like researcher Victor Strecher at the University of Michigan (Strecher, 2019). He sees a direct connection between having a purpose in life and how we behave, particularly in terms of choices that affect our health. For Strecher, lacking a sense of purpose is just as great a health risk as any other (e.g., smoking, obesity, etc.). He believes that when we start thinking "bigger than ourselves" (self-transcendence) we behave in ways that result in great health.

Clarifying our values is a key step to developing our sense of meaning and purpose. Strecher cites research showing that cigarette smokers who affirm their core values are more open to anti-smoking messaging and less defensive about it. He also found that people are more likely to participate in diabetes risk assessments if they have just completed their values list (Falk, 2015).

Evidence of the connection between health and having meaning and purpose continues to mount. Strecher and other researchers at the University of Michigan "...found that people with greater senses of purpose in life were more likely to embrace preventive healthcare: things like mammograms, prostate exams, colonoscopies, and flu shots" (Kim ES1 S. V., 2014).

The work of Kim, et al. (Kim, et al., 2013) (Kim, et al., 2010), found that greater purpose in life reduced the risk of myocardial infarction (heart attack) and reduced the incidence of stroke in older adults.

The connection between longevity and meaning and purpose has increasingly found support as well. Dr. Patricia Boyle, a neuropsychologist at the Rush Alzheimer's Disease Center and an assistant professor of behavioral sciences at Rush University Medical Center in Chicago, studied 1,238 older adults using a sense-of-purpose evaluation. When comparing scores, Boyle found that those with a higher sense of purpose had about half the risk of dying during the follow-up period as did those with a lower sense of purpose. And she said that was true, even after controlling for such factors as depressive symptoms, chronic medical conditions, and disability.

"What this is saying is, if you find purpose in life, if you find your life is meaningful and if you have goal-directed behavior, you are likely to live longer," she said (Boyle, 2010).

Though much other research has found that having a purpose in life is crucial to maintaining psychological wellness and can be important for physical health as well, Boyle said she believes the new study is one of the first large-scale investigations to examine the link between life purpose and longevity" (Boyle PA, 2010).

A study at the Mayo Clinic by Rasmussen, et.al., showed that lower purpose in life satisfaction was associated with higher hemoglobin A1C scores in diabetic patients. The study recommended that:

> The primary care clinician is encouraged to consider screening for purpose in life satisfaction by asking a single question such as "Do the things you do in your life seem important and worthwhile?" The patient's response will assist the clinician in determining if meaning or purpose in life distress may be interfering with diabetes self-care. If this is the case, the clinician can shift the conversation to the value of behavioral and emotional health counseling (Rasmussen, 2013).

The purpose of life is not to be happy. It is to be useful, to be honorable, to be compassionate, to have it make some difference that you have lived and lived well.

— **Ralph Waldo Emerson**

The Coach's Take-Away—Meaning and Purpose

Despite the recognition of the importance of meaning and purpose in personal and professional growth, and numerous studies linking it to the previously mentioned health benefits, the topic is often absent in health and wellness promotion programming. Such programs often use a less-than-holistic approach that focuses on concrete, measurable, and objective goals (such as weight loss, health-risk reduction, etc.). Unfortunately some health and wellness coaching work is done the same way. While the rigor of a behavioral approach is appropriate, we must not forget the whole person. This may be where it is good to remember that wellness coaching or health coaching is really a part of life coaching. Our best work comes forward when we help our client to improve their *lifestyle* by helping them improve their *life*.

Such whole-life coaching can include helping our clients to create a Wellness Plan that is based upon their values. In helping people get clear about what they truly want in life and develop a Well-Life Vision, we help them get more in touch with what their sense of meaning and purpose is. Such a Vision guides them in co-creating with their coach a Wellness Plan that will best serve them.

Masterful Moment

When the client lacks clarity about their values and sense of meaning and purpose (again, no matter how simple it might be) it will be harder for them to see an imperative motivational link between the goals they are attempting to achieve to improve their wellness and the action steps they are taking to get there.

Helping Your Client to Discover Their Sense of Meaning and Purpose

Getting in touch with one's meaning and purpose is not something that can be artificially injected into a coaching process. People arrive at clarity about meaning and purpose at many different stages in life. Some folks find it in their youth, others not until the golden years. What a coach can do, however, is help their clients make the seeking of meaning and purpose more of a conscious process. For many it is a matter of getting in touch with the meaning and purpose that they already have.

1. **Help your client to get in touch with and clarify their values.**

   Powerful questions in the coaching conversation can challenge a client to look a little deeper. "What would it look like…" questions are very effective here. "So, what would your life look like once that weight loss is accomplished?" "What would your life be like smoke-free?" "If there was nothing in the way and you could spend a day doing exactly what you want, what would that look like?" "Who else would benefit from you managing your diabetes at a truly effective level?" Also explore "What really energizes or excites you?"

A Values Clarification Exercise

A fun exercise to help your client get in touch with values is to have them describe what they would do on a vacation of their choosing. Present the exercise in a way like this: *"Let's say you have two weeks to take a vacation and there are no obstacles in the way. You can afford it easily. You won't get behind at work. No problems. You are just doing what you would like to do for two weeks. Describe for me, in detail, what your vacation would be like."* Each person's vacation story will tell so much about them. While one person would backpack the Appalachian Trail, someone else would take an organized bus tour of the Civil War Battlefield sites in the Mid-Atlantic States. From this conversation draw out what values showed up.

2. **Ask them to what degree they feel they are living their life in accordance with their values.**

   The Institute of Stress at McGill University (where Hans Selye did his pioneering stress research) says that the greatest source of stress we can have in our lives is to be living our lives out of accordance with our values. Be prepared for some sadness and possibly regret. Empathize and help your client explore the compromises they have made, the trade-offs, and what they are ready, or not ready, to do about this. Help them to identify what steps they may be ready to make to live the life they really do want to live. This process may have a tremendous and positive effect on their Wellness Plan.

3. **Help your client to live their life on purpose.**

   As you explore what is important to your client, help them construct experiments that can help them to be more in contact with what brings them joy. The pet lover may want to volunteer at an animal shelter. The nature lover may want to see what environmental action organizations are in their community. The closet writer may benefit from taking a risk and joining a writers group.

4. **Encourage self-reflection.**
Busy lives end up lacking in time for self-reflection. Putting one foot in front of the other, caring for a family, developing a career, etc., we often get out of touch with our true self. As your client values the process of exploring meaning and purpose, encourage them to keep a personal journal. Encourage them to read books that will help with self-exploration and personal growth. (Victor Frankl's classic *Man's Search for Meaning* heads the list.)

Solo time is a self-reflection practice that can have tremendous value. This may be as simple as setting aside an afternoon to spend quietly alone as you set all work aside. Or it may take on the commitment of a personal quest adventure. You might also introduce your client to the idea of a "technological Sabbath" where they go dark for a day (no media of any kind, internet, texting, or even phone use) and spend the time more purposefully.

5. **Make the development of a greater sense of meaning and purpose a conscious part of the Wellness Plan.**
Instead of seeing meaning and purpose as something that just evolves on its own, help your client to engage in a purposeful quest to achieve a greater sense of meaning and purpose. Through the coaching process experiments and action steps can be set up to carry on this exploration. The goal is not to attain clarity on any particular timeline, but to begin the journey and do it consciously!

It may seem challenging to fit a personal exploration of meaning and purpose into a wellness program, or into a coaching process, but if *lasting* lifestyle improvement is what we are after, it may be one of the most valuable endeavors we can pursue.

Food for Thought—Meaning and Purpose

Do people with greater meaning and purpose have a different way of viewing the world? Are they less reactive to stress? Does greater meaning and purpose and all of the cognitive and emotional functioning that goes with it serve to buffer the individual from the effects of stress? Does this way of thinking and feeling result in less perceived stress, functioning as a filtering mechanism as we are exposed to potentially stressful experiences? Is this really what we are talking about when we speak of resilience?

The mystery of human existence lies not in just staying alive,
but in finding something to live for.

— Fyodor Dostoyevsky, *The Brothers Karamazov*

Transforming Wellness Coaching

In the following chapters we will be equipping you to be a better wellness coach by focusing on effective ways of being and doing in the coaching process. It is our intention to foster your deeper development as a craftsperson in the artistry of wellness coaching.

Wellness coaching as an integral craft—we will look at how the coach's own personal growth and transformation on the path to mastery can better equip them to provide more effective coaching. We will look at how the coach can develop their craft more deeply and employ a gentle self-vigilance that keeps them serving their client well.

REFERENCES

Allen, J., Ardell, D. (2016). Leading for Purpose: How to Help Your People and Your Organization Benefit From the Pursuit of Purpose. Healthyculture.com.

Ardell, D. (1977 Rev. 1982). *High Level Wellness: An Alternative to Doctors, Drugs and Disease.* Rodale Press, 1977

Ardell, D. (1982). *14 Days to Wellness: And a Lifelong Pursuit of Whole Person Excellence.* New World Library.

Bandura, A. (1977). Toward a unifying theory of behavioral change. *Psychological review*, 84(2), 191-215.

Boyle, P.A., Buchman, A.S., Barnes, L.L., & Bennett, D.A. (2010, July). Effect of a purpose in life on risk of incident Alzheimer disease and mild cognitive impairment in community-dwelling older persons. *Archives of general psychiatry*, 304-310. http//10.1001/archgenpsychiatry.2009.208

Buettner, D. (2012). *The blue zones: Nine lessons for living longer.* (2nd ed.). National Geographic.

Cashman, K. (2017). *Leadership from the inside out: Becoming a leader for life.* (3rd ed.). Berrett-Koehler Publishers.

Collins, J. (2004). *Good to great: Why some companies make the leap...and others don't.* Harper Collins.

Conley, C. (2007). *Peak: How great companies get their mojo from Maslow.* Josey-Bass.

Deci, E. A., & Ryan, R. M. (2000). Self-Determination theory and the facilitation of intrinsic motivation, social development and well-being. *American psychologist. 55*(1), Jan. 2000, 68-78.

Dunn, H. L. (1959, June). High-Level wellness for man and society. *American journal of public health*, 49(6), 786-792.

Falk, E. B., O'Donnell, M. B., Cascio, C. N., Tinney, F. Yoona, K. Lieberman, M.D., Taylor, S. E., An, L., Resnicow, K., & Strecher, V. J. (2015, February 17). Self-affirmation alters the brain's response to health messages and subsequent behavior change. *Proceedings of the National Academy of Science USA.* 112(7). https://doi.org/10.1073/pnas.1500247112

Frankl, V. (2012). *Man's search for meaning.* Rider.

The Free Dictionary. (n.d.). http://www.thefreedictionary.com/evocation

Harinath, B. (2010). *SVYASA Yoga University, Bangalore.* Convocation Address. SEVAMED: A Journal with Judicious Blend of Spiritual & Medical Science.

Hill, P. L. (2014). Purpose in life as a predictor of mortality across adulthood. *Psychological science*, 1482–1486 .

Kim ES1, H.S. (2015). Purpose in life and incidence of sleep disturbances. *Journal of behavioral medicine,* 590-597.

Kim ES1, S.V. (2014). Purpose in life and use of preventive health care services. *Proceedings of the National Academy of Science.*

Kim, E.S. (2013). Purpose in life and reduced incidence of stroke in older adults: The health and retirement study. *Journal of psychosomatic research.* 427-432.

Kim, E.S. (2010). Purpose in life and reduced risk of myocardial infarction among older U.S. adults with coronary heart disease: A two-year follow-up. *Journal of behavioral medicine.*

McClelland, D. (1988). *Human motivation.* University of Cambridge Press.

Merriam Webster's Dictionary (n.d.). https://www.merriam-webster.com

Milton, J. P. (2019). home page. *The way of nature: Spiritual fellowship.* http://sacredpassage.com

Papanicolaou, G. (2019). *The Framingham heart study.* National Heart, Lung, & Blood Institute & Boston University. rhttps://www.framinghamheartstudy.org

Ory, M. L., Matthew Lee Smith, Nelda Mier, & Meghan M Wernicke (2010). The science of sustaining health behavior change: The health maintenance consortium. The *American journal of health behavior,* 647-659.

Pink, D. (2009). *Drive: The surprising truth about what motivates us.* Riverhead Books.

Prairie B. A., Scheier, M. F. Matthews, K. A., Chang, & C. H. Hess, R. (2011). A higher sense of purpose in life is associated with sexual enjoyment in midlife women. *Menopause,* pp 839-844.

Prochaska J. O. & Prochaska M. J. (2016). *Changing to thrive: Using the stages of change to overcome the top threats to your health and happiness.* Hazeldon Publishing.

Rasmussen, N. S. (2013). Association of HbA1c with emotion regulation, intolerance of uncertainty, and purpose in life in type 2 diabetes mellitus. *Primary care diabetes.* pp 213-221.

Rutledge, P. (2011, Nov. 08). Social networks: What Maslow misses. Retrieved 2-11-19. *Psychology Today.* https://www.psychologytoday.com/blog/positively-media/201111/social-networks-what-maslow-misses-0

Strecher, V. (2019). home page. Retrieved from *On purpose.* http://www.dungbeetle.org

Travis, J. (2004). *The Wellness Workbook* (3rd ed.). Celestial Arts.

The trick to real and lasting lifestyle changes *HEALTHbeat*(n.d.). Harvard Health Publishing https://www.health.harvard.edu/healthbeatat/the-trick-to-real-and-lasting-lifestyle-changes

PART ONE

TRANSFORMATION

Chapter 2—Transformation of the Coach: Wellness Coaching as an Integral Craft

CHAPTER 2

Transformation of the Coach: Wellness Coaching as an Integral Craft

If one really wishes to be master of an art, technical
knowledge of it is not enough. One has to transcend
technique so that the art becomes an "artless art"
growing out of the Unconscious.

D.T. Suzuki – Introduction to *Zen in the Art of Archery*

Any master musician, master psychotherapist, or master coach is grounded in theory. This grounding allows them to think on their feet because they know the science, whether it is music or mathematics or behavior. When the coach works with their client, they operate from this base of theory and let the art lead the way. The art transforms the science into a craft. When a coach, in particular, does not understand this "in their bones," as the Coaches Training Institute likes to say, they come across as impersonal. They are not connecting person to person at the level they could.

Since 1965, the American Academy of Psychotherapists has been publishing the journal *Voices: The Art and Science of Psychotherapy*. Written quite purposefully in a personal rather than academic tone, the journal had a deep influence on me in my formative years as a psychotherapist. I realized that the way in which we deliver our science-based knowledge is just as important as the knowledge itself. Witnessing the work of master psychotherapists in action, I quickly was in awe of the art they displayed. Observing an accomplished therapist like Laura Perls, or Joseph Zinker, at the Gestalt Institute of Cleveland was like experiencing pianist Arthur Rubinstein perform Beethoven's "Moonlight Sonata." Rubinstein's contemporary was Van Cliburn. While the ultimate technician, Van Cliburn lacked the heart and soul that somehow came through when Rubinstein played. As one musician friend of mine said, "When Van Cliburn plays the 'Moonlight Sonata,' you are impressed. When Rubinstein plays it, you weep at the beauty."

In this evidence-based world, the "art" is often forgotten or dismissed. Yet, the application of science in clinical and coaching practice requires art. The transition of art and science into practice becomes a craft. The development of a craft is part skill and technique, but just as we spoke in analogy about musicians, the real craft comes by developing something beyond technique.

Becoming a craftsperson is a concept that can be applied to any endeavor. We can look at the work of a potter, a weaver, a singer, or a web designer and say, "Now that's a craftsperson!" Such a person is often called an *artisan*. Even in a huge, modern grocery chain store, surrounded by industrialized, pre-packaged foods, we are drawn to the artisanal bread and similar items, and are willing to pay more for such items. Quality is appreciated, and rewarded.

A finely executed piece of work (or performance, delivery of a service, painting, etc.) shows us a dedication to quality. Quick shortcuts are avoided and more purposeful steps are taken. Part of what is evident in the work of an artisan or more masterful coach is creativity and imagination. From this comes innovation. I recall witnessing health promotion pioneer Dee Edington tell his audience, "If all you do is evidence-based, you'll never innovate!" Of all the times jazz legend Miles Davis played the tune "So What," it's safe to say it was never played exactly the same way twice. Creativity and intuition are present in the work of the craftsperson coach fitting the work to the unique person at this unique moment in time.

The craft of wellness coaching is not, however, free-form abstract art. Fine craftspeople work within structure, respecting the laws of physics, the nature of their materials, their subject matter. Likewise the coach who has elevated their work to a craft honors the value of structure, proven methodology, and effective skills and tools. Our clients make so much more progress when they have co-created, with their coach, a well-designed Wellness Plan.

Witnessing the craftsperson in action we see a continuous desire to improve. This is the truly professional waiter/waitress studying the food production and delivery systems, the seating floor plan, and the nature of the clientele in the restaurant to calculate their most efficient table delivery routes and provide the best customer service experience. This is the university professor studying how to teach, not just learning more about their subject matter. This is the wellness coach spending hours listening to recordings of their own coaching and reviewing where their competencies need improvement. This is about the transformation of competencies into proficiencies and beyond.

Most wellness coach training is aimed at developing competencies. Competency implies an adequate and acceptable level of skill and knowledge. Every client certainly wants his or her coach to be competent. Yet, wouldn't every client want their coach to be not just competent, but truly proficient or even masterful at his or her craft? How does a coach move up a notch to a level where they are coaching beyond the basics, where they are fluidly implementing what they have learned and can now think on their feet, dance in the moment, and be creative?

Masterful Moment

Who do I want to be as a coach?

How do I create a default mind of curiosity?

How can my values shape my desire for mastery?

How can I be inspirational?

Apprentice, Journeyman, Master

Since the Middle Ages there have been traditional systems of study to learn crafts. Someone skilled at a craft, say blacksmithing, would take on a young apprentice who would work for years and years at the master's side, doing the menial tasks of assistance and watching closely. At some point they would be permitted to pick up the tools of the trade and begin trying their hand at the beginnings of the craft. Starting with projects that risked little to the business, doing supplemental production work the journeyman learned directly by doing, by practicing.

When we think of master craftspeople, often the Japanese masters come to mind. The work of master potters, sword builders, and other artisans sometimes astonishes us with their perfection. The Japanese system of master-apprentice had Chinese origins as the custom of master-apprentice found its way to the islands of Japan from China, often via Korean immigrants around 300 A.D. The Japanese formalized these customs and added the concept of *Kaizen*, or continuous improvement. "As generations passed these institutions and rituals were strengthened by the introduction of the Zen principles of dispensing with the superfluous and harmonizing life and nature, resulting in masters who could actually achieve virtual perfection in the arts and crafts" (Mente, 2009).

Today wellness coaches usually go through no such apprentice-like process. If they are working for a company or organization that provides coaching, they are often thrown into the deep end of the pool and expected to coach as soon as trained. It is a combination of training and learning-by-doing. Hopefully there is an emphasis on self-evaluation, listening to recordings, etc., and working with a coaching supervisor or mentor. Independent (self-employed) coaches may be able to transition to higher levels of proficiency more gradually as they continue to further their coaching education through advanced classes mentoring and experience.

The Four Stages of Competence

The Four Stages of Learning (also known as The Four Stages of Competence) is a theory posited by psychologist Abraham Maslow in the 1940s. Then in the 1970s Noel Burch brought this forward as The Four Stages of Competence (Exceptional Leaders Lab, 2019). Let's examine how they apply to the learning journey of the wellness coach.

1. Unconscious Incompetence: This stage can be simply described as *you don't know what you don't know*. This is like the health-care professional who has been assigned to be a wellness coach without any training or introduction to what wellness coaching actually is. Most likely they will attempt to coach by doing what they have done before in their profession—educate, diagnose and consult, etc. They think they are doing a good job, but are truly unaware of what effective coaching is really all about.

2. Conscious Incompetence: You don't understand or know how to do something, but you do recognize that the deficit exists. For example, I may have played a trumpet in high school band, but I have no idea how to play a chord on a guitar. There's nothing wrong with that, I just don't know, but I realize this and want to learn. This would be the wellness coach that we described above when they realize that their old way of educating or consulting just isn't getting the behavioral change job done. They seek out wellness coach training.

3. Conscious Competence: You understand or know the how, but demonstrating this skill or knowledge requires your concentration. Our budding guitarist has taken lessons and is continuing to practice. As they do, they have to engage in more effortful concentration, perhaps watching music charts, looking at their finger placement on the fretboard. At this stage our developing coach is equipped with skills, tools, and methodology but has to practice with real focus on the coaching process.

4. Unconscious Competence: You have had so much practice that the skill or knowledge becomes second nature and can be performed easily. Fingers move fluidly as our guitar student glides easily through chords and finger-picking. They can reach whatever note they want whenever they want it. They probably migrate to playing jazz! Our coach can now think on their feet. Theory is so ingrained, skills so well practiced that a wide variety of coaching responses are easily accessible. This more masterful coach inherently trusts the coaching process and is free to be creative and spontaneous. They dance in the moment like they absolutely love being out on the dance floor!

Coaching and the Mastery Path

Becoming a masterful wellness coach is much akin to developing a masterfully healthy lifestyle. It is not an event, a training, an experience, a certification, or a degree, but rather a lifetime journey. We craft a wellness lifestyle and then must practice it—live it! We craft a profession as a wellness coach, and then practice it, and grow it.

In his classic book *Mastery: The Keys to Success and Long-Term Fulfillment*, George Leonard describes the path to mastery as one of short bursts of increased performance followed by slowly ascending plateaus (Leonard, 1992).

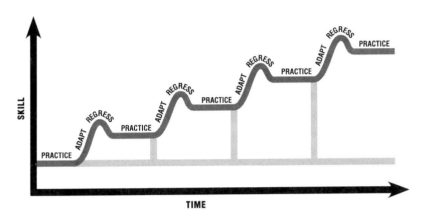

FIGURE 2—THE MASTERY CURVE, Adapted from the book *Mastery* by George Leonard

The key is to learn to enjoy the plateaus and know that eventually there will be progress. We live most of our life in these plateaus. Regardless of what we are trying to master, whether it is losing weight, smoking cessation, or deepening our professional skills, the journey is fraught with plateaus. It is full of the mundane. The musician practices scales over and over. The martial artist goes through their *katas* endlessly. Great musicians, golfers, yogis, all learn to love the practice. Living a wellness lifestyle is really practicing a way of living...over and over again.

Our coaching practice can also become mundane. To keep it alive we have to notice. Noticing—being aware and mindful of the here and now—allows us to discover intrinsic joy through our senses and our emotions. Noticing is my own term for mindfulness.

It is easy to allow the process of coaching to become rote, routine. The independent coach may specialize in a certain area and fall into a template-like way of working with most of their clients. The busy coach in the disease management company or employee wellness program may have a routine prescribed by the system in which they work where checking the boxes of completed tasks may become paramount. Your challenge is to still notice, to still engage.

Leonard's Five Keys to Mastery

In his book *Mastery*, George Leonard describes five keys to mastering anything, be it music, tennis, computer programming, or, in our case, developing into a masterful coach. He points to:

1. Instruction
2. Practice
3. Surrender
4. Intentionality
5. Pushing the edge

Let's look at each of these as they relate directly to your development as a health and wellness coach.

1. Instruction

a. Look for coach training that is approved by the National Board for Health and Wellness Coaching and the International Coaching Federation.

b. Look for programs approved by a good variety of health-related professions for continuing education credit. Ideally such training includes what we know from the fields of health and wellness promotion, not just life coaching.

c. Get great foundational wellness coach training, but then, just as importantly, look for advanced training in wellness coaching. Look for courses that take your learning further and deeper, beyond basic competencies. Continuing education should be part of professional life. Some companies supply CEs for their professional employees. If your firm does not, seek CEs out on your own.

d. Finding a great mentor, who specializes in wellness coaching in particular, can be the key to your transformation as a masterful wellness coach. One of the central advantages of mentorship is that it is a feedback process that focuses on your actual practice of coaching.

e. Your continuing education needs to be a blend of the intellectual, the theoretical, and the practical.

2. Practice

Practice, practice, practice. Certainly, there is no substitute for increased experience. Yet, something we are learning about practice is that it is not all the same. There is a myth about the number of hours that produces mastery. It is sometimes called the *Myth of the Ten Thousand*. A commonly held idea or belief is that practicing most any skill or craft for approximately 10,000 hours, or times, leads to mastery. It is thought that this applies to almost everything: playing guitar, practicing karate, or coaching. New research on the development of expertise, however, is giving us the proverbial answer of "it depends" (Jenkins, 2012).

Not all practice is the same. When we sit down with our guitar and play the same music we usually play repeatedly we may develop more facility at playing those songs, but, we're finding out, we don't really get that much better at playing the guitar. Musicians who instead looked at their performance and identified the specific aspects of their skill that needed improvement and repetitiously practiced exactly that, truly improved. They work on what musicians call their difficult licks. These are the musicians who amaze you in concert. When you have a chance to complement them and say something like, "Your playing was amazing. You just have such extraordinary, God-given talent!" they will retort with, "Thanks, but what you heard wasn't all about talent. That may have sounded spontaneous, but it's the result of practicing six hours a day for fifteen years!" Not just hard work, but smart work, trumps talent.

The Coach at Practice

While a musician may work on intonation, finger dexterity, or, say for a brass player, diaphragm strength and embouchure, the coach has their own set of skills to develop. Here are some suggestions for expanding your expertise through effective practice.

a. **Coach a Great Diversity of Clients**. Often, I encounter coaching students who are passionate about coaching people who are on a wellness journey very similar to their own. They say they want to coach clients who are essentially just like themselves: same gender, age, socio-economic group, etc., who are working on improving their lifestyle in the same ways that they have. If, on the journey to do this coaching, they have not worked with clients who are different than themselves in every way, they will have learned so much less about how to be a truly effective coach, compared with the coaches who sought diversity in their clients. Our clients are our greatest teachers. A wide range of clients will cause you to reach down and draw upon the foundations of effective coaching. They will challenge you to provide the kind of coaching presence and powerful listening that familiarity will never bring out. Without diversity, the danger is that you will get good at playing the same old songs over and over and never progress at your craft. You want clients who will stretch you, challenge you, and make you think! You want clients who will leave you puzzled, even frustrated at times. These same clients will also, as they conquer their fears, make progress and create success in their lives and will give you some of your most rewarding coaching experiences.

b. **Self-evaluation: Listen to Your Coaching.** As you sit behind the wheel and steer your development as a wellness coach, listening to recordings of yourself in action is like twisting your head around and looking into the blind spot between your rearview and side-view mirrors on your car. You may be jolted into sudden awareness of habits and patterns you didn't know you had. *"I can't believe it! I'm saying 'okay' after almost everything my client says!" "I missed that shift in their tone of voice completely!" "Wow! Now that would have been the perfect place for a great question and I just paraphrased." "I'm forgetting to paraphrase, and my client is just rambling!"*

We don't know what we don't know until we discover it. Going over recorded sessions (with your client's complete permission, of course) can be a real eye-opener.

Listen for your expression of coaching presence as well as your use of techniques and methods. Are you sounding natural, genuine, and fully engaged? Do you come across like you're trying too hard? How many suggestions did you make in a 30-minute appointment? Did you travel down your client's favorite rabbit hole again? Are you working with a coaching mindset or have you slipped into your consultant style again? And, don't forget, perhaps one of the most important self-examining questions of all: What am I doing well? What's working? Have I improved in the specific areas that I'm focusing on improving? Use the self-evaluation tool in the Appendix to help with your learning.

c. **Ongoing Evaluation/ Practicing During Performance.** Talk with professional musicians who play a regular gig; that is, they are busy performing, say at a fine restaurant or club, most every night. They will tell you that their rehearsal, their practice, is really in the performance itself. For a lot of us coaches, our practice is very much the same thing. We practice as we coach.

Naturally, musicians like the kind we've referred to here put in thousands of hours of practice privately over the years before they were good enough to score a regular job as we described above. They will also take you aside and admit to hours of work behind the scenes, going over new arrangements, practicing their difficult licks, and then putting it all together that night at the club.

The musical analogy with coaching is a pretty solid one, especially if you are talking jazz. There are compositions, arrangements, but there is also improvisation. Masterful coaching showcases improvisation. The dynamic and creative nature of coaching allows coach and client to dance in the moment and create something that is perfect for the task at hand. We can only play the music that our instrument will allow, but we can arrange the notes in an infinite number of ways. Coach and client catalyze each other in creative thought. Insights emerge and creative solutions appear. It may be an old riff that we haven't played for a long time, but it works here, as well. It may be something we've never tried before, but holds true to solid coaching principles. There's studio work, and there are live performances. Most of the time, it's the live performance recordings that capture the magic.

Coaches benefit from looking at how they can improve their coaching while they are working with actual clients. Effective coaches learn to bravely ask their clients to process the process with them and see how it may be improved. What is working well in the coaching process and the coaching relationship? What would work better? Hopefully there is enough trust with your client that they can honestly give feedback and ask for what they need. Are they finding that the way accountability is handled is not very effective for them? Is there a way that education and coaching can be blended better? Perhaps the coach is blindly ignoring a client need that is only subtly being expressed. Clients can sometimes become compliant but not genuinely invested in the coaching when there is no real congruity between how the coach is proceeding and what the client really wants. Don't wait until coaching has terminated to evaluate and get feedback. Coaches often retain clients longer when they are on the same page and when they adjust the course in the middle of the journey.

d. The Practice Mindset. One can approach practice with either a mindset of the imperative or the volitional. As a junior high school student, I often approached my trumpet lessons under the imperative mindset. I would sometimes avoid practicing all week and then a night or two before my lesson I would get in a couple of 20-30-minute practices starting with those boring scales and exercises. I did want to be in the high school band, my parents had bought this shiny trumpet for me and were paying for the lessons, so…. As I got older, I found that I enjoyed the sense of accomplishment as I mastered my lessons and could play tunes I relished. Playing in the actual band, and especially the jazz band, was completely fun and spurred me on. Today whenever I think of a professional musician, like trumpet-master and bandleader Wynton Marsalis, I think of the thousands of hours of practice that got him to where he is today. Think of a famous martial artist, the Bruce Lee type. How many times did they do their repetitious *katas* to get to where they could draw upon any move in a nanosecond and execute it perfectly? To get there, at some point they practiced because they wanted to — the volitional.

A volitional approach to improving our coaching comes more from a place of personal growth and self-actualization. We truly do want to be the best we can be. We seek out further education, we record sessions, and we listen to our work over and over again, searching for ways we can be a better listener, sharper at using questions, providing the coaching presence that engages our clients maximally. I've often said that when a wellness coaching client discovers that wellness is primarily about personal growth, they really make progress. The same is true for the coach seeking to master their profession.

3. Surrender

When we surrender to trying new things, to allowing ourselves to perhaps even appear foolish, we often discover rich rewards. Overcoming our initial fear and getting out on the dance floor, trying a food we can't pronounce at first try, allowing ourselves to ask for support, etc., can open amazing doors.

Surrendering is not giving up. Here we are talking about surrendering our ego, our persona. What unnecessary limitations do we put on ourselves that hold us back from new opportunities? How hard do we work to maintain some kind of image we have of ourselves? Can we try something that seems foreign to our own background or training? Can we let go of coaching by-the-book? Think of all the pleasing surprises that have awakened new interests, new skills, new tastes, and new opportunities in your life.

We all want to be the best coach we can be. If we allow this positive intention to become an overriding concern about avoiding mistakes, we may find ourselves holding ourselves back. Such a student coach may avoid volunteering to coach in a workshop for fear of not doing it perfectly in front of others. We will make mistakes. Fortunately, in wellness coaching, our missteps seldom do any damage. We and our client can simply acknowledge that something is not being productive, back up, and try a new approach. Surrendering means acknowledging this reality and being self-compassionate. We can then let go of our fear of appearing foolish and allow ourselves to grow.

— — —

A Foolish Learning Story

Many years ago I was fortunate enough to attend a workshop with George Leonard. Leonard was the former editor of *Look* magazine, a famous educator, and true pioneer of the human potential movement. He had grown up a tall, awkward, geeky sort of guy, but now, as he stood before the workshop crowd with a high-level black belt in Aikido around his uniform, he presented a very different picture. He moved like a panther in his Aikido demonstration, mesmerizing all with his skill. Yet what he talked about was the subject that had driven him to write his groundbreaking book *Education and Ecstasy*. (Leonard G., 1968) The story from that day that stuck with me was his tale about what he'd discovered about learning at a California hippie festival back in the 1960s.

George was walking around the festival, set in the hills of California, enjoying the people playing music, dancing, selling food and flower-child paraphernalia. The sound of bongo drums drew him to a young, bearded hippie sitting cross-legged on a blanket with a second set of bongos there on the ground—an open invitation for someone to join in. Leonard was tempted to do so, but held back when he pictured his long legs awkwardly trying to hold a set of bongos and when he imagined being heard attempting to play in front of a circle of listeners. He walked away and explored more of the festival for a while. Before long, he was drawn back and decided to take the young bongo player up on his invitation.

Settling in gracelessly onto the blanket, George positioned the bongos and looked over at his grinning hippie music instructor. Commencing by mimicking the hippie's simple thumps on the bongos, the pair traded drum strikes, creating an accelerating rhythmic crescendo. Now the crowd gathered around clapping, dancing, and thoroughly loving the jam session. Their drumming finally climaxed in a wild finish and, George, almost out of breath and laughing with, yes, ecstasy, looked over at his jam session companion. The hippie laughed and said to him, *"Ya' know man. You're a good learner!"* Hearing this, George's professional educator side was piqued. *"What do you mean I'm a good learner?"* he asked. *"Well man, you're willing to be a fool."*

— — —

According to Leonard, the path to mastery means surrendering to the path and to the requirements of our profession. It means sacrifice and dedication to learning, to practicing, setting aside easier routes to remain on a path that will truly serve us. It may mean surrendering our limited thinking about who we are. Taking some learning risks may result in discovering that we are more of a people person than we thought. We may discover that we can allow our warm and empathetic side to show through and reap rewards instead of injuries.

Surrendering means allowing ourselves to let go and to experiment. It may mean letting go of our preconceived notions of how we should coach. It may mean allowing ourselves to ask for help and guidance so that we may truly grow.

4. Intentionality

It joins old words with new—character, willpower, attitude, imaging, the mental game—but what I'm calling intentionality, however you look at it, is an essential to take along on the master's journey.
— **George Leonard**

For both coach and client the way forward to living our lives better works best when we do it with full intentionality. Envisioning our best life possible and laying out a concrete plan to get there works much better than just mustering willpower and plowing ahead. Seeing us living our well-life vision can provide a motivational tipping point that pulls us towards practicing all of the day-after-day, mundane steps that make up a wellness lifestyle. Setting our intentions positively is a proven process that leads to success. Creating a well-life vision that motivates and then creating an actual Wellness Plan to get there gives us a road map for achieving the life we truly desire.

Leonard speaks about the power of visualizing the outcome you want, be it in golf, Aikido (like him), or achieving most any goal. He even quotes Arnold Schwarzenegger speaking about how the vision creates the "want power" that drives motivation, as it did for him seeking and winning the Mr. Universe title.

As a professional wellness coach, what is the outcome you are seeking? What is your professional desire? What are the goals you want to achieve? Is it to be adequately competent to get a job, or is it to become a truly masterful coach? Implement one of Steven Covey's *Seven Habits of Highly Effective People* and "Begin with the end in mind" (Covey, 2013).

> *If you have built castles in the air, your work*
> *need not be lost; that is where they should be.*
> *Now put the foundations under them.*
>
> **— Henry David Thoreau**

5. Pushing the Edge

Finally, pushing the edge means extending our efforts just a bit further than we thought we could at the start. It means walking even though it is raining; going the extra mile; taking a step that is safe, but for us very bold. Leonard speaks about the paradox we find in those we call masters. While they are dedicated to relentless practice of the fundamentals, "At the same time—and here is the paradox—these people, these masters, are precisely the ones who are likely to challenge previous limits, to take risks for the sake of higher performance…" (Leonard, 1992).

The key here may be distinction. Life in our comfort zone may live up to its name, but, as it is said, "Nothing grows there." Think about most of what you've achieved in your lifetime and your reflections will show that at some point success required vacating your comfort zone. We want to move into what is for us a stretch. For the coach it may be honoring your intuition and risking a question that pushes, that stretches your client.

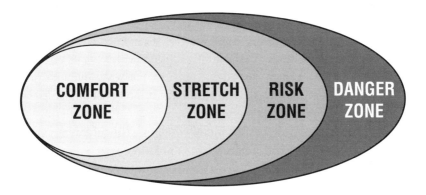

FIGURE 3—PUSHING THE EDGE

The challenge is distinguishing between a *stretch* and a *risk*, or even a *danger*. The stretch may be coaching for the first time a client who has a chronic illness yet realizing that by staying true to the coach approach you can still be helpful. It may be applying a newly learned coaching technique, or coaching around emotion more thoroughly.

Sometimes a well-considered risk pays off. It may mean asking permission to explore a sensitive area for our client. Perhaps we share an observation about a connection we are noticing. Our client suddenly gains significant insight about how they are holding themselves back.

When a risk crosses over into the area of danger it is usually when we have pushed beyond our scope of practice and ethics. It may also be when we urge our clients to move forward too fast into territory they are not prepared to deal with.

I would say that the best experience of pushing the edge comes from a centered and grounded place. The reason that the martial artists can try some extreme acrobatic move is the foundation of training in the fundamentals that they have practiced before. The reason that Frank Lloyd Wright could design such outrageous buildings that seemed to defy gravity was his solid grounding in the theories of physics. He just stretched them to their limits! A great jazz musician may play a few discordant notes but knows when to return to harmony.

Similarly, that more masterful coach can take the risk of courageously confronting their client—but only does so when there is a solid, trustful alliance in place. That same coach is willing to process the process with their client and ask what can and needs to be improved in the coaching relationship and method of working together.

The practice of coaching is not as critical as surgery. A nicked artery is a major disaster. A coaching experiment that went nowhere is easily repaired. Coach and client can stop, reassess, and start over in a new and more productive direction, most likely accompanied by sheepish grins and mutual laughter.

When we are firmly on our journey of professional development and have both our vision and intrinsic motivation working for us, we push through more barriers. We get more comfortable with stretching. The confidence we gain from our risky successes reinforces the practice of wisely pushing the edge.

Self-Mastery and the Self-Vigilant Coach

As the coach travels this path of learning through the different stages, they must maintain a vigilant level of self-awareness. The helping professions often speak of getting yourself out of the way. How are our own values, beliefs, preferences, and even agendas interfering with the coaching process and relationship?

In wellness coaching we may, without even realizing it, subtly promote our own favorite package of dietary, exercise, and stress management advice. It is not usually about ego getting in the way, but rather about the zeal the coach feels for certain wellness approaches. They really believe that certain diets, fitness programs, or stress reduction methods are really fantastic, and they want to share this with heartfelt conviction! Coaches can also fall into the trap of promoting their own favorite ways to be well when they stray from the coach approach and feel that if they just tell clients what to do it will save so much more time.

A well-known motivational interviewing trainer often begins his talks by extolling each of the audience to "Give up your job!" He argues, as do I, that holding on to thinking that you can be successful while attempting to convince or persuade people to be well is about as self-defeating as the client behaviors we are attempting to change. Yet many of us in the health and wellness promotion fields and medical professions find ourselves spending years doing just this. The exasperation that finally comes from this fruitless way of working with clients and patients is often what drives folks to look for a better way, and what often leads them to coaching. Tired of pushing or pulling people up the mountain of lifestyle improvement, one finally asks, "How's this working for me?"

Beginning coaches also have to be vigilant about how their own path to wellness may interfere with their client work. Some wellness coaches were attracted to the fields of healthcare, human helping, and wellness because they were able to meet and overcome a serious health challenge by, at least in part, improving their own lifestyle. They may have an allegiance to some sort of holistic health path or wellness formula that helped them and now they feel the need to proselytize.

"What worked for you?" clients often ask. Here the coach has to proceed very carefully. We can use some appropriate self-disclosure but rather than answer the question directly, the coach might ask, "What are you hoping to learn by hearing about my experience?" Often that client's question is coming out of a place of low self-efficacy. They have had little lasting success at lifestyle improvement, so they are looking to you, the expert, to show them a better way. We have to determine if this is a time to provide some information/education, make an effective use of self-disclosure, or is it a time to empower the client to continue to seek their own answers. The vigilance comes in when we catch our own tendency to slip into the expert role.

Part of mastering wellness coaching is narrowing down our blind spots as much as possible. Some lack of awareness, some self-deception may still remain, but our job is to increase our awareness both in retrospect and in the moment. We make great headway with this when we accept responsibility for our own feelings and reactions. The values and lifestyle of our client may be 180 degrees different than our own. We may be appalled at the self-defeating behavior we see the client exhibiting and rush to judgment. We may have a personality that pushes us to straighten out a client's way of operating in this life. Part of our effective vigilance is noticing when we are pressing a client about how they ought to live. Can we allow the client to live their life without our interference? Coaching should never interfere with someone's life, unless it is a situation of safety (see below).

When we blend in some wellness/health education, how neutral do we stay when it comes to any of the numerous, and often controversial, healthy living debates? "Saturated fat is fine. Enjoy!" "Saturated fat will kill you!" Can we act like a true professional and coach our client to find out their own answers from a variety of trusted, evidence-based sources?

Masterful Moment

Experiment with entirely eliminating the phrases
"You need to…"
"You ought to…"
"I want you to…"
from the way that you coach with people.

Distinguishing Between Our Agenda and Client Safety

Coaches are not responsible for the choices their clients make. However, if your client is riding his wellness bicycle towards a known cliff, we do have an ethical obligation to share what we know about the landscape ahead. Consider this ethical quandary: Let's say your client says, "Hey coach! I'm going to start the Twenty-Seven Grapefruit A Day Diet! All I have to do is eat nothing but 27 grapefruits for a month and the pounds will just drop away like magic! Will you support me in this coach?" We love to say that in coaching the client's agenda is THE agenda. This does not mean, however, that we can't operate with one important caveat—the safety of our client. Now, unlike the obvious cliff our grapefruit-dieting client is headed for, most of our clients present more ambiguous situations and questions. For example, there are a number of immensely popular diets out there, which promise extraordinary weight loss results, but have more recently been shown to present medical risks and/or have an abysmal record of sustainable results. What is the coach to do when the client presents a plan to follow such a diet?

Our first step is to monitor ourselves and ask if our desire to have our client think twice before they launch forth with a potentially self-defeating, if not self-destructive course, is motivated by what we know of the facts, or our own prejudices. Are we aware of evidence that puts their course of action in serious doubt, or are we instead simply favoring some alternative that we are fans of?

The second step would be to inquire what the client knows about this course of action (diet, or whatever wellness/health promotion idea). How did they become aware of it—through what sources? What do they know of the integrity of this action course? Are they aware of contradictory evidence regarding this way of attempting to be well? The coach can strongly recommend that the client check this out with their treatment professionals or trusted educational professionals. The coach can help the client to carefully examine their options. If the client insists on carrying out a course of action the coach truly feels is detrimental to the well-being of the client, they can directly share that with the client. If the client still persists on moving ahead with their plan, the coach can share with the client that they will not be able to support the client in doing this as part of their journey together.

Finding Your Path

Backpacking's popularity rose rapidly in the 1970s as gear improved and the youth culture embraced its adventurous nature. A classic book that informed newbies was *The Complete Walker*, by Colin Fletcher (Fletcher, 1968). Fletcher's style was engaging, entertaining, quirky, and frankly a bit obsessive-compulsive! You might call him the James Michener of backpacking with his attention to detail, even minutia. This really struck a chord with some folks, none more so than the young man I met in the Great Smoky Mountains National Park.

He was hiking the Appalachian Trail end to end, all the way from Stone Mountain, Georgia, to Mount Katahdin in Maine, 2,184 miles! Resupplying in Gatlinburg, he was hitchhiking back to the "AT" when I gave him a ride to a trailhead. The moment I saw him I knew he was a younger, but absolute clone of Colin Fletcher, from precise model of shorts, hat, and backpack down to his four-foot-long bamboo walking stick. Conversation confirmed this and evidently it was working for him quite well to follow what we could call *The Hiker's Bible* according to Fletcher chapter and verse.

As people begin learning about wellness, they often start out following the path that was forged by others before them. They follow the procedures where they work. They rigorously follow the training methodology that they learned in their wellness coach training. They read my book or others and look for guidance for every step. Just like the young man on the Appalachian Trail, they think that if they are going to venture into the wilderness of working one-on-one with people about lifestyle behavioral change, they had better do it carefully, so following a manual or a guidebook is where they start. It's all very understandable and can be viewed as a natural developmental stage. As the coach progresses, they learn that they can integrate more of their own style build upon the foundation they gained.

As our young backpacker logged more miles down the trail, however, I'm sure he started to build confidence in himself and his ability to not only survive, but also thrive. Now perhaps his personality was such that holding on to every little detail of his mentor's methods continued to please him. I'm guessing, though, that as his experience broadened and his belief in his own abilities improved he started to modify his equipment and his style. Perhaps he discovers that a solid five-foot walking stick is better than Fletcher's hollow bamboo. He finds a pack that is actually better for him than the one Colin used. Innovations in equipment give him a lightweight water filter that Fletcher never had. He starts to realize it is not only okay, but actually preferable, even vital, to find his own path and walk it.

Finding our own path is not about the path itself, but who we are on it. Self-mastery in coaching is about integrating who we are with the work we do as a coach. It's blending the tasks, skills, and presence of coaching with our authentic nature. The result is as many different types of coaches as there are people doing the coaching. The common threads of the profession, the science and the craft tie all of us together, but we all have our own unique expression.

As we become more comfortable with the process and skills of coaching, as our practice makes certain moves more spontaneous and accessible, we are freer to allow our own nature to show through. We are less in our heads trying to figure out what to do next, and instead can be in the moment, listen much better, and respond more dynamically. Our own personality can show through. Some of us will be more lively, others more calm and steady. We discover that there are varying degrees of directiveness that are more appropriate for some clients over others, and are more in line with our own style. We experiment with allowing some of our own unique gifts to come through and discover that they enhance the coaching instead of detract from it. We realize that we don't have to be like the coaches who trained us, but we do still have to be a coach.

Our own personal growth journey fuels our ability to be the best coach we can be. Greater self-awareness and understanding can be achieved in a myriad of ways. The point is to make it a conscious process. Life throws many personal growth experiences at us whether we seek them or not. We grow through challenges and blessings alike. It is when we take the time to self-examine, reflect, and determine where our growing edge is, and then commit to sharpening it, that we leap forward in a direction that truly serves us well.

Coaching expects a lot from people who study to become coaches. How many other professions require such self-awareness? We want our surgeon or dentist to have supreme focus as they take blade or drill to our bodies, but does it require much self-reflection? On the other hand, look at how, for coaching to be effective, the coach has to be quite self-aware and on top of their game throughout the coaching process.

My Professional Coaching Vision

Plant the Seed

Begin thinking about what you really want your professional coaching career to look like. Turn it over in your mind again and again. Write about it whether you like to journal or not. Talk with friends and fellow coaches about it. As you speak to them, don't just listen to their visions; ask them to help you consider yours. Reflect. Take some time by yourself to process this.

Consider the Possibilities

Who do I want to be as a coach? What aspects of coaching work will give me the greatest satisfaction? What types of coaching will give me the most meaning and purpose? Are there particular health challenges I see myself working with to a greater extent? Do I see myself operating my own coaching business? Do I see myself working within some sort of an organization? Don't get lost in the details of possible outcomes, but ponder enough to paint a clear picture of where you are going.

Eliminate the Negative

Dreaming, imagining can trigger the inner critic. Catch yourself when it is the "Gremlin" talking, and not the cautious part of you that cares about you. When you share it with others, it's an opportunity for the naysayers in your life to chime in with your own self-doubt and derail your efforts to actualize your vision. Seek out more positive allies to discuss your vision with, avoiding the cynics.

Write It Down

We know that when intentions are put to pen and paper (or a digital file) they take on much more power than just thoughts in our brain. For one thing, in order to write it down a certain amount of clarity has to be achieved. Writing it down requires adequate structure of thought, and therefore some organization to those thoughts. From such organization it is easier to put a plan in motion.

Visualize It

In one of his signature plays on words, psychologist Wayne Dyer was fond of saying, "You'll see it when you believe it." Manifesting what we want in life begins with our own belief in its possibility. When we literally take the time to relax and create images in our mind of living out that set of intentions (dreams, if you like), we set in motion some type of motivating force that helps drive us towards that outcome. Positive mental rehearsal is a proven commodity in the world of sports and performance. It's even been shown to increase our intrinsic motivation (Plessinger, 2018). Indeed, to build a career/business and succeed, we need to enjoy the process and be intrinsically motivated to put in the time and effort.

Record It, Refresh It, Remember It

Keep track of your progress towards your goals. Write down your steps along the path. Go over your master plan frequently and refresh it with changes driven by your own processing and by the changing landscape as you encounter it. Keep it alive by talking about it with others. Perhaps make a mentor or business/career coach part of your way to stay on track and succeed in creating the professional life you want.

The river is constantly turning and bending and you never know where it's going to go and where you'll wind up. Following the bend in the river and staying on your own path means that you are on the right track. Don't let anyone deter you from that.

— **Eartha Kitt**

Thoughts to Ponder on the Mastery Path

Self-reflection has an aspect of balance to it.

Do I tend to be so self-reflective that I am often held back from action?

Do I avoid being self-reflective?

What am I afraid I will discover?

In this chapter we encouraged the coach to look at their own transformation. How does the coach move from competency to proficiency and on to mastery? We looked at what it means to develop one's craft as a more masterful coach and delved into George Leonard's Mastery

Path. That path includes a great deal of self-vigilance as the coach learns how to be mindful that their own attitudes and beliefs do not get in the way of effective coaching.

Next we begin Part Two of our book—How to Be—with Chapter Three: Being and Doing. We will explore how our coaching presence, our way of being is just as important as any technique or methodology we employ. We will see how vital an understanding of awareness is and how to help our clients to become more aware of themselves. We will bring in the philosophy of Taoism and see how concepts from it apply with full congruity to coaching.

REFERENCES

Covey, S. (2013). *The 7 habits of highly effective people: Powerful lessons in personal change,* (2nd ed.). Simon & Schuster.

Fletcher, C. (1968). *The complete walker: The joys and techniques of hiking and backpacking.* Alfred A. Knopf.

Jenkins, B. (2012). Deliberate practice: How to develop expertise. *Scientific learning.*

Leonard, G. (1968). *Education and ecstasy.* Delacorte Press.

Leonard, G. (1992). *Mastery: The keys to success and long-term fulfillment.* Plume/Penguin Group.

Mente, B. L. (2009). *Amazing Japan: Why Japan is one of the world's most intriguing countries!* Phoenix Books.

Plessinger, A. (2018). The effects of mental imagery on athletic performance. *Health psychology home page,* Vanderbilt University. http://healthpsych.psy.vanderbilt.edu/HealthPsych/mentalimagery.html 4.23.18

It's time to give Noel Burch some credit. (2017, July 11). Exceptional Leaders Lab. https://exceptionalleaderslab.com/its-time-to-give-noel-burch-some-credit/ [...]

PART TWO
How to Be

Chapter 3—Being and Doing

CHAPTER 3

Being and Doing

The most precious gift we can offer others is our presence.
When mindfulness embraces those we love,
they will bloom like flowers.

—**Thich Nhat Hahn**

How to be with your client is equally important to what you do with them. In fact, it may be of even greater importance. Knowledge and skills can be learned. Much of it can even be programmed into a machine. But, what is offered by human connection is irreplaceable. In virtually all the research on human helping relationships the differentiating factor of success is, time and again, the nature and quality of the relationship itself.

Common factors such as empathy, warmth, and the therapeutic relationship have been shown to correlate more highly with client outcome than specialized treatment interventions. The common factors most frequently studied have been the person-centered facilitative conditions (empathy, warmth, congruence) and the therapeutic alliance. Decades of research indicate that the provision of therapy is an interpersonal process in which a main curative component is the nature of the therapeutic relationship. Clinicians must remember that this is the foundation of our efforts to help others. The improvement of psychotherapy may best be accomplished by learning to improve one's ability to relate to clients and tailoring that relationship to individual clients (Lambert, 2001).

Coaches are not clinicians and psychotherapy is not coaching, but it is easy to feel confident in saying that the coaching relationship is the critical factor in how well coaching works. Large disease management and health coaching companies discovered early on that the best results occurred when the client received coaching from the very same coach every time instead of experiencing a "coach du jour."

To build that coaching alliance we need to hone our craft of being as much as our craft of doing. In this chapter let us work with developing your own awareness, your own personal wellness foundation, and your own mindfulness. We'll look at how you can develop the awareness, centeredness, and groundedness to allow you to be more masterful with your coaching client.

The Coach's Personal Wellness Foundation

Achieving high levels of awareness and being truly present with our clients requires a good degree of what we might call functioning wellness on the part of the coach. Staying sharp, having the stamina for the kind of work described here comes so much easier when we are living a wellness lifestyle to the best of our ability. One might ask, how physically fit does a person have to be to sit and talk on the phone with someone? Yet, fatigue and lethargy even at a desk job can sap our concentration, our focus, and numerous aspects of our mental functioning. Coaches working in some settings may see four clients per hour! It requires sustained energy for such endurance. So we might ask, does the diet of the coach help them maintain their energy throughout the day? Are they getting enough rest to replenish their energy supplies?

Wellness, of course, is not just about diet and exercise. We coach better when we are getting our emotional needs met as well. Are we connecting with friends enough to really satisfy us? Are we content with a sense of meaning and purpose in our lives? Are we living in ways that allow us to express our values, our creativity? If you love to dance, are you dancing? If you love to hike, are you hiking?

Many people who enter the human helping professions tend to be focused on the care of others. Too often they tend to be rather poor at self-care. Minimizing self-care activities, not getting our own needs met is a formula for burnout.

Coaches don't have to be perfect to be effective in their work. We are all doing the best we can at the moment. However, when we focus on what our own mind, body, and spirit needs, we can connect better with others and be of greater service to them.

Our dedication to our Wellness Plan demonstrates integrity. It's not about achieving an appearance that lands us on the cover of *Fit* magazine. It's about working on our own wellness goals and maintaining the health and wellness we have. Our modeling comes through in the course of a coaching relationship.

The best coaches believe in the concept of self-actualization and are constantly striving to achieve more of their own human potential. Making personal growth a priority is imperative if we are really on the path towards mastery. This path can take many forms, and usually ends up containing many twists and turns. We always need to temper our zeal for growth, however, with self-compassion.

There are endless resources on the topic of "how to be well." That is not the focus of this book, however. Seeking out the best resources for you, creating your own Wellness Plan, and perhaps engaging with a wellness coach will not only serve you well, it will help you understand your client's journey.

Awareness

Reality is nothing but the sum of all awareness as you experience it here and now.

—Frederick S. (Fritz) Perls

When we work as any kind of human helper we are living on two levels at once. There is the role and function of being the ally for our client, and yet there is always the inescapable essence of who we are present at the same time.

To bring mindful awareness to our work with someone, or even to a precious moment with a friend, we have to get ourselves out of the way by setting our own issues and our own agenda aside. Then we can be fully present, mindful of our own experience, but focused on our client.

Coaching begins with self-awareness but quickly moves into awareness of your client on many levels. Here your own powers of observation need to be honed. To really become your client's ally, the first challenge is just to observe, to notice...just to notice. Leave judgment out of it. Don't play detective looking for the real meaning of those arms folded across your client's chest. This is about listening with your whole person, not just your ears. Notice your client's non-verbal signals (even the vocal ones that come through on a phone or computer connection) and, rather than interpret, either file them away for future reference or feed them back to your client. "I notice that each time you've referred to your boss today your voice gets louder and sharper." You'll also find that when you just notice without judgment, or trying hard to figure it all out, you naturally are less critical and your client feels more supported.

Be aware of your client's context. Did they just rush to see you after begging their reluctant supervisor for the time? Are they not entirely present with you because of stress and worries about what is next? Do they have a condition where they could be in some level of physical pain? Inquire so you will understand where they are coming from. Affirm their experience, be compassionate, and check out their ability to engage with you right now.

As your client tells their story and checks in on commitments they made for the week, be aware of patterns that emerge and feed those back to your client. This is often where great insights are born.

Be aware of your client's expression of energy. What are they passionate about? What sounds flat? Follow the energy by paraphrasing and reflecting what you are hearing (matching the energy in your own voice as you do) and by asking powerful questions where the energy is highest or lowest.

Be aware of your client's emotional expression. This is partly about following the energy (an old axiom of Gestalt therapy) but also a barometer of motivation and perhaps even the need for referral. Sustaining motivation for lifestyle improvement is a long-term challenge. If your client's enthusiasm for an area of focus has faded, if they don't seem to have the energy for it anymore, check it out. You'll be tipped off by your own awareness of their emotional expression regarding that area they are working on.

> *Drink your tea slowly and reverently, as if it is the axis on which the world earth revolves — slowly, evenly, without rushing toward the future. Live the actual moment. Only this moment is life.*
>
> —Thich Nhat Hahn

Awareness of Self: Coaching from the Inside Out

Call it what you will, self-awareness, consciousness, or mindfulness. Regardless of term, we are talking about the degree to which you, the coach, are aware not only of your client and your surroundings, but of what is going on inside your own skin. Coaching from the inside out is about being cognizant of:

- Your bodily sensations
- Thoughts
- Feelings
- Intentions

Body Awareness

What is happening in your own body from head to toe, and what is it telling you? It's about noticing the tightening in your stomach when your most difficult client calls, instead of ignoring that sensation. It's scanning your bodily awareness periodically throughout the coaching session instead of getting lost in your head thinking about what to say next. It's practicing body awareness techniques and methods such as tai chi, yoga, qigong, dance, etc., to help you connect with your body more, to identify with your whole person, not just your cerebral cortex. It's about being aware of your body and it's position in space much like a dancer would in the middle of the dance. When you've danced often enough you automatically are maintaining that awareness without giving it any conscious attention. You hold your frame in a centered way that allows you to be even more sensitive to the movements of your dance partner. It's body, breath, posture, movement, all combined in an amazing living wholeness.

The How-To of Body Awareness

1. **Notice.** Don't jump into interpretation or the paralysis of analysis. Just notice and take note of what you've become aware of. File it away and see if a pattern develops. Does your breathing become short and shallow each time your client pushes back and rejects a suggestion of yours?

2. **Be centered physically.** This is part posture and part being centered in your life. Perhaps you notice that working with this client actually has you back on your heels. Sit up! You'll be amazed at how dif-

ferent you coach when you are consciously aware of your posture and sitting (or standing) up, feeling grounded. Think of the martial artist in their horse-riding stance, knees slightly bent. The purpose of this stance is to be able to respond to absolutely anything that comes at them with 360 degrees of choices. Being centered in your life is about being engaged in a process of living a true wellness lifestyle that is fulfilling in all areas of your life (and accepting that you are working on that process to the best of your abilities at this time in your life). Let's face it, when you don't feel well physically, when you're emotionally going through a crisis, it's hard to be in the here and now and give it your very best. Ask yourself what do you do on a regular basis to get your needs met, to come into the present moment, to return to a state of balance. I know that I am a better coach when I've had more exercise, more rest, more contact with friends, and with the natural world. Do what centers you in your life, be it gardening, reading fiction, writing, hiking, meditating, praying, connecting with dear friends, etc.

3. **Get centered for your appointment.** Do this on a practical and mental level (as we'll discuss below), but also on a physical level. Break your routine. Stand, stretch, move, and breathe. Do more than review case notes. Develop little rituals that help you prepare for your next client so you will be with them as though they are the one and only person you see that day (even if they are the eighth).

Self-Centering Before a Client Session

- **Shift**—A few minutes before your next appointment shift away from whatever you have been doing. Stop completely, close your eyes for just a moment, and breathe.
- **Breathe Deeper**—Take a couple of deep, slow and full breaths.
- **Scan**—Scan over your body from head to toe and check in on how you feel physically. Notice tension and where it is located.

- **Focus**—Focus your awareness wherever tension resides and imagine that your next breath actually breathes into that area. Allow yourself to relax and let go.
- **Question**—Ask yourself what you need to do to be fully present for your next appointment.
- **Prepare**—Reacquaint yourself with your upcoming client by going over your coaching notes.

Awareness of Thoughts, Feelings, and Intentions

Being present in your body helps you to be more present in your mind, but it takes more than that to be a good coach. Before your client arrives or calls, become conscious of your own intentions in coaching this person. Get grounded in your intention to be your client's ally in their wellness journey. Review client notes. Affirm your coaching mindset as the ally, not the expert; as the guide, not the guru. Get grounded in your own confidence to be that ally, remembering the training and experiences that have brought you here. Recall the facilitative conditions of coaching that need to just be a part of who you are in the coaching process: empathic, non-judgmental, warm, compassionate, genuine/authentic. This is what adds up to coaching presence.

Sit in gentle vigilance regarding your own issues and filters that might get in the way. When your thoughts lead you into your own world (your past, your worries, your favorite wellness recommendations, etc.) you leave the world of your client. When your own prejudices, stereotypes, and opinions surface, gently refocus on your client. Focus on the present moment. Other than a limited amount of note-taking eliminate all other multi-tasking. Be totally with your client. This is a great part of what makes a powerful listener. This is not chess. Don't be thinking two or three moves ahead. It's OK to be developing a strategy to facilitate what is happening with your client but, you need to trust the coaching process and not over-think it. As you do focus on the present, note your own emotions. What feelings come up for you as your client speaks? Don't be afraid to connect with these feelings and learn from them. At times, an appropriate self-disclosure of one's own feelings may be very beneficial to your client. We will explore this in the next chapter.

Mindfulness and Wellness Coaching

In the 1960s the Western world started to look beyond its own insular thinking and search for new ideas from the ancient sources in the East. The increasing interest in philosophy that emerged in that era sought out wisdom from Buddhism, Hinduism, Taoism, Zen, and practices like meditation, yoga, tai chi, and Eastern martial arts. This dovetailed beautifully into the popular human potential movement and the rise of humanistic psychology. All of this laid a foundation of practices and philosophy that has more recently re-emerged as Mindfulness. Today, the work of Jon Kabat-Zinn and others has provided validating research that has allowed such practices to enjoy widespread use (Kabat-Zinn, 2013).

As wellness coaches look for ways to live and practice coaching in more centered and mindful ways, we can benefit a great deal by looking at the concepts central to the philosophical side of Taoism.

The Tao of Wellness Coaching

When I let go of what I am, I become what I might be.

—Lao Tzu

History and Context of the Tao

It is said that the legendary Chinese sage, Lao Tzu, rode off on the back of an ox when leaving the Middle Kingdom. Before a sentry guard would let him pass out of the city gates, he asked the sage to write down his teachings for the good of all. The result was the seminal text, the *Tao Te Ching*. Lao Tzu then rode off into the wilderness, never to be heard of again.

The wisdom of this book was never lost from those times (5th-6th Century BCE), but instead spawned a philosophy that holds real merit for our lives today. Our challenge is to bring the Tao, or The Way, into those busy lives and, ultimately, into every aspect of our being. When we do, we operate very differently. We engage in our work in a different way. We experience stress but respond to it more effectively. We can, potentially, coach differently.

The Tao is a concept cloaked in mystery for most of us. Sage sayings that sound like one conundrum after another leave us puzzled.

> *Those who know do not speak.*
> *Those who speak do not know.*
>
> *Yield and overcome; bend and be straight.*
>
> —Lao Tzu, Tao Te Ching

Yet, there is a strong appeal because we often covet the apparent peace of mind of practitioners of the Tao. They seem so centered. They seem to have a quiet confidence that guides them. They appear to know just what to do.

When we speak of the Tao and wellness coaching we are not implying that to know the Tao and make use of it one must study and adopt the more religious form of Taoism. We will, instead, focus on the philosophy. Taoism is most often defined as a philosophical tradition that is all about living in harmony with life, or literally translated, *The Way*. One can pursue living in harmony as a way of life without necessarily becoming involved in a religious pursuit, per se. Carolyn Myss tells us that living in harmony with the Tao is a way to "… reduce the friction inherent in most of life's actions and to conserve one's vital energy" (Myss, 2019).

The bookstores of the world are packed with titles such as *The Tao of Business*, *The Tao of Golf*, *The Tao of Leadership*, *The Tao of Physics*, and infinite variations on this theme. Clearly many find value in this ancient wisdom and have found ways to make it relevant and advantageous. Psychologist Wayne Dyer worked on translating the meaning of the Tao for an entire year. He provided us with a profound resource with his book *Change Your Thoughts—Change Your Life: Living the Wisdom of the Tao* (Dyer, 2009). There are many translations of the *Tao Te Ching*, but for the Westerner, Dyer's book may be the best introduction because it explains so many of the concepts in ways we can apply to our everyday and professional lives.

What Centers Us in Life

There are many things that center us in our lives. Being centered is about living our lives in a healthy balance and getting our needs met so that we have vitality. Many things do this for us. Ask yourself, "What keeps you in balance, what centers you?" You may say getting regular exercise, gardening, reading fiction, connecting regularly with friends, getting out in nature, getting enough rest, etc. All of these activities and more help us to be more in balance, to live a wellness lifestyle, to be in harmony with the tao. When that balance is missing we find it more difficult to function at the same high level.

Our wellness lifestyle forms the foundation for this centered way of living, but any number of mindfulness practices can help us take it further for even more benefits. Practicing yoga, various forms of meditation, mindfulness based stress reduction, contemplative prayer, and other methods can all help center us and not only teach us the ways of the tao, but actually alter our psychophysiology in a positive way. All of these practices have the potential to help us shift our nervous system more into what is know as the relaxation response (Benson, 2000), the activation of the parasympathetic branch of our autonomic nervous system. This results in a lowering of heart rate, blood pressure, etc., and therefore makes it easier for us to be calm and less reactive to stress; in other words, more centered.

The Tao in Movement

Tai chi is a taoist inspired soft martial arts practice, a moving meditation actually, that embodies many principles of the tao. The health benefits of tai chi are well documented.

> Tai chi is often described as meditation in motion, but it might well be called medication in motion. There is growing evidence that this mind-body practice, which originated in China as a martial art, has value in treating or preventing many health problems (Harvard Health Publications, 2019).

The benefits one can derive from such a practice, however, go well beyond the psychophysiological. For me personally, practicing tai chi has been a non-cognitive way to study the tao. It is centering practice. I was fortunate in the late 1980s to learn the short form of the *Yang Style of Tai Chi* taught by a physician from China. My practice since then has been consistent, if not as frequent as I would like. The result of regular practice is a centered way of moving, and, to an increasing degree, a centered way of being. This is living in harmony with the tao. For me it has been a 30-year journey in body-centered learning.

When we move from the center we are always in balance. Think of the martial artist in action, such as a practitioner of karate, aikido, or Tai Chi Chuan. For them to be effective in combat or competition, they must move from center. If they aggressively lean too far forward they land on their face, or if they are too afraid and lean backwards they end up on their backside. Think how this same principle applies to a salesperson attempting to make a sale, an instructor attempting to get a point across, an encounter you may have attempting to resolve conflict with someone. Think how this applies to our coaching. The metaphor holds up. If it did not go well, we might realize that we weren't very centered.

Centered Coaching: What the Tao Has to Teach Us

When I observe masterful coaching the style of the coach may vary, but one thing is always present: centeredness.

A centered coach speaks less and listens more. They can dance in the moment effortlessly, going wherever the client needs to go, no matter how unexpected. They are not attached to outcome, but are focused on results. A centered coach can shift into new directions, but remains grounded in structure and the foundations of coaching. Such a coach has no need to impress or appear powerful. They don't work at being powerful, yet they are. Centered coaches do not push their own agenda, yet they do not collude with their client, either. They know when to push, to confront, and have the courage to do so. They also know the power of yielding.

Mastering others is strength. Mastering yourself is true power.

—Lao Tzu

Essential Concepts of the Tao

When the best leader's work is done the people say
"We did it ourselves."

—Lao Tzu

Effective wellness coaching is, inherently, very much in harmony with the tao. Let's look at two key taoist concepts and how they apply to wellness coaching.

Yin-Yang Balance

Fundamental to Taoist thought and foundational to Chinese medicine is the concept of yin and yang. These are the polar opposite, yet complementary, forces of the world that, for health and well-being to exist, must be in balance. The yang forces are active, positive, hot, overt, masculine, light, and hard. The yin is passive, yielding, negative, cool, quiet, feminine, dark, and soft. In the classic symbol the yang rises to the top and is represented by the light area with the black dot in it, while the yin sinks to the bottom and is represented by the black area with the white dot in it.

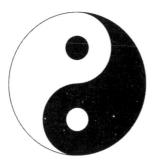

FIGURE 3—YIN/YANG

The key is to understand that the two elements are opposite, yet interdependent, complementary, and interconnected. When we experience having too much of one and not enough of the other, we experience dysfunction whether it is at the physical, psycho-emotional, or behavioral and practical level. Regaining balance becomes the return to a level of healthy balance.

The goal of achieving a healthy balance is paramount as coaches work with clients to achieve a wellness lifestyle. We must rest, but not become lethargic. We must move and exercise, but not to the point of exhaustion and fatigue. We must find a way to take in sufficient calories, but find the right level for our optimal health, etc.

As coach and client co-create a Wellness Plan the concepts of yin and yang can be very useful. Our culture tends to reinforce and pro-mote the yang forces while not supporting those of the yin. We are urged to be productive, work hard, play hard, achieve, accomplish, try harder, and push. Wellness is often portrayed in highly vigorous ways with images of runners, spinning class cyclists sweating profusely, etc. Seldom are we reinforced, much less accommodated for self-care ac-tivities such as getting adequate sleep, relaxing, taking time to get a massage, meditate, or enjoy our leisure. In fact, we may face criticism for such indulgence.

Many components of a Wellness Plan involve greater frequency of self-care activities. As clients look at their health and well-being through a more holistic lens, they often see the value of taking more time to meet these needs to balance their lives. Often these same cli-ents have been admonished by their healthcare providers to engage in more self-care activities in order to improve their health. Many times wellness coaches work with clients who have been foregoing their medical self-care, such as taking time to do self-testing (e.g., diabe-tes), following up on medical appointments, doing rehabilitation ex-ercises, etc. Instead they have been consumed and distracted by the yang-style demands of their work and their own belief systems.

When wellness coaches work with their clients to construct ways to manage stress more effectively, they are inevitably working to achieve yin-yang balance. Without ever speaking of the terms (yin and yang), we might consider how all actions possess either yin or yang energy and help our clients to decide how much to include in their lives. There may be great stress management wisdom in exploring strategically with our clients when it is best to push and when to yield.

A coach's job is to remind people that they have choices.

At a fundamental level our clients are often in a state of ambiva-lence about change that displays the push-pull of yin and yang forces. Should I, the client, change my way of living, or not change? When we carefully examine the ambivalence resolution methods of motiva-tional interviewing (MI), we can see a taoist stance taken by the ther-apist or coach. The coach does not pull for one path to be taken over the other. Instead, they neutrally allow the client to explore and expe-rience both energies; change and no change. The coach using this MI approach remains as centered and non-judgmental as possible, helping the client to weigh the pros and cons (again a yin/yang process).

Wu Wei—Effortless Effort

Living in harmony with the tao is about letting nature take its course and not interfering with the natural order of things. The concept of wu wei conveys the idea of non-doing, non-action, or non-intervention. This concept seems antithetical to Western thinking. In Western culture we are taught to make things happen. In Western medicine the expert seeks to find the best intervention and implement it as soon as possible. To accomplish a desired outcome by allowing things to simply be and progress on their own seems either too slow or doomed to failure. Yet think for a moment. Have you ever needed to relax and unwind and the harder you tried to do so, the more anxious and tense you got? There is only one way to relax; you have to allow yourself to do so. When we intervene medically to treat a wound, the actual healing that follows is something we have to patiently allow to happen.

Wu wei is perhaps best thought of as living in a state of effortless harmony and alignment with the natural cycles and ways of nature. We are truly going with the flow, and able to respond to whatever comes our way. As coaches allow such a way of being, our ability to dance in the moment is maximized. We aren't there to intervene or to fix things. We are not attached to a therapeutic agenda or to a treatment-oriented course of action. The client is in the lead and we are able to effortlessly dance with them.

Keeping It Client-Centered

At the heart of all coaching is the client-centered approach. From the psychotherapeutic roots of Carl Rogers, this person-centered way of interacting has become the basis for the coaching alliance.

There have been parallels made regarding Carl Rogers' person-centered theory and the way of doing nothing in taoism (Hermsen, 1996). Rogers suggested that the most therapeutic counseling occurred when the therapist was authentic and real in the relationship and placed trust in the client to discern what was best for himself without interference from the therapist (Hayashi, 1998). A central concept of taoism is doing nothing and being natural. Both Rogers' theoretical beliefs and tao philosophy maintain that when these conditions are achieved successfully in therapy, the human organism will develop almost spontaneously (Hayashi, 1994).

An excellent review of this concept is found in *East Meets West: Integration of Taoism Into Western Therapy* by Rochelle C. Moss and Kristi L. Perryman (Moss, 2012).

Coaches following these principles get themselves out of the way and trust in the wisdom of their clients. We see our work as helping to bring forth, or evoke, the inner wisdom of our clients. When we are not attached to rigid protocols, yet operating out of grounded principles and methodology, we can serve as guides to help our clients learn and grow.

> Coaches and clients walk down a pathway together at night in the forest. The coach's job is to hold the flashlight and illuminate what is before them. The client's job is to choose how the path will be followed.

Neutrality allows the coach to operate without bias and without their own judgments and prejudices. This is where wellness coaches must adhere to the ethics of coaching and not guide or push their client in directions that the coach favors. This allows the client to be in the lead, making their own choices.

The highest virtue is to act without a sense of self.
The highest kindness is to give without a condition.
The highest justice is to see without a preference.

—Lao Tzu

Knowing When to Yield

Coaches who find value in the concept of wu wei see the value in yielding. In Western society yielding is often seen as failure, as giving up. Yet some of the most storied successes on both Eastern and Western battlefields came because of strategic retreat. In wellness coaching this may take the form of allowing a client to set their own levels of accountability. For example a client may state that they can perform a certain behavior, such as walking, five times in the coming week. The coach may suggest that going from not exercising at all to doing so five times a week may be less likely to be successful. The client insists that they can hit this target of five times a week. The coach then patiently allows the client to go ahead with their experiment rather than argue, and let the client experience what Adlerian psychologists would call natural consequences. The client feels supported by their coach and realizes that their coach does not have to have it done their way. The client often discovers that the target was harder to hit than they thought. With their coach's support they reset their level differently the next week.

The power of yielding may also be something for our clients to discover. Often people approach situations with only one option in mind: to win! The wise person approaches any situation wanting to have all options at their disposal. In dealing with conflict, in managing stress, the option of yielding often pays off better than pushing for one's initial desires.

At the heart of both the coaching process and Maslow's theories of self-actualization and personal growth is the principle stance that human beings are inherently moving towards health and wholeness. With barriers removed and balance achieved, people will naturally make progress towards their highest good. The continually accumulating evidence from the positive psychology research substantiates this position. Such a way of looking at human beings and their experience in life is in complete alignment with taoist principles of the interconnectedness of all things, synchronicity, and the let it be attitude of wu wei.

The Centered Wellness Coach

Drawing upon philosophical taoism the wellness coach can find wisdom that does not necessarily contradict any other beliefs they, or their client may have. What we find is real alignment with the principles of growth and self-actualization that form the foundation of the wellness field. What we find as well are very functional guidelines for practicing as an effective coach.

1. Practice What Centers You in Your Life

The wellness of the coach is the foundation all else is built upon. When we embrace whole-person wellness that includes body, mind, spirit, and our relationship with our environment, we practice a lifestyle that moves us towards optimal functioning. The key here is the word practice. Coaches are usually very caring people who place the needs of others far above their own. That can easily result in a lack of self-care, a neglect of the very wellness practices that we encourage in our clients. Find what centers you and practice it with regularity. Connect with friends, read novels, garden, hike, bike, walk, dance, meditate, do yoga, tai chi, go fishing, enjoy your grandchildren, play with your photography or poetry, pray, volunteer at a non-profit, scrapbook, quilt, take your neighbor's child for a day in the park. Do whatever gets your healthy needs met and gives you meaning and purpose.

When you get knocked off-center, accept that this is simply part of the normal human experience. The centered person does not tiptoe through life as though they were on a balance beam. The idea is that of reducing our center-recovery time. If we are practicing what centers us in our lives we can come back to center more quickly.

2. Practice Effortless Effort

The primary mistake I notice when I observe coaching students who are learning the craft is that they work too hard. The coach is working much harder than the client. When coaching does not go well it is usually when the coach is trying to make things happen. The coach is busy fixing the situation and/or the client, instead of facilitating the client to do their own work. The coach is busy attempting to convince or persuade the person to be well. The centered coach is patient.

3. Embrace Paradox

By trusting their coaching methodology, and by trusting their client, the coach is able to offer a coaching presence that is: calm, yet lively; supportive, yet challenging; accepting and nonjudgmental yet discerning; empathic, yet not colluding; compassionate, yet firm. Again, it is from this centered stance that such paradox can exist.

4. Know When to Push and When to Yield

We have a culture obsessed with interventions—with taking action. The Tao teaches us that there is a time for both action and non-action. Nothing is gained by pushing for action whether the client is ready or not. When we use Prochaska's readiness for change theory we are actually acknowledging the reality of the energetic state our client is in. An old Gestalt Therapy expression is, "Don't push the river." But, we also know the need to paddle when we are in a dead-calm lake! There is a time in coaching to forward the action through request. The Tao is as much about taking action as it is about pivoting and moving with no resistance. Again, the coaching metaphor of dancing in the moment means know when to push and when to yield.

5. An Effective Wellness Plan Is About Balance

A well-crafted Wellness Plan, co-created with our client, would resemble the yin/yang symbol of Taoism. Ideally there would be as much involvement in active steps to build energy as there would be for more passive steps to help one relax, replenish energy, and achieve more balance. One side would balance out the other.

The reality is that as coaches we have been practicing the Tao of wellness coaching all along whether we called it that or not. Taoistic principles have already been infused into psychology, psychotherapy, business, leadership, and more. Being more conscious in their application expands the coach's repertoire of options and helps them nurture their own wellness as well.

Masterful Moment

How open am I to learning from a source of information outside of my own culture?

How easy or difficult is it for me to both push and yield?

What are three steps I can take to become more centered?

This chapter began our look at how to be in coaching and how equal it is in importance to all that we do. Our way of being with our clients influences the coaching alliance and eventually affects the success of the coaching. We explored how multi-layered awareness is and how to help our clients to increase awareness. Drawing upon the philosophical aspects of Taoism we demonstrated its usefulness in the coaching process.

In Chapter Four—Building the Coaching Alliance—we will emphasize the foundational role that the coach's mindset plays in all that we do in coaching. We will define coaching presence as the provision of the Facilitative Conditions of Coaching and deeply explore the concept of empathy and how to convey this to our clients. We'll look at all aspects of the influence the Client-Centered model has had upon coaching. The relevant theory of Appreciative Inquiry will be explored and the field of positive psychology and its contributions to coaching will be covered. We'll then look further at the role a directive —non-directive continuum—plays in how we individualize coaching.

REFERENCES

Benson, H. (2000). *The relaxation response. (Expanded ed.).* William Morrow Paperbacks.

Dyer, W. (2009). *Change your thoughts—change your life: Living the wisdom of the Tao.* Hay House.

Hayashi, S.K. (1994). A reevaluation of client-centered therapy through the work of F. Tomoda and its cultural implications in Japan. *Third International Conference on Client-Centered and Experimental Psychotherapy.* Gmunden, Austria

Hayashi, S. K. (1998). Client-centered therapy in Japan: Fujio Tomoda and Taoism. *The Journal of Humanistic Psychology.*

The health benefits of Tai Chi. *Harvard Women's Health Watch.* http://www.health.harvard.edu/staying-healthy/the-health-benefits-oftai-chi

Hermsen, E. (1996). Person-centered psychology and Taoism: The reception of Lao Tzu by Carl C. Rogers. *The International Journal for the Psychology of Religion,* 107-125.

Kabat-Zinn, J. (2013). *Full catastrophe living: Using the wisdom of your body and mind to face stress, pain, and illness,* (2nd ed.). Bantam/Random House.

Lambert, M. J. (2001). Research summary on the therapeutic relationship and psychotherapy outcome. *Psychotherapy: Theory, research, practice, training.* pp 357-361.

Moss, R. P. (2012). East meets west: Integration of Taoism into western therapy. *American Counseling Association.* https://www.counseling.org/knowledge-center/vistas/by-year2/vistas-2012/docs/default-source/vistas/vistas_2012_article_33

Myss, C. (2019). *Philosophical and religious Taoism.* Retrieved from Caroline Myss https://www.myss.com/free-resources/world-religions/taoism/philosophical-and-religioustaoism

PART TWO
How to Be

Chapter 4—Co-Creating the Coaching Alliance

CHAPTER FOUR

Co-Creating the Coaching Alliance

Building the Coaching Alliance

What does it mean to be an ally? There is a practical side to building the coaching alliance: Creating agreements instead of expectations, clarifying roles, defining boundaries, determining the best format for coaching meetings, and clarifying the age-old question of who is responsible for what. There is, however, a deeper, more interpersonal side to answering the question, *"What does it mean to be an ally?"* If we are to become truly proficient, even masterful at our coaching, how do we connect with our clients in such a way that we become true allies? How could we become the kind of ally that you would want with you on the most perilous journey of your life—someone you would want on your lifeboat?

Honestly, the coaching alliance is a bit one-sided. In other spheres such as friendships or international political alliances, the allies support each other in a mutual and reciprocal fashion. In coaching, we are signing on to be of assistance to our client in their quest. The client is not there to assist us in ours. This agreement is the nature of human helping professions. As coaches, we willingly sign on for this. So, in this context, how do the expert coaches that we admire manage to quickly establish and maintain an alliance of trust and support? This is a very subjective realm, but what we can point to is an answer that begins with the coaching mindset, being client-centered, and providing the facilitative conditions that Carl Rogers always spoke of. Let's take a deeper look at all of this.

The Coaching Mindset

A mindset is our way of operating, our way of viewing the world. Definition.org defines it as "A fixed mental attitude or disposition that predetermines a person's responses to and interpretations of situations." To me the key word here is *predetermines*. When we view the world a certain way, or we view ourselves a certain way, we are locked into that way of thinking. The way we respond and/or interpret the situations before us becomes heavily influenced by not only our perception of reality, but also our thoughts about it.

The award-winning work of Stanford University psychologist Alia Crumm "...focuses on how changes in subjective mindsets—the lenses through which information is perceived, organized, and interpreted—can alter objective reality through behavioral, psychological, and physiological mechanisms." One of her most famous studies showed how providing one group with information that shifted their mindset about how much exercise they were already getting in their job resulted in weight-loss, blood pressure reductions, and more (Crum, 2007).

We are just beginning to see the power of how our mindsets influence all that we do. When coaches work with their clients the professionally operational mindset they hold is critical. Most coaches come into their work operating out of either a "prescribe and treat" mindset or an "educate and implore" mindset. Their challenge is to shift to a coaching mindset of being the ally instead of the expert consultant, to adopt a mindset of "advocate and inspire." Coaches sometimes struggle with abandoning their own default setting that their professionally operational mindset is stuck in. Behind this "stuckness," I believe, is a sincere desire to help. The scenario below describes what often occurs.

> We meet our coaching client with the very best of intentions. We want to help. And help sometimes means slipping into doing what the client seems to have been unable to do for themselves up to this point—figure out solutions. Instead of empowering our clients to come to their own solutions, we seek to fix it for them. We draw upon our knowledge,

our wisdom, our intelligence, and put effort into guiding the conversation to this goal of helping the client to live better and be healthier. We take on more than our share of responsibility for the outcome. Imagine when your client is speaking about a very challenging situation in their complex life. You are fully engaged—in trying to figure it out. You are curious, in a detective sort of way. Your internal chatter is racing: "What's going on here? How can the client handle this better? What should the client do? The client is not dealing with this effectively. The client is engaging in self-defeating behavior or irrational thinking."

So, you ask questions: really good questions. You delve deeper into the problems. You seek solutions. You analyze. But, you're not coaching. The more you think the less you feel. The more you analyze and use deduction, the more you step away from your client and all that they feel and all that they are. You, the coach, forget to empathize. You forget to neutrally help your client explore and to do the work themselves. You have become your client's consultant, taking on the work that belongs to your client.

As James Prochaska (internationally recognized for his work as a developer of the stage model of behavior change) loves to say about change, making the shift to the coaching mindset is a process, not an event. The shift did not become locked in place on the day when you completed an initial coaching course. We all keep going back to our default setting, be it treatment provider, educator, or consultant. What reinforces the old mindset is that many of our clients expect us to be the consultant, the trusted expert. They are used to working with consultants and practitioners of every stripe and they often come to coaching with feelings of low self-efficacy and seek the guidance of experts who can point the way for them.

Up in Our Heads

The more we are in our own heads, the more we miss about what is going on for our client. Our analyzing and wondering about where to go next removes us from what is happening right here and right now.

Perhaps our client is talking about what they had for breakfast, and the greater context is that they are having breakfast alone for the first time after their children have gone to live with their former spouse. We are missing the undercurrent in their voice of loneliness. We miss inquiring about their emotions, and, instead, focus on the cholesterol content of what was on their plate. We miss reflecting on our client's feelings because we don't notice what they were feeling. We miss an opportunity to express empathic understanding. Dealing with those emotions may have more impact on our client's present and future dietary habits than all of the nutritional information we could have shared.

Trust the Coaching Process

To quit our consulting job and truly coach we must trust the coaching process. It is a leap of faith to let go of our urge to help and instead to assist. We have to trust not only the coaching process—that it is valid and potentially effective—but also trust our client. As the Coaches Training Institute teaches, when we feel it in our bones that the client truly is naturally creative, resourceful, and whole, we can finally coach. When we apply this cornerstone of coaching we don't rescue our client. We don't provide for them what they may actually be capable of creating themselves (Kimsey-House, 2018).

Back to Center—Back to the Present

So, how do we stay in the moment with our client, yet provide the structure that is an absolutely essential part of effective coaching? It comes down to the proverbial dancing in the moment that coaches are so fond of referencing, but it also acknowledges that we have made an agreement with our client about the music.

An effective coach operates within an evidence-based, theoretically grounded coaching structure. We provide a methodology that allows facilitation of the client's success at improving their lifestyle and, therefore, their life. As we follow that music (our agreed upon coaching structure) we put our attention into the process of awareness. We listen with ears, eyes, and heart. We pick up on the nuances of speech that reveal what may be going on beneath the surface. We explore without preconceived notions of what the client's experience is. We may simply say to the client as we observe their tight voice and the furrowed brow, "Are you aware of your forehead right now as you say that?" Let them do the work.

Client Centered

The *sine qua non* (essential condition) of a coaching mindset is the concept of operating in a client-centered way. Until we truly view our clients as the one in the driver's seat, not us, we haven't really arrived at the level of interaction that could be called coaching. To understand this concept of working with others we must reach back to the work of one of psychology's giants (Kimsey-House, 2018).

As time marches on it is easy to put the contributions of Carl Rogers into the seldom-read chapters of psychology history books. We thereby miss an important appreciation for the etymology of how the way we work with people today, in both psychotherapy and in coaching, came to be. When Rogers began his work as a psychologist and psychotherapist the theories of psychoanalysis dominated. The therapeutic relationship was seen as either a non-factor, or a blank slate upon which the patient (not client) would project their issues. As Rogers worked with children, families, and adults he found great value in the newer relationship theories and related work developing in the 1930s. In 1942 he crystalized his new take on how to work with people in psychotherapy with the publication of his groundbreaking book *Counseling and Psychotherapy* (Rogers, 1942). It was actually Rogers who popularized the term "client," urging, even then, a mindset shift away from treating people in therapy like patients.

Initially in the 1940s and 1950s, Rogers' non-directive methods assiduously avoided asking questions, making suggestions, giving advice, or any other directive methods. It relied on skillful listening and reflecting feelings back to the client without judgment, allowing them to explore and work with those feelings more deeply. He soon realized that even more important than the techniques used was the attitude of the counselor/therapist. Feelings needed to be reflected with genuine acceptance and conveyed with empathic understanding for therapy to be effective. Thus, Rogers began development of the core conditions that would become known as the facilitative conditions of therapy: genuineness or congruence, empathic understanding, unconditional positive regard, and warmth.

What clients need is not the judgment, interpretation, advice, or direction of experts, but supportive counselors and therapists to help them rediscover and trust their own inner experience, achieve their own insights, and set their own direction (Kirschenbaum, 2018).

Rogers continued his work through the 1960s, 1970s, and 1980s and his *Person-Centered Approach* continued to contribute to the flourishing human potential movement and was completely congruent with the self-actualization work of Abraham Maslow and others. Rogers' influence on our field of coaching is extensive and inescapable. Many of his students and colleagues took this foundational work and evolved other client-centered approaches often used in coaching today, such as appreciative inquiry, nonviolent communication, and motivational interviewing.

The Coach Approach Grew Out of Being Client-Centered

The pioneering work of the authors of *Co-Active Coaching* (Kimsey-House, H, Kimsey-House, K, Sandahl, P. Whitworth, L.) (Kimsey-House, 2018) was steeped in the client-centered tradition. Their foundational cornerstone of coaching (that the client is held to be naturally creative, resourceful, and whole) orients the coach to a mindset that is non-judgmental, accepting, and relies on the inherent drive towards self-actualization of which Rogers spoke. It puts the client in charge of the agenda. It introduces the concept of co-creation to the coaching process.

Coaching Presence — Providing the Facilitative Conditions of Coaching

As a counseling psychologist much of the foundation of my education was grounded in the research that looked at what allowed therapists of many different theoretical schools to get effective results. In the late 1960s and early 1970s, three academics, Robert Carkhuff, Bernard Berenson, and Charles Truax, took the work of Carl Rogers and made it objective enough to study through behavioral science (Carkhuff, 1967) (Carkhuff R. R., 1967). What they found was that regardless of what approach to therapy someone took (psychoanalytic, behavioral,

Gestalt, client-centered, etc.), their effectiveness came down to their ability to provide what Rogers called "... the facilitative conditions of therapy." When a therapist provided empathy and unconditional positive regard, and was authentic and genuine in their interactions with the client, the therapy worked, regardless of theoretical orientation. Since those days we have seen other more recent research substantiate this and point to the therapeutic relationship as the key determinate of therapeutic effectiveness. Hazler and Barwick summarize much of this in their book, *The Therapeutic Environment: Core Conditions for Facilitating Therapy* (Hazler, 2001).

As the field of coaching has evolved the term *coaching presence* has often been used to describe this way of being as opposed to the techniques of doing. The ICF defines coaching presence as: *"Ability to be fully conscious and create spontaneous relationship with the client, employing a style that is open, flexible, and confident"* (International Coach Federation, 2020). The Federation goes on to define coaching itself in a way that also gets at the concept of coaching presence. *"ICF defines coaching as partnering with clients in a thought-provoking and creative process that inspires them to maximize their personal and professional potential"* (International Coach Federation, 2020).

When we see masterful coaching what is often coming through is largely the facilitative conditions of coaching. These are the same elements that Rogers called the *Facilitative Conditions of Therapy* (Rogers, 1942).

- Empathic understanding
- Unconditional positive regard
- Genuineness, authenticity

Coaching Presence

To me coaching presence is providing, through your way of interacting with your client, the conditions that allow them to maximally open up to their own growth process.

Great coaching presence allows your client to feel safe, and to feel understood. They feel connected to you, their coach; accepted and receiving compassion.

Unconditional Positive Regard

When we come into contact with the other person,
our thoughts and actions should express our mind of
compassion, even if that person says and does things
that are not easy to accept. We practice in this way until
we see clearly that our love is not contingent upon
the other person being loveable.

—Thich Nhat Hahn

Buddhist monk Thich Nhat Hahn provides a powerful description of unconditional positive regard. We meet our client where they are without judgment. We notice, we observe, and we don't judge. This is the separation between who a client is and what they do. We often observe our clients engaging in behavior that is truly self-defeating. We may challenge them to look at how a particular attitude, belief, or behavior is working for them or against them, but we are still accepting them as a person on the journey of growth.

> When our coaching clients experience complete acceptance of who they are, without judgment, when they feel prized and understood, great things can happen.

The suspension of judgment is a real challenge for many people. To keep ourselves safe in the world we have learned to make distinctions. Our ancestors needed to quickly appraise the behavior of an animal and know whether to ignore it, hunt it, or climb a tree very quickly! Today we can certainly protect ourselves by being wary of the suspicious salesperson (or website) pushing the deal that sounds too good to be true. We can hold on to our right to choose whom we associate with. Drawing distinctions is not the same thing as making judgments, but sometimes we get the two confused.

Our first distinction as a coach may be between the person who is our client and their behavior. Perhaps as our client recounts a tale of moral ambiguity, we may get a picture of someone who may behave in ways that are contrary to our own personal values. But can we suspend judgment, listen deeply, connect with the person telling the tale, and help them feel heard? If we show in any way our disapproval of them or communicate that they are a bad person for having behaved as they have, their defensive walls will go up. If we receptively stay with them and allow their story to unfold, we may be surprised at how our perception of both them and their behavior changes.

Sometimes passing judgment occurs when we are in the diagnostic mindset of trying to figure out the other person or fix them. When we don't understand another person's actions or motivations, we may fill in the blank with a theory of our own, sometimes based in judgment. It is so tempting to make sense out of our client's behavior by trying to imagine what we would do, and when it is different, to pass judgment. When we coach like this, despite our own efforts to convince ourselves that we are merely figuring out the person's characteristics, we are usually being judgmental.

The most devious aspect of judgment is that we often aren't aware we are doing it. We need to do our best at self-monitoring and then choose how we want to interact with others. Once again, providing unconditional positive regard, being non-judgmental is a coaching skill of *being* rather than *doing*. It is not a technique. Techniques come from the head rather than from the heart.

For Rogers, unconditional positive regard was just that—acceptance without conditions, and he held this acceptance to be a basic human need. Unconditional positive regard is about respect without strings. The other person need do nothing at all to deserve it.

Can we accept all aspects of the person's behavior, even those aspects that they don't want to change? For the health and wellness coach or any wellness professional, this is a critical point. Can we accept the fact that our client does not want to quit smoking? It is not okay that they smoke. It is not good that they smoke. We know it is bad for their health (as they probably do, too). We don't give permission to smoke. However, can we suspend judgment on that behavior and work with the whole person, accepting them fully as a person, and becoming a true coaching ally? Experienced coaches tell of many times when they accepted the foibles of their clients, they eventually chose to quit the negative behavior on their own later in the coaching process.

To Stay Out of Judgment

Judgment, self-deception, and attachment to an outcome may go hand-in-hand. To better self-monitor to keep from your judgment emerging and become more self-aware consider these ideas:

- Notice if you are reaching conclusions about your client before you have all the information you need.

- Are you coming to conclusions about their level of motivation early in the coaching?

- Notice if you are engaging in diagnostic thinking, analyzing your client's situation and thinking that you quickly understand. Notice if you have begun to develop solutions to your client's problems.

- Facilitate your client exploring more by using the active listening skill of requesting clarification.

- Ask yourself how attached you are to a certain course of action and outcome. Do you want to see your client behaving a certain way?

- Remember, you are not a consultant. You do not need to figure things out for your client. You are the facilitator who keeps your client on the path of discovery and insight.

- Instead, maintain a mindset of curiosity. Receive information, especially about your client's lifestyle practices, home environment, etc. with a sense of "Oh! Isn't that interesting!" Pursue elaboration. Provide empathic understanding first. It is harder to slip into judgment when you engage in empathy.

Expectations

The Samurai of ancient Japan had a saying: "Expect nothing, be prepared for anything." The saying entreats us not to hold the expectation that nothing will happen, but rather to have no expectations whatsoever.

Expectations are the flipside of the same coin where judgment resides. Our expectations limit our awareness and ultimately our experience of the other person. In coaching we create agreements rather than holding expectations. My client and I create an agreement whereby they will track their activity each day for the next week. If I simply expect these things to happen, I may be disappointed and have no real way to confront the client if they fail to follow through on my expectations. If I expect the client to behave in certain ways, I am putting my own "shoulds" onto them.

In Al Ritter's book, *The 100/0 Principle* (Ritter, 2010), we see how essential a lack of expectations and judgment is to all of our relationships. Our relationships are in fact the biggest factor in our success and satisfaction in life. Ritter proposes that by taking 100% responsibility for our relationships and expecting 0% back in return we can transform our lives by creating solid relationships all around us. He outlines three simple steps:

1. Demonstrate complete respect and kindness whether you believe the other person deserves it or not.

2. Expect nothing in return, absolutely nothing.

3. Be persistent; we often give up too soon.

Sounds like he's been reading Carl Rogers.

Empathic Understanding

Empathic understanding is a very direct way to express this unconditional positive regard, and one more of the facilitative conditions of therapy/coaching. Empathy is conveying to the other person that you know, at least to some degree, what it is like to feel what they are feeling. You may have never had their exact experience (e.g., having a heart attack, being obese, etc.) but you know what it is like to feel fear, loss, shame, regret, etc. You put yourself in their place and see the world from their perspective, tapping into your own feelings so as to connect with them deeply.

Empathy and Sympathy – A Crucial Distinction

Struggling to understand the distinction between empathy and sympathy is natural enough. The root of both words is the Greek word pathos, meaning suffering/feeling. We express sympathy for a person when we feel sorry for their loss, or what they are going through. We regret that they have to suffer. We commiserate with them about their loss, etc. Expressing sympathy in coaching is entirely appropriate when there is a loss to be grieved, when we regret our client's suffering, and, in a show of compassion, express this to them.

It is quite possible to experience both sympathy and empathy for and with another person. Our client may have just lost a loved one. In addition to expressing our regret, condolences, and such, we may also express our empathy because of our own awareness of what it is like to feel such loss, or perhaps because we get in touch with losses like this that we have had.

When it is empathy that our client needs and it is sympathy that we deliver, the coaching relationship can take a setback. When our clients are struggling, they don't want someone feeling sorry for them. They resent it, possibly vehemently. They may take this as a message that they are perceived as weak, or somehow inadequate. When empathy is called for, our client is really looking for an ally, not someone who seems to be placing themselves above them, doling out sympathy.

Imagine that your new client is challenged by diabetes. They come to coaching hoping to manage it better and become healthier overall. Your own experience has never involved facing any type of serious chronic illness. You have never had to monitor your diet so severely, much less engage in any kind of daily self-testing and self-care like your client. How do you empathize?

This is where you, the coach, can connect on the common human experiences that you inevitably share. Have you ever experienced a serious loss in your life? Your client has gone through feeling like they have lost a huge part of their health, or even more. Have you ever had to self-monitor in any way and keep close track of your behavior? Have you shared with a person you are close with a health journey that might be as challenging as the one your client is going through? That becomes the level where you connect with your client. We don't have to identify with our client's challenges to be compassionate with them. Psychologist Daniel Goleman, the author of *Emotional Intelligence and Social Intelligence: The New Science of Human Relationships*, speaks from his conversations with the famous psychologist and researcher Paul Ekman about empathy. Goleman reports that this enlightening connection led him to understand that there are three types of empathy: cognitive, emotional, and compassionate empathy or empathic concern (Goleman, 2007).

Cognitive Empathy—I Understand

Cognitive empathy is being able to understand what the other person, our client, is going through. We aren't necessarily feeling the same feelings, but we truly get it, we understand how upsetting something is, how bitter the feelings are, how deep the loss may be. Cognitive empathy is "perspective taking." I can take on this person's perspective and see the world through their eyes and understand (mentally) what that experience would be like.

Emotional Empathy—I Feel

Emotional empathy, or affective empathy, is when we actually experience the same emotion as our client. Upon recounting a story of tragic loss the client begins to cry. We are deeply touched by the story and find tears welling up in our own eyes. Their experience is not exactly the same as ours, but the feelings generated are very similar. We feel the other's distress. It's upsetting to them, and it's upsetting to us. We are feeling right along with our client and what happens is sometimes labeled emotional contagion. Empathy is no longer contained in the head; the heart is touched. We are in tune with our client, we are walking along with them. It's like we are experiencing the other person's feelings without really experiencing them. We struggle for analogies in the world of empathy: seeing through another's eyes, walking as though in the other person's shoes, or walking a mile in their shoes.

According to Hodges and Myers in the *Encyclopedia of Social Psychology*, emotional empathy consists of three separate components:

> The first is feeling the same emotion as another person.... The second component, personal distress, refers to one's own feelings of distress in response to perceiving another's plight.... The third emotional component, feeling compassion for another person, is the one most frequently associated with the study of empathy in psychology (Hodges, 2007).

The risk of emotional empathy is that if we are not skilled at managing our own emotions it can lead to emotional exhaustion and burnout. Think of the social worker hearing one tragic story after another as they work with a severely disadvantaged population. We hear this referred to as compassion fatigue.

Empathic Concern—I Understand, I Feel, and I Want to Help

This is where you not only understand what the other person is going through, but you are spontaneously moved to help. "Yes! I hear what's happening here for you. Let's work together and do something to make it better!" Paul Ekman refers to this as compassionate empathy, while Goleman uses the term empathic concern. As Goleman shares from his interview with Ekman: "Paul told me about his daughter, who works as a social worker in a large city hospital. In her situation she can't afford to let emotional empathy overwhelm her. My daughter's clients don't want her to cry when they're crying," as he put it. "They want her to help them figure out what to do now—how to arrange a funeral, how to deal with the loss of a child" (Goleman, 2007).

The Sound of Empathy

The presence of empathic understanding facilitates the coaching experience greatly, but what about the expression of empathy? How do we communicate our empathy to our client? Much of it is certainly achieved nonverbally. Perhaps, like many communication researchers say, the vast majority of the impact of a message is nonverbal. It comes across in our body language, the look in our eyes, and in gestures. It comes across vocally through modulations in the volume, tone, and rapidity of our voice.

When Marshall Rosenberg, the founder of Nonviolent Communication, was asked about empathy this exchange ensued:

Question, "Is it speaking from the heart?"

Rosenberg, "What? Empathy? In empathy, you don't speak at all. You speak with the eyes. You speak with the body. If you say any words at all, it's because you are not sure you are with the person. So you may say some words. But the words are not empathy. Empathy is when the other person feels the connection to what's alive in you."

The essence of empathy is conveyed not so much in the words we say, but in how we say them. In respectful disagreement with Rosenberg, we do need to learn what words to say. Much of coaching is done over the phone where our visual cues will not transmit. Even when we coach in person, there are words and phrases that convey our empathy directly to our client. If we are in touch with our own emotions the words will most likely come easily. Empathy can be expressed in many ways, but it always sounds genuine, sincere, and real.

Sounds like...

Sounds like phrases are mostly conveyed as an affirmation of the other person's experience, perhaps reflecting the feeling that the client may be experiencing.

> *"Sounds like it was so frustrating for you to just sit there while your boss criticized you!"*
> *"Sounds like you've had so much disappointment with weight loss."*

That must be...

> *"That must be so discouraging to not see progress on the scales!"*
> *"That must be painful to see your children get into trouble like that!"*

Combined...

> *"Sounds like you've had to be really patient to see progress like this. That must feel really good!"*
> *"Sounds like you're already much too familiar with resuming smoking. That must be really disappointing."*

In Question Form...

We can even convey empathy by putting our empathy into a question form, such as this example where we show our astonishment and concern.

> *"Wow! What's it like to be in pain like that every day?"*

Simple and Direct...

Empathy doesn't have to be high prose. Sometimes just a few words, delivered with sincerity in the right tone of voice and in the right context, can do the job very well.

> *"Yes! That does suck!"*

"I hear you."
"I'm with you on that."

Genuineness and Authenticity

Authenticity and genuineness are not techniques, they are ways of being. Sincerity cannot be faked. If your heart is not in the coaching process, don't coach. Take a day off, or if it's not just a temporary experience, look for a new career. Most people, including all of our clients, have terrific B.S. detectors and know when someone is just going through the motions of being a helper. Likewise, when they experience you being your authentic self it gives clients someone they are attracted to working with and feel safe enough to trust with their feelings, hopes, dreams, and fears.

In wellness coaching, our clients have often tried and failed at lifestyle improvement before, sometimes many times. For them to go further towards success they have to feel as though they can truly trust the ally who is journeying with them. They have to believe that this ally genuinely cares about them, completely accepts them as a person, understands their experience, and is not afraid to go wherever the journey takes them. The coaching relationship is the heart and soul of the coaching process. A competent coach has skills, techniques, tools, and methodology to help the client on their journey, but it is the coach's way of being that is the crucial difference. The client/coach connection is omnipresent and foremost in the client's mind.

"The privilege of a lifetime is to become who you truly are."

—Carl Gustav Jung

Opportunities to Empathize: F.A.V.E.
First Acknowledge, Validate, and Empathize

Some new coaches and some coaching models plow ahead with immediate problem solving while ignoring their client's affective state. Coaches, for various reasons, simply miss opportunities to empathize and bring the benefits of that empathy into the coaching process.

Contrasting Coaching Conversations

Our client:

A middle-aged woman who had been very athletic all of her life. Now, with chronic bursitis in her hip, she had not been able to exercise for months. Every day she experienced significant chronic pain. She gained weight as she became much more sedentary. She naturally found this huge shift in her lifestyle very frustrating. She shared her story with you and waited for your response.

Coaching Conversation One—Missed Opportunities

Coach One: *So, tell me more about your bursitis.*

Client: *Well, I'm not sure what there is to tell. I'd never had anything like it before. It really hurts more than I could have anticipated.*

Coach One: *And, how long has it been since you've been able to exercise?*

Client: *Oh, it's been months! I used to go running about four times a week, played volleyball, all kinds of things.*

Coach One: *Wow! You were really active! So, have you tried water aerobics, or less strenuous exercises?*

Coaching Conversation Two—Empathy in Action

Coach Two: *So tell me more about your bursitis.*

Client: *Well, I'm not sure what there is to tell. I'd never had anything like it before. It really hurts more than I could have anticipated.*

Coach Two: *Wow! What's it like to be in chronic pain every day? That must be so difficult.*

Client: *Yes, it is. I used to think I was pretty strong, kind of tough, really. This has really brought me down.*

Coach Two: *It must be so difficult to go from being so active to not being able to exercise at all.*

Client: *Exactly! I miss all the things I used to do so much. The friends I used to play volleyball with were so much fun.*

Coach Two: *So, it's impacting your connections with other people too. Talk about frustrating!*

These two coaching conversations illustrate how opportunities for expressing empathic understanding can be missed or maximized. Coach One is concerned about getting the facts straight and may be trying to understand the client's situation better. This could be done, but first an empathetic response to the client's experience could take the conversation in a whole new direction that may yield even more information, as we saw in the work of Coach Two (social connections). Coach One pursued solutions quickly, suggesting a less strenuous exercise. The coach and client could eventually reach the step of seeking strategic solutions, but first building the coaching alliance and honoring the client's feelings could allow for a richer coaching process.

The experience of coaching teaches about the power of relationship, of person-to-person connection, because all the evidence from coaching and psychotherapy shows that this is the critical factor in determining success. We each need to feel truly heard by others that we are attempting to be in a relationship with. When we share our lives, our experiences, and our feelings we truly want to have acceptance, acknowledgment, and validation.

If your client shares that they have been in pain since an injury and it is breaking their heart that they can't get out and enjoy the physically active things they love to do, they don't want someone consulting with them about a solution. They want someone to say, "Wow! That must be so terribly difficult for you to be unable to exercise." They want their coach to "get it" that they are not only in pain, but are frustrated, angry, stuck, depressed, and feeling a loss. Once they feel like their experience is understood at that heart level, that their feelings have been affirmed, that what they have gone through has been acknowledged, and it's been conveyed that it's okay for them to feel the way they feel, then they will be more open and likely to launch into some great strategic thinking about seeking solutions.

When coaches convey the facilitative conditions of coaching clients feel the validation, acceptance, and acknowledgment. Coaches have to find the words to convey empathy, acknowledgment, unconditional positive regard, warmth, and genuineness and they have to remember to do that *first*, before they jump to solution seeking.

As our client's story unfolds, tune into it with the mind of compassion, the mind of understanding, and the mind of connection. Some of what works is relaxing into the coaching process and realizing that just by being true to our naturally warm and empathic way of being, we are providing that "safe container" that allows the client to open up. We "hold sacred ground" for our clients to do the exploration they need to do. When we attempt to find a solution without adequate exploration, the path taken is often unproductive at best and counterproductive at worst.

So you haven't been able to run or bike ride for three months now. How tough it must be to go from being so athletic to hardly exercising at all! Tell me more about what that has been like for you.

As you do this you validate their experience and their emotions. Your unconditional positive regard (and therefore lack of judgment) makes it possible for the client to feel that it is okay for them to feel the way they feel. You are affirming that what they have told you has been their reality. You help the client feel that their story is validated, and as you coach further, with that accepting and yet at times challenging coaching presence, you help them learn that they are not their story. As you acknowledge, affirm, and validate, you help them feel well heard. You help them explore their experience and express their feelings so they can let go of it, put it in the rear-view mirror, and realize they are not trapped by their story.

Our most powerful vehicle to convey this acceptance and affirmation, this sense of support, is the expression of empathic understanding. That kind look in the eyes, your thoughts of compassion are very sweet, but they are not enough. We have to put it into words (think telephonic coaching) and convey our empathy.

So when you have free time you just have to sit there and wish you were able to move like you used to. How challenging! You must miss being active very much. It sounds like you've tried to deal with this as best you can, but it's got to be a real loss for you.

It takes courage on the part of the coach to practice FAVE. You've got to be okay with emotion, not afraid of it. Empathy is not trying to cheer the person up, not quickly reassuring them that everything will be all right; in essence rescuing them. FAVE is getting down in the mud, or up riding high in the sky with our client—meeting them where they are at, not where we want them to be. It is important to remember that when we allow our clients to feel the way they feel, they usually do so and move through the emotions more fluidly. When they are not able to do that, even after our repeated attempts at providing our best facilitative conditions, it's probably time to consider referral to a mental health professional.

So, **FAVE**! First of all, acknowledge your client's experience. Paraphrase, restate, and reiterate what they have said. Remember to reflect their feelings. Help them feel that it has been recognized that they have been experiencing the emotions they have been living. Acknowledge the courage it takes to share. Acknowledge the self-caring it takes to seek help and assistance. Acknowledge the depth of your client's challenges and their strengths.

Masterful Moment

How easy or difficult is it for me to feel empathetic towards others?

Do I have old beliefs about how other people should be that get in the way of me connecting on an empathic level?

Is there some fear within me of connecting that closely with another person's emotions?

How easy or difficult is it for me to connect with others?

What gets in the way?

Sensitivity to Our Client's World: Multiculturalism and Coaching

Many coaches today are working with very diverse populations. Large organizations often have employees from several different countries at varying degrees of acculturation. Our coaching client today may be a woman from Pakistan, a man from rural Appalachia, a woman from a small town or a huge metropolitan area.

To be a true ally to our client we must see them in the context of the world they live in. The coach's challenge is to never assume that we know that world like our client does. Instead we seek to be educated by our client, to be informed of their experience, their beliefs, their values, and their own challenges. Do not assume you understand the client's circumstances. Instead, inquire. Ask about your client's access and ability to find the food they need for a healthier diet. What kind of support do they have for making healthier food or exercise choices? How do they feel about seeking out a second opinion about their medical condition? Are there safe places to walk or exercise in their area? When we operate on assumptions our client's efforts may not only result in failures, but also the coaching alliance can be impacted in a negative way. While there is so much that unites us all, we must honor the differences among us. Sometimes we are primed to do so by more pronounced differences, such as race or gender. At other times we miss the subtler, but potentially profound differences such as urban vs. rural, social class background, ethnicity, generational, etc.

Our client may have a cultural background that has different beliefs about health and medicine. They may be more inclined to seek out a native healer than to consult a physician. They may have a family that has powerful prohibitions against seeking help from others, even professionals. The effective coach is continually operating from a stance of curiosity, requesting to be informed about our client's experience. Instead of making a simple suggestion about how they might pursue one of their goals, we ask how they think they could implement the ideas we've talked about in coaching in their situation, in their family, in their world.

In my first years as a therapist, I worked in a counseling center at a university known as a "Public Ivy." Many of the students there were from upper middle to upper class homes. Despite my graduate school education, my own steel-mill town, working-class background made it difficult for me to empathize with some of their suffering at first. When I heard about their dysfunctional families, I was tempted to minimize their difficulties and their pain. After all, they had such great advantages of wealth and status. As I listened

> *more to what they went through, I began to see that pain is pain, that we all bleed real, red blood. I no longer held back on my expression of empathy and I became a better therapist.*

When we co-create with our clients instead of prescribing, when we present ourselves as ally not expert, when we treat our clients with the utmost respect, we make a huge leap toward the kind of sensitivity that embraces differences and empowers instead of weakening others. The coach approach is in itself inherently more multiculturally sensitive than many other ways of relating in the helping professions. However, our great downfall is our inevitable ignorance about our client's world that can be rooted in bias we are not even aware of. We must learn, we must inquire, we must invite our client to educate us about that world in order to build the strongest alliance possible and serve our clients maximally. The topic of multiculturalism in coaching is worthy of books of its own. Bringing health and wellness coach training to a number of predominantly underserved populations in the United States and to several foreign countries has taught me a great deal about the need for coaching allies throughout the world. These allies need to be just that, real partners in their client's journey to health and well-being.

Relevant Theory
Appreciative Inquiry—Positive Mindset and Reframing

The collaborative process called appreciative inquiry is entirely congruent with the positive way coaches build the coaching alliance in a client-centered way. Developed by David Cooperrider and Diana Whitney, its aim is "liberating the human spirit to consciously construct a better future." Appreciative inquiry, or AI, was designed as a collaborative process to improve organizations, but it beautifully supports the principles and methodology of both life coaching and health and wellness coaching.

In this quote below, written for the organizational context, you can see how AI aligns with Maslow's theory of self-actualization, the work of humanistic psychologists, such as Rogers, the modern positive psychology movement, and the foundations of coaching laid out by Whitworth, et.al. in the book *Co-Active Coaching* (Kimsey-House, 2018).

> In AI the...task of intervention gives way to the speed of imagination and innovation. Instead of negation, criticism, and spiraling diagnosis, there is discovery, dreaming, and design. AI seeks fundamentally to build a constructive union between a whole group of people and the massive entirety of what they talk about as past and present capabilities: achievements, assets, unexplored potentials, innovations, strengths, elevated thoughts, opportunities, benchmarks, high point moments, lived values, traditions, strategic competencies, stories, expressions of wisdom, insights into the deeper corporate spirit or soul—and visions of valued and possible futures (Cooperrider, 2005).

When applying the principles of appreciative inquiry to health and wellness coaching, we focus away from the problem: what isn't working. Instead of trying to fix, we focus towards evoking the qualities of the client's "inner core." That is, that which connects our clients to life, energy, possibilities, and thriving. There is an amazingly rich palette in every client for client and coach to draw upon to define, discover, dream, design, and forge into destiny (the 4D cycle of appreciative inquiry).

Within the context of health and wellness coaching sometimes the appreciative inquiry 4D cycle is expanded into a 5D cycle where the additional first step is:

Define: the topic or focus of inquiry. This may be the client's overall area(s) of focus for coaching, the focus of the session, or the focus of an inquiry that the coach leaves with the client at the end of the session. Client and coach co-design a positive life-sustaining focus. Coaches follow the client's energy to pursue exploration of what is life-giving to the individual.

The 4D Cycle of Appreciative Inquiry:
Discover, Dream, Design, and Destiny
Health and wellness coaches can apply the 4D cycle in the following way:

Discover: Inquire into stories that are life-affirming. It is a whole person inquiry into the "positive change core." We appreciate all that contributes to and makes up the positive core in the individual.

Dream: Imagine what could be by identifying themes that appear in the stories and exploring topics for further inquiry. Create a vision in relation to the discovered qualities and client potential, and ask questions that elicit intrinsic motivation. (For example, who is your inner self calling you to become?)

Design: Determine what is wanted by creating an image of a preferred future; defining possibility propositions that tap into the positive core and are in alignment with the new dream.

Destiny: Create what will be by exploring and identifying ways (goals and action steps) to create that future, strengthening and affirming self-efficacy, building mometum around a deeper purpose, and orienting the client towards taking action, learning, adjustment, and improvisation.

The Five Basic Principles of Appreciative Inquiry and Their Application in Health and Wellness Coaching

According to Cooperrider and Whitney, even as the process of appreciative inquiry is underway with their organizational clients, the question what to do with the real problem arises. This is as relevant to clients in health and wellness coaching as it is to organizations attempting to make change (Cooperrider, 2005). To address this question, they point to "the five principles and scholarly streams considered central to AI's theory-base of change."

The Constructionist Principle

The Simultaneity Principle

The Poetic Principle

The Anticipatory Principle

The Positive Principle

1. The Constructionist Principle: Positive conversations and interactions. Essentially, we "construct" or create our beliefs and truth collaboratively through language and discourse with those around us, over time, based on our collective observations and experiences. From the coaching perspective: positive energy and emotions generate positive conversations.

This principle honors the *influence of social connection*. It acknowledges that one's social connections and environment have a huge impact on beliefs, understanding of the world, and possibility thinking. The coach can facilitate awareness of positive and negative beliefs held by the client, and the influence and role of social norms and other social forces on those beliefs. Through positive inquiry and exploration, coaching can help to strengthen positive social influences, past and present.

The Constructionist Principle also focuses on the *importance of "the story."* There is a saying, "If you want to change your life, change your story." The coach can help their client gain awareness of what their story is and its negative or positive impact. The coach can also promote awareness of the negative or positive impact of others on the client's story. And, most importantly, through positive inquiry, the coach can facilitate creation of a new and/or different positive story.

This principle also acknowledges the *importance of self-talk*. Self-talk is the inner conversation, which is every bit as influential as social conversations and connections, if not more so. It's what feeds, nourishes, and perpetuates the negative or the positive story. The coach can facilitate identification of negative self-talk and how to address it and promote positive self-talk (e.g. the client's story, personal mottos, well life vision statement, reminders, etc.)

Lastly, the Constructionist Principle addresses the importance of the coaching conversation. In the same way that family, friends, culture, and work life factors influence a client's story, the coaching alliance and the quality of the coaching conversation can have a defining impact. In AI it is critical to be focused on positive inquiry and reflections. It's equally important for the coach to honor and respect the client's autonomy. That entails inclusion and integration of all the different aspects of the core self, and the client's freedom to choose which aspects of self to highlight their story and how it unfolds.

2. The Simultaneity Principle: Change begins in the inquiry—including the conversations, questions, and reflections. The moment we ask a question, we begin to create change.

> Inquiry and change are not...separate moments, but are simultaneous. Inquiry is intervention...The questions we ask set the stage for what we "find," and what we "discover" becomes the...material and the stories out of which the future is conceived, conversed about and constructed (Cooperrider, 2005).

The importance of the coaching mindset comes through again. As coaches we want to be very aware that change begins the very moment we initiate inquiry. This principle reminds us that anytime we begin to analyze something, that very thing we are analyzing is affected and in some way changes. Therefore, the more masterful coach understands that it is important that we are mindful in our inquiries and are focused on asking what AI calls "unconditional positive questions" and using positive requests for clarification. We want to use open questions that allow the client maximal freedom to explore and answer what is true for them. While perhaps no question can be completely without influence, we try our best. The only tilt to the questions is their positive nature.

Examples of Unconditional Positive Questions and Requests for Clarification

- Describe the most energizing moment, a real "high" from your life. What made it happen?
- Without being humble, describe what you value most about yourself.
- Describe your three wishes for the future.
- Describe a time when you were...
- What made it possible to...?
- What made it an exciting experience? What gave it energy?
- What was it about you—the unique qualities you have—that contributed to the ...?
- Who were the most significant others in your life?

- What made them significant? What were the qualities you saw in them?
- What were the most defining moments in your life?
- What were the most important factors that helped to make it a meaningful experience?
- What was a peak moment in your life?
- In what ways did you contribute to the creation of (a past success)?

3. The Poetic Principle: Positive attention and focus on the here and now. By exploring *what is* in a positive and thorough way, we begin to see *what could be!* This is what coaching calls possibility thinking at its best. Very similar to the inquiring process of Gestalt therapy or existential approaches to therapy and philosophy, the poetic principle has us stay centered in the here and now, the present moment of existence.

> Positive attention to the present leads to positive anticipation of the future (anticipatory principle), which in turn leads to positive questions and reflections (simultaneity principle), resulting in positive conversations and interactions (constructionist principle), which culminates in positive energy and emotion (positive principle) (Dossey, 2014).

Contrast this positive approach with the usual analysis of what's wrong with a situation. A focus on what is not wanted will perpetuate the creation of the same. A focus on what is wanted will result in creating just that.

4. The Anticipatory Principle: Humans move in the direction of their image of the future. "When a positive anticipation is held, positive outcomes become possible. When positive outcomes are anticipated, individuals and groups become more resilient, hopeful, and creative about the future" (Dossey, 2014). The positivity theme of AI continues strongly in this principle. Coaching has always been a strengths-based, positive psychology approach. People need positive motivation to pull them forward towards the kind of healthy life they really want to live. Coaches use questions in a positive way that helps the client to describe the outcome that they want to see. AI emphasizes this using questions such as *What would it look like?* This principle keeps the focus on creating a positive future and the coaching is designed to help the client to not only identify it, but to foster belief that such a future is possible.

5. The Positive Principle: Positive energy and emotion. Whether we see this principle as the culmination of the AI process (as Dossey, et al. state above), or the core that runs through all of it, building positive energy and emotion is very different from how we often approach "helping" people. Instead of the *What's wrong and how can we fix it?* mindset that we spoke of earlier in this chapter, this principle moves us from fixing what's wrong to helping people grow.

> Positive actions overcome an imbalance in energy and are stimulated by positive energy and emotion. Conversely negative energy and emotion, which are part of finding fault or correcting weaknesses, lack the force needed to move in new, positive directions (Dossey, 2014).

Cooperrider and Whitney draw upon their work with groups and businesses to state:

> It has been our experience that building and sustaining momentum for change requires large amounts of positive affect and social bonding—things like hope, excitement, inspiration, caring, camaraderie, sense of urgent purpose, and sheer joy in creating something meaningful together. What we have found is the more positive the question we ask in our work, the more long-lasting and successful the change effort (Cooperrider, 2005).

> The Positive Principle asserts that positive energy and emotion disrupt downward spirals, building the aspirations of people into a dynamic force for transformational change. Positive energy and emotion broaden thinking, expand awareness, increase abilities, build resiliency, offset negatives, generate new possibilities, and create an upward spiral of learning and growth (Moore, 2015).

For me, what appreciative inquiry does is underscore the strength of the coach approach. AI should not be confused with a naive Pollyanna way of viewing the world. A positive approach does not mean wearing blinders to the challenges of life. Rather, it fortifies the rationale for coming at our challenges with a different mindset. It reframes our view of what is and enables us to see what could be, and then we work towards that. You may find some real value in the 4/5 D Cycle of Inquiry to help guide your coaching process. You may find that if you are steeped in the client-centered approach, grounded in positive psychology, and well-trained in the Core Competencies of Coaching (International Coach Federation, 2020), that the way you coach is already entirely congruent with Appreciative Inquiry.

Positive Psychology
and Wellness Coaching

While the practice of both professional life coaching and health and wellness coaching is thoroughly infused with a positive psychology approach, there is much to be learned from attending to the academic study of positive psychology. Positive psychology has become a field of professional study defining itself as *the scientific study of the strengths and virtues that enable individuals and communities to thrive*. This field is founded on the belief that people want to lead meaningful and fulfilling lives, to cultivate what is best within themselves, and to enhance their experiences of love, work, and play.

As life coaching developed, it was the work of the humanistic psychologists and authors such as Abraham Maslow (who first coined the term positive psychology in the 1950s), Carl Rogers, Virginia Satir, Sidney Jourard, Rollo May, and many others who influenced coaching's founders. Coaching took on the tenets of the humanistic perspective and viewed humans as being in the process of moving towards greater levels of self-actualization and realization of their potential. The coach approach became a strengths-based approach instead of a remedial, treatment-oriented way of both viewing people and working with them. Coaches, like the humanists, embraced the centrality of human values and meaning, and saw individuals as possessing the capacity to be creative, resourceful, and capable of overcoming obstacles to their growth.

While the humanistic psychologists laid a strong and positive foundation that influenced the practice of counseling and psychotherapy, it did not build a large evidentiary base. They tended to use qualitative research rather than the scientific methodology found in most experiments and laboratory settings. What has been a fascinating and a quite ironic development in recent years is how the newly developed field of Positive Psychology has used these same scientific methods to, in fact, validate much of what the humanists touted, and that life coaching embraced.

Positive Psychology Today

Positive Psychology's birth as a domain occurred in 1998 when Martin Seligman selected it as the theme for his term as president of the American Psychological Association. Mihaly Csikszentmihalyi, Barbara Fredrickson, and Christopher Peterson are also hailed as progenitors of this field. It built on the humanistic movement, but integrated creative research to substantiate it. Seligman's groundbreaking book, *Authentic Happiness: Using the New Positive Psychology to Realize Your Potential for Lasting Fulfillment* (Seligman, 2004), introduced the field to many. The work of Barbara Frederickson (Frederickson, 2009) and her book *Positivity* is another central resource. Positive psychology is not a singular method, theory, approach, or question. It can better be understood as a large field of study that is, in many ways, complementary to traditional psychology, and not a replacement for it.

While many psychologists have largely focused on studying, diagnosing, and treating mental illness, psychologists within the field of positive psychology focus their time and efforts on systematically investigating well-being and human flourishing (Seligman, 2012). To clarify, the study of positive psychology is built on a foundational assumption that the absence of mental illness is not equivalent to mental health or well-being. And, while a more traditional medical approach within psychology remains vitally important, researchers and practitioners within positive psychology assert that investigating the causes and correlates of flourishing within individuals, organizations, and communities should be considered at least equally as important.

The Value to the Coach

By reviewing studies within positive psychology, wellness coaches can leverage nuanced empirical findings to inform their approach and improve their effectiveness. Understanding what research has to say around topics like goal setting, inquiry, emotion, mindset, behavior change, resilience, etc., can equip wellness coaches with greater knowledge and help to increase the probability that they are providing the most informed and valuable coaching they can to their clients. Simply put, positive psychology may bolster the reliability of certain coaching approaches or methods by taking some of the guesswork out of the equation (Biswas-Dieners, 2010).

Positive psychology researchers are continually coming up with new exercises, interventions, methods, and tools that may be useful for wellness coaches to incorporate into their coaching. Reading their research can engender curiosity in the coach that helps them understand psychological theory and human behavior even better.

Barbara Frederickson pointed to the importance of going "beyond happiness" to "focus on flourishing" (Frederickson, 2009). Flourishing includes doing good and not just feeling good, having a sense of meaning and purpose, and arriving at resiliency in the face of negativity.

In his book, *Flourish*, Seligman outlined his theory of PERMA™ (Seligman, *Flourish: A Visionary New Understanding of Happiness and Well-being*, 2012) and the five building blocks that enable flourishing:

- **Positive emotion**

- **Engagement:** One example of engagement is the experience of a flow state. "Engagement is an experience in which someone fully deploys the skills, strengths, and attention for a challenging task." (University of Pennsylvania, 2019)

- **Relationships:** The presence of friends, family, intimacy, or social connection are fundamental to well-being.

- **Meaning:** Belonging to and serving something bigger than one's self.

- **Achievement:** Achieving goals and ambitions that give us a sense of accomplishment.

Looking at the building blocks of flourishing, we can see that each of these elements contributes to the kind of lifestyle that supports health and wellbeing. In particular, when wellness coaches work with clients on *connectedness*, building *relationships* that support their wellness, they are supporting flourishing. Coaches help clients to feel more *engaged* in their own life through connecting with what motivates their efforts at lifestyle improvement. Coaching works with clients to reframe their experience in more *positive* ways yielding more *positive emotions*. Effective coaching helps clients connect with their values and discover greater *meaning and purpose*, which we know is correlated with better health in many ways.

Barbara Frederickson is probably best known for what she calls *The Positivity Ratio* (Frederickson, 2005). This research showed that our ratio between positive and negative thoughts and emotions will help determine one's odds of languishing or flourishing. While most of us experience a ratio of two positive emotions for each negative emotion (and for more depressed individuals the ratio may be more like 1-1 or lower), those who reach a 3-1 ratio seem to hit what Frederickson calls a *tipping point* where the odds of flourishing increase dramatically.

Frederickson is also quick to point out that the way to increase positivity is not to adopt a Pollyanna slogan of "be positive." It is the realistic facing of our negative emotions that keep us grounded in the reality of our lives; that serve, as she likes to say, like a sailboat's keel holding us steady on course. As coaches help their clients to embrace these more negative emotions and work through them with process coaching, clients can access and express more of a full range of emotions. The humanistic psychologists we've referred to call this *full-feeling* reactivity and saw it as a quality of more self-actualized people.

A *mindset* of positivity, Frederickson contends, is the best pathway to increasing your positivity ratio. To develop and hold such a mindset, she entreats us to:

- Be open
- Be appreciative
- Be curious
- Be kind
- Be real

These strategies describe the kind of mindset that coaches strive to operate with. By being role models for our clients and encouraging this type of mindset in our clients, coaches can, hopefully, engender the increased positivity ratio that supports flourishing (i.e., personal growth).

> The boundaries between you and not-you—what lies beyond your skin—relax and become more permeable. While infused with love you see fewer distinctions between you and others. Indeed, your ability to see others—really see them, wholeheartedly—springs open (Fredrickson).

Client-Centered Directiveness Is an Oxymoron But It Works

At its very foundation, coaching is client-centered. The work of Carl Rogers profoundly influenced the founders of the life coaching profession. Beginning coaches take the client-centered foundation of coaching very seriously. Yet the question of how directive or non-directive to be remains an area of unsureness and anxiety for many wellness coaches. In fact, they are often hesitant to offer their own perspective, to challenge their clients, or to make any suggestions. They sometimes over-compensate by being overly client-centered and non-directive. Effective and more experienced coaches have found a way to remain true to these client-centered roots as they integrate more directive methods with their coaching.

Coaching Practice, in Reality, Is More Directive Than You Might Think

Coaches do ask questions, plenty of them. A question directs a client toward a specific line of inquiry.

- As coaches we share our observations with the client. Sometimes referred to as "Saying what is so," we point out patterns in our client's speech, actions, and affect that we observe. For example: "Have you noticed that each time you speak about taking time for yourself to exercise, that you immediately go into a story about your partner?"

- Coaches challenge their clients. When our client offers a commitment of practicing a mindfulness or meditational method only once a week, the effective coach will ask if that will produce the results the client desires, rather than simply accepting what the client has offered.

- Coaches use tools. The moment we suggest using a coaching tool we are being directive, even if we've asked our client for permission to make the suggestion. The tool, whether it be something as simple as a Wheel of Life, or as complex as a Health Risk Assessment, comes from the recommendation of the coach. It is their idea, not the client's.

- Wellness coaches often make the suggestion of resources for healthy living information, for practicing various stress-management methods, for seeking out social support for their goals, etc. The challenge for the coach is to know just how directive to be, and with whom!

The Sound of Effective Directive Coaching

- "Have you considered keeping track of your behavior?" (A question, yet really a suggestion.)
- "When my clients write it down on a calendar or enter it into an app they are often more successful."
- "What I see you doing here is…"
- "Let me give you my best thinking here…"
- "I have a coaching tool here you may find value in…"
- "Have you ever worked with www.myplate.gov?"
- "What is your well-life vision?"
- "If you only practice relaxation twice a week, will that really give you the results you want?"
- "Tell me what another perspective on that would be?"
- "If you could work your best possible day, what would it look like?"

The Directive/Non-Directive Continuum

When we examine the work of both beginner and master coaches we see them all operating somewhere on a continuum from non-directive to very directive.

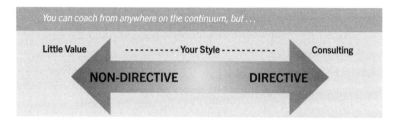

FIGURE 4—THE DIRECTIVE/NON-DIRECTIVE CONTINUUM

Operating as a coach on the extreme non-directive end of this continuum is probably more theoretical than actual. In some way coaches will demonstrate at least a degree of directiveness. On the other extreme of complete directedness, coaching transitions from coaching to consulting or teaching. We are no longer coaching; we are being the expert/consultant who is advising and directing. In between the extremes there is lots of room for variation that still can qualify as effective coaching.

Where the coach operates on this continuum is, in part, determined by the personality and style of the coach themselves. "Be yourself" in coaching is very important to authenticity. Watch films of some of the great psychotherapists of our time and you'll see that to a great degree their approach in therapy reflects simply who they are. Rogers really was a kind and gentle soul. Fritz Perls, while actually much more caring and empathic than many may think, was a truly irascible fellow, while Albert Ellis really was a brash New Yorker. Likewise, great coaches let their true selves work for themselves and for the benefit of their clients. So, give yourself permission to let your own gifts show through. However, never think that being yourself is an excuse for not serving the client well. The timid coach may need to stretch themselves and be more actively involved. The domineering coach may need to realize when they are taking direction too far and self-regulate.

Overly Non-Directive Coaching

When coaches take being non-directive too far, they end up not providing as much as they can for their clients. Without any structure or guidance, many of our clients flounder seeking direction. In an extensive workshop with James Prochaska I once asked him about just how client-centered a coach needed to be. He said: *"Be client-centered. But, don't be so client-centered that you are not helping someone as much as you possibly can"* (Prochaska, 2016).

The overly non-directive coach
- Doesn't share observations about their client and the coaching process.
- Doesn't say what is so.
- Doesn't make any suggestions (even with permission).
- Doesn't challenge their client.
- Provides little if any structure.
- Doesn't share what has worked for others.

The overly non-directive coach essentially is not providing as much value and structure to the client as they could be. We might even go so far as to say they are avoiding responsibility for contributing anything to the coaching process that might influence it.

Overly Directive Coaching

The overly directive coach is usually operating out of a consulting mindset whether they realize it or not. They may still be relying on an educational/informative model. Perhaps their background is more of a health educator, or a holistic health practitioner who is still being quite prescriptive. Perhaps they have a business-consulting background and believe that their clients want to be told what to do.

The overly directive coach
- Acts more as a consultant/expert.
- Provides solutions (instead of coaching for the client to find their own solutions).
- Has a ready-to-go Wellness Plan for their client.
- Makes many suggestions. Is often rigid about structure instead of co-creating it.

- Presents lots of opinions instead of observations.
- Often doesn't listen well and fails to include the client's point of view.
- Sometimes thinks falsely that being directive saves time.

Almost all of the techniques and methods that coaches use fall somewhere on the "Coaching Spectrum."

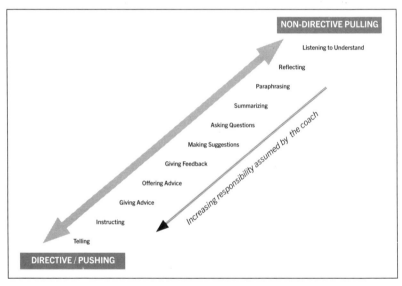

FIGURE 5—THE COACHING SPECTRUM,
Effective Modern Coaching, Miles Downey

As you can see in this illustration, the more directive the coach becomes the greater the level of responsibility they take for where the coaching goes. Shifting more and more into the consulting role at the directive end of the spectrum, the consultant assumes more and more control if the client does not resist. In any given coaching session, a coach will be moving about within this spectrum, at times simply listening, paraphrasing, etc., and at other times asking questions, all the way to occasionally, with permission, providing some education. The coach needs to be aware of their patterns and overall tendencies across a number of sessions.

How to Keep Directive Coaching Client-Centered

- Maintain the coaching mindset—(The client is held to be naturally creative, resourceful, and whole.)
- Facilitate the client's process—evoke inner wisdom.
- Don't rescue! Work with the client to help them explore more instead of providing suggestions prematurely.
- Introduce suggestions so the client truly knows they can decline them.
- When clients decline, respect their decision. Explore it, but go with it.
- Clients are always accountable to themselves, not to you.
- All planning and accountability is co-created! Every bit of it.
- Record your sessions periodically for review and count how many suggestions you made.
- Have a rationale for any suggestion you do make.
- A ready-to-go wellness program is wellness, but not wellness coaching!

Adapting the Coaching to Your Client

Effective health and wellness coaching adapts in many ways to our client. As we assist a person in finding ways to live a healthier life there are many adjustments that need to be made to deliver a customized experience that will work best for that individual.

Wellness coaching clients vary tremendously on mental/emotional and environmental variables. One client may be highly motivated to improve their lifestyle and very open to and welcoming of coaching. They may have abundant resources at their disposal and great support from other people in their lives. Or they may be the mirror image of all of these qualities. Some of our clients may be familiar with coaching from experiences with business/life coaching, or from having had some form of telephonic wellness coaching as a benefit from their employer or insurance company. Many, of course, will be very unfamiliar with wellness coaching and how it works.

One way to adjust to what our client needs is to see where they fit into the following matrix:

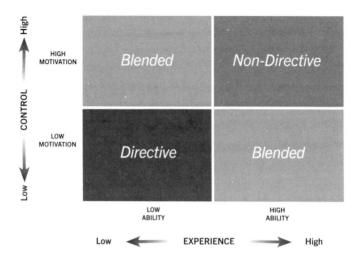

FIGURE 6—CONTROL / EXPERIENCE APPROACH

If we just look at the variables of *Experience*, *Control*, *Motivation*, and *Ability* we can see how we might work with these combinations in either more directive, less, or non-directive and blended approaches. *Experience* may refer to more or less experience with coaching or with the process of changing lifestyle behavior. *Control* may refer to the client's own need for control, or how "in charge" they like to be. *Motivation* may refer to motivation to engage in the coaching process, and/or motivation to improve one's lifestyle. *Ability* may refer to intellectual ability or to environmental circumstances that limit the client's ability to engage in lifestyle improvement efforts.

The matrix is not perfect. We could, for example, have a client who is of low ability and low motivation, but who has high needs for control. In such situations we would have to decide which variable trumps the others. In this case, I personally would recommend honoring the high need for control as paramount.

Perhaps this illustrates that someone will always have their own unique position in the matrix and require us to adjust the degree to which we are directive or non-directive. We might imagine their location being plotted like somewhere on a graph, as in our example, near the top of the Directive Quadrant, closer to the border with the Blended Quadrant. In other words, we are not advocating a simplistic four-quadrant approach to coaching, but again, honoring the unique position of each of our clients on the matrix.

Examples—Ronaldo and Hazel

Our client, whom we'll call Ronaldo, is an industrial design team leader who has had some experience with leadership coaching. He's struggling with stress, sleeping well, and his biometric markers have hit an alarming borderline zone with his blood sugar, blood pressure, and blood lipid levels. He's very concerned about this and highly motivated to engage in coaching and make some positive and immediate lifestyle improvements. He clearly fits somewhere in our non-directive quadrant on our matrix. Coaching with Ronaldo will most likely proceed, as it would with all of our clients, building a strong coaching alliance, using an effective coaching methodology and structure. Ronaldo will want to feel like he is definitely the one with his hands on the steering wheel. All of our steps together will be *co-created*. Ronaldo will need little in the way of suggestions or even education, but he may benefit tremendously from a great ally to strategize with, a strong system of support, and what we might call "gentle" accountability.

Another client of ours, we'll call her Hazel, is a hardworking housekeeper with a large hotel chain. She has never had any experience with coaching and is unfamiliar with what it can offer. She's finding that despite her high level of physical activity she still continues to gain weight. She is also very discouraged from many failed attempts at crash dieting. Accurate information about how to eat better has been lacking for her. She finds learning new systems difficult and doesn't really like change. Her family situation also contributes to making lifestyle improvement challenging.

Hazel would fall somewhere more into our Directive Quadrant. Again, we would be treating Hazel with the same high level of honor and respect that we would with all of our clients in building a powerful coaching alliance. We would avoid stereotyping Hazel or making assumptions about her abilities. We would, however, be realistic in meeting her where she is. It's quite likely that Hazel would actually appreciate a more directive approach. She may benefit from recommendations for nutrition education resources. If the coach is a qualified dietician or nutritionist, they may want to create an agreement to combine these roles into the coaching that is done and "wear two hats." The coach may take on a role where they are guiding the client through the coaching methodology more carefully, yet keeping it client-centered, with Hazel still being in charge of choosing each step that she wants to do. Accountability agreements may need to be adjusted more closely to make sure that Hazel is clear about the agreements and sees the value in them for her.

"Just tell me what to do!"

There are times when clients more like Hazel really ask the coach to simply tell them directly what to do. How should I exercise? What should I eat? Usually such clients are discouraged by past failure experiences and their own self-efficacy is so low that they have no faith in their own ability to create an effective way to change. They seek consultation more than coaching. They want a real "expert" to direct them on the right path. A great coaching response to such requests goes something like this:

> *So, when you've asked the experts about what you should do, and followed their advice, how did that work for you?*

Almost always the person will think for a moment, sigh, and then have to admit that while such expert advice may have worked for a short amount of time, eventually it didn't work at all. That's when you can lightheartedly suggest that you and your client defy the so-called definition of insanity—doing the same thing again and expecting different results! We need to meet our client's request for complete direction (to the point of consultation, not coaching) with empathy and understanding. Keeping them in charge, remaining client-centered can still be done, even though we may coach them in a more directive style.

Staying True to the Coaching Mindset

No matter how directive or non-directive we are with our client, we still will be coaching from a stance where we hold them to be naturally creative, resourceful, and whole. Our task is still to evoke our client's inner wisdom. Some of our clients may be at the point of doubting they even have such wisdom and strength. This is where it is good to remember the famous quote from Goethe.

> *If you treat an individual as he is, he will remain how he is.*
> *But if you treat him as if he were what he ought to be and*
> *could be, he will become what he ought to be and could be.*

> —Johann Wolfgang von Goethe

Masterful Moment

How comfortable do you feel being more directive?

Are you at ease allowing the client to take the lead?

How can you develop your coaching craft to where it feels like you always have the option to be more or less directive?

Getting Started—What Shapes the Coaching Alliance

Beginning coaches often feel awkward initiating the coaching conversation. Clients come through our door or arrive for their online and/or phone coaching session sometimes unsure how to get started as well. A lesson from anthropology will tell us that social greeting behavior is expected, normal, and helps everyone relax. It's not only okay to exchange what we might call pleasantries, talk about the weather, etc., it grounds us in a more comfortable and familiar interaction from which to proceed. The key is to keep it brief.

The Essential Role of Structure in the Coaching Session

While every coach is free to develop their own coaching style, and is probably a better coach because of it, consciously following a basic coaching structure will help ensure that sessions are as productive as desired. Clients engage with coaches in order to accomplish what they have not been getting done in their lives. Much of the help that coaches provide is in helping clients to become better organized, to plan, to commit, and to be accountable to themselves, thereby producing the results they want to see. Health and wellness coaching clients are often attempting to change very specific, daily behaviors. This requires a consistent approach that usually involves effective tracking and accountability. Structure allows this to happen in a more reliable way.

While coaching sessions benefit from a structure that is flexible and adaptive to current circumstances, it is also a template for both coach and client to rely upon. Here is a very approximate breakdown of how a session may be divided up. Forwarding the action takes time. Leave 1/3 of the session for it.

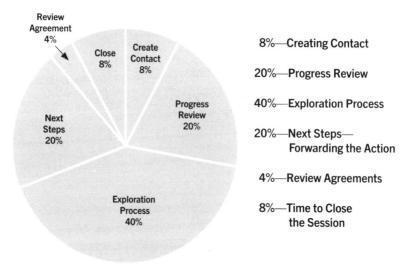

8%—Creating Contact

20%—Progress Review

40%—Exploration Process

20%—Next Steps—
Forwarding the Action

4%—Review Agreements

8%—Time to Close
the Session

FIGURE 87—SESSION BREAKDOWN

1. **Creating Contact**—Casual and friendly greetings. Brief small talk. This helps put clients at ease and normalizes the conversation.

2. **Progress Review**—Begin by checking in with what went well. Then report on progress and challenges to committed action steps. Save processing for next step. Consciously co-create the agenda of today's session (see below).

3. **Exploration Process**—Helping client draw out learning and understanding of the current situation. Examining internal and external barriers to change. Exploring dynamics, sources of support. Develop insights, develop new strategies.

4. **Next Steps**—Forwarding the Action—Partnering with your client to co-create strategies and stage-appropriate action steps towards progress. Agreements for committed action. Inquire who/what else can be sources of support for these efforts. Make sure client understands a motivation connection between what they want to accomplish and what they are committing to doing.

5. **Review Agreements**—Go over agreements made for next steps. Clarify any details about strategy, tracking, etc.

6. **Close the Session**—Summarize or have the client summarize the session. Identify any "take-aways" for the client (what they learned). Reinforce and acknowledge their progress and way forward. Certify next appointment arrangements.

Co-Creating the Agenda—Every Time

Coaches help their clients to get clear about what they want to accomplish in coaching. They consciously partner with their client to co-create the coaching alliance. They hold the client's agenda to be the agenda, but that does not mean starting a session with the often-disastrous invitation "So! What do you want to talk about today?" Make your coaching sessions more productive and satisfying by using the following steps as part of your coaching session structure.

Ten Steps to Structuring Great Wellness Coaching Sessions

1. **Preparation.** Begin working on the session before it happens. Have your client use a Coaching Session Prep Form to list their wins, address their commitments to action steps, and share what is important to process. Do your own homework on this client by reviewing notes, and getting mentally and physically prepared for the session.

2. **Acknowledge and...** When a client comes bursting through the door, so to speak, with an important issue to discuss handle it like this:

   a. Acknowledge their experience.

   b. Reflect their feelings about it.

   c. Emphasize the importance of being sure to talk about this issue today and ask what else the client wants to be sure to include in today's agenda.

3. Dealing with crisis. Realize that when a client comes to the session in the midst of an immediate crisis that the empathic understanding and support of the coach may be all that "gets done" today, and that is totally okay. Create an agreement to just focus on helping them to express themselves about this issue and perhaps do some immediate problem solving, such as helping them find additional resources to deal with the crisis (this could include referral to medical resources, mental health resources, or other possibilities).

4. Wins! An energizing way to begin most sessions is by checking in on what has gone well for the client since the last session. Looking at Wins! first is a positive psychology approach that coaching is famous for. It works! A win is either something that the client accomplished (such as completing action steps), learned, or realized since the last session. It may also be a positive opportunity that is coming up, such as a friend who likes to be active coming to visit. You also may want to go over a Session Preparation Form together.

5. Consciously co-create the agenda for the session. Create an agreement about what will be worked on in this particular session. This should be relevant to the client's overall Wellness Plan, or to the development of that plan. Following a map ensures that we will get where we want to go. Remember that co-creation means that you, the coach, can also contribute to the agenda. Coaches often can point out items such as key elements of the client's Wellness Plan, that need to be discussed.

6. Drawing out learning and processing. Explore the client's experience with those action steps, with internal and external barriers that have come up. Coach for realization, insight, and deeper understanding of self and environment. Connect with motivation. Coach for possibilities. This often takes up the bulk of the coaching session, perhaps about 40% of the time you have together.

7. Next steps—Forwarding the action. Leave about one-third of the session available for "Where do we go from here?" Drawing upon what was gained in the session co-create next steps for the client to take in applying what they are learning. Look at previous commitments to action steps and either *recommit* (to the same action steps), *reset* (adjust the action steps to a different level or threshold), or *shift*

(shift to new action steps). Set up mutually agreed upon accountability regarding each action step.

You may also want to co-create an inquiry for them to work on in the coming week—something for them to think about, journal and/or converse about that is relevant to what came up in the session.

8. Review and agree. Summarize the essence of the session. Review exactly what the client's understanding of the way forward is, and agree upon specific action steps to which the client commits. Reinforce the motivational connection between the steps and how they will help the client achieve what they want in their Wellness Plan.

9. Wrap it up and close. Leave the client with inspiration, acknowledgment, and clarity about the next meeting time.

10. Notes and self-care time. Finish up your notes, including notes about information you need to find (such as knowledge about a medication your client is taking) and any action steps that you have committed to doing. Then, take a little time for your own self-care, on a mental, emotional, and/or physical level.

Feedback from students in our advanced wellness coaching competencies classes and our mentoring coaching program tells us that implementing the co-creation of an agenda for the session, Step #2, has completely changed and improved how they coach with their clients. Step #3 has often helped them to stick to this structure and meet the client where they needed to be met.

Structure often serves to paradoxically increase our freedom. Instead of wandering or even floundering on our coaching path, we find we cover more ground, and discover more along the way by having a map to follow. Adhering rigidly to structure can be counter-productive. Effective coaching is that balance that allows for "dancing in the moment" while appreciating the guidance of a co-created design for our coaching work. Being client-centered does not mean passively following the client in conversation wherever they may lead. It means facilitating the client's own process, keeping them in the driver's seat, but traveling down the road to where the client wants to go.

In this chapter we saw how foundational a role the coach's mindset plays in all that we do in coaching. We defined coaching presence as the provision of the facilitative conditions of coaching and deeply explored the concept of empathy and how to convey this to our clients. We saw how the client-centered approach to therapy has had a profound effect upon coaching. The relevant theory of appreciative inquiry was explored and the field of positive psychology and its contributions to coaching were covered. How to remain client-centered and yet be directive in our coaching can be a real challenge. We looked further into how to do that and at the role a directive/non-directive continuum plays in how we individualize coaching.

In our next chapter—Being Isn't Always Easy—we will discover how to provide the compassion our clients need yet be detached enough to serve ourselves and the coaching relationship well. We'll grapple with how to coach clients who appear resistive and difficult. How much to self-disclose is often confusing for coaches. We'll explore an effective way to do that and address the thorny issue of collusion.

REFERENCES

Biswas-Dieners, R. (2010). *Practicing positive psychology coaching*. Wiley.

Carkhuff, R. R. (1967). *Beyond counseling and therapy*. Holt, Rinehart and Winston.

Carkhuff, R. R. (1967). *Toward effective counseling and psychotherapy: Training and practice*. Aldine Publishing Co.

Cooperrider, D. A. (2005). *A positive revolution in change: Appreciative inquiry*. Case Western Reserve University, The Taos Institute.

Crum, A. J. (2007). Mindset matters: Exercise and the placebo effect. *Psychological science*. 137

Dossey, B. M. (2014). *Nurse coaching: Integrative approaches for health and wellbeing*. International Nurse Coach Association.

Frederickson, B. (2005). Positive affect and the complex dynamics of human flourishing. *American psychologist,* 60, 678-686.

Frederickson, B. (2009). *Positivity*. Harmony.

Goleman, D. (2007, June 12). *Blog*. Daniel Goleman: http://www. danielgoleman.info/three-kinds-of-empathy-cognitive-emotional-compassionate/

Hazler, R. J. & Barwick, N. (2001). *The therapeutic environment: Core conditions for facilitating therapy*. PDF Open University Press. McGraw Hill Education https://www.mheducation.co.uk/openup/chapters/0335202829.pdf

Hodges, S. D. (2007). Empathy. *SAGE Knowledge.* http://sk.sagepub.com/ reference/ socialpsychology/n179.xml

International Coaching Federation. (2020). Core competencies. *The gold standard in coaching - ICF - International Coach Federation.* https://coachfederation.org/ core-competencies

Kimsey-House, K. K. (2018). *Co-Active Coaching, (Fourth ed.): The proven framework for transformative conversations at work and in life.* Nicholas Brealey.

Kirschenbaum, H. (2018, April). The history of the person-centered approach. *The Association for the Development of the Person-Centered Approach.* http:// adpca.org/content/history-0

Moore, M. J. (2015). *Coaching psychology manual, (*2nd ed.). Lippincott, Williams & Wilkins.

Medium.com. https://medium.com/achology/carl-rogers-and-the-core-conditionsof-counselling-a87167028905

Ritter, A. (2010). *The 100/0 principle: The secret of great relationships.* Simple Truths.

Rogers, C. (1942). *Counseling and psychotherapy: Newer concepts in practice.* Houghton Mifflin.

Seligman, M. (2004). *Authentic happiness: Using the new positive psychology to realize your potential for lasting fulfillment.* Atria Books.

Seligman, M. (2012). *Flourish: A visionary new understanding of happiness and well-being.* Atria Books.

PART THREE

What to Do

Chapter 5—Being Isn't Always Easy

CHAPTER FIVE

Being Isn't Always Easy

It's not easy being green.

—Joe Raposo as sung by Kermit the Frog

Being of service to others is both full of reward and fraught with difficulties. It gives us meaning and purpose to help others on their journey and to see them grow. We revel in their accomplishments, in their joy, and in their triumph. Our compassion feels the pull of sadness when our clients' struggle, when they fail, and when they suffer. We attempt to be that reliable, centered, solid ally, yet we are vulnerable to all of the challenges that come with being human.

How do we maintain a coaching presence that both benefits the client and retains our own wellbeing? How do we relate effectively with clients who present themselves as reluctant, conflicted, resentful, and difficult to coach? How can we become aware of how we are contributing to these difficulties? How can we avoid our own burnout and not become a victim of compassion fatigue? How much of ourselves do we share, and how?

Operating from a Coach Approach

When we see ourselves as our client's ally, not their doctor, healer, priest, or therapist, we take a stance of closeness and caring but with less of a feeling of responsibility for their solutions and cure.

In wellness coaching, instead of operating on a *problem du jour* model, we work with our clients to help them take stock of their current health and wellness, create a vision of their best life possible, and then co-create with them an effective Wellness Plan. When we realize that doing so is our job we can allow for more of a healthy, compassionate detachment to take place.

Compassionate Detachment

We practice compassionate detachment for the benefit of our client and for our own benefit as well.

> *Compassionate detachment is respecting our client's power enough to not rescue them while extending loving compassion in the present moment. Simultaneously, compassionate detachment is also respecting ourselves enough to not take the client's challenges on as our own and realizing that to do so serves good purpose for no one.*

Compassionate detachment is an honoring of our client's abilities, resourcefulness, and creativity. We remain as an ally at their side helping them to find their own path, their own solutions. We may provide structure, an opportunity to process, a methodology of change, and tools to help with planning and accountability, but we don't rescue. As tempting as it is to offer our suggestions, to correct what seem to be their errant ways, to steer them toward a program that we know works, we don't. We avoid throwing them a rope and allow them to grow as a swimmer. Sure, we are there to back them up if they go under or are heading toward a waterfall. We are ethically bound to do what we can to monitor their safe passage, but we allow them to take every step, to swim every stroke to the best of their ability.

To be compassionate with a client we have to clear our own consciousness and bring forth our non-judgmental, open, and accepting self. We have to honor their experience.

> *Only in an open, nonjudgmental space can we acknowledge what we are feeling. Only in an open space where we're not all caught up in our own version of reality can we see and hear and feel who others really are, which allows us to be with them and communicate with them properly.*
>
> — **Pema Chodron,** *When Things Fall Apart*

Compassionate detachment is also about giving ourselves permission to protect ourselves. Being in proximity to the pain of others is risky work. There are theories about the high rates of suicide among physicians and dentists based on this phenomenon. Compassionate detachment is also about being detached from outcome. We want the very best for our clients and will give our best toward that goal, but we give up ownership of where and how our client chooses to travel in the process of pursuing a better life. Their outcome is theirs, not ours.

Compassionate detachment is not about distancing ourselves from our client. It is not about becoming numb mentally, emotionally, or physically. It is not about treating our clients impersonally.

> *Compassionate detachment is being centered enough in ourselves, at peace enough in our own hearts, to be profoundly present with our clients in their pain, and in their joy as well.*

The Quandary of Closeness and Compassion in Coaching

"Don't get too close to your clients." It may have been my junior year of being an undergraduate psychology major when a professor offhandedly gave this warning to me and a couple of other students. There is always this question about therapeutic distance. Therapists may wall themselves off from connecting too closely to protect themselves from the pain of their client's suffering. At the same time, therapists are exhorted to empathize, to connect genuinely, authentically — to allow a therapeutic closeness to grow. They are often left in this ambivalent quandary of just how close to be to their client. This is true in the coaching relationship as well.

The coaching relationship is not intended to be a therapeutic one, even though it may contribute to a client's own healing. Many experiences are therapeutic and the experience a person has with coaching may be just that. However, our intent is not to heal the old wounds of our client, but to be their assistant in their personal growth. The coach's quandary is similar to that of the therapist, but also different. We are not our client's treatment provider or friend. We are their ally and support. We will hear stories of suffering. How do we protect ourselves from feeling their pain as our own?

In studying people who could be considered very compassionate, research professor Brenee Brown discovered something that they all had in common: boundaries. They tended to have very well-defined boundaries with other people and fully expected, even insisted, on others having good boundaries with them. This seemed to free them up to be very compassionate. Brown sees compassion as a belief system where we have made a commitment about how we are going to treat ourselves and other people (Brown, 2020).

Brown's research caused her to notice that the most compassionate people she found were excellent at setting clear boundaries. She believes that such strong boundaries allow us to express our compassion and avoid resentment. It is like the presence of clear boundaries allows us to relax and have the healthiest and most functional of relationships.

Boundaries in coaching are formed on two levels: external and internal. The external level is part of the coaching structure, part of consciously co-creating the coaching relationship. We make it clear to the client that we are serving them as a professional and with that comes ethical boundaries. We clarify that our role is not to relate to them like a personal friend, even though we will be warm and friendly. We set boundaries when we clarify what we will do for our client and what we will not, such as sending them reminders to exercise, or responding to their emails on a weekend.

The internal boundary setting is where the coach must engage in their own self-monitoring. Boundaries work both ways and clients benefit from professional and respectful boundaries as well. This self-monitoring means directing the coach's awareness to how they are interacting with their client. The coach is treating their client like they truly believe in the cornerstone of coaching: that their client is naturally creative, resourceful, and whole (Kimsey-House, 2018). When we do so we treat our client with the utmost in respect. We respect their integrity, their intelligence, their abilities, and their personhood. In doing so we do our best to catch ourselves if we begin to treat them in a parental way, in a way to rescue them, or in a way based more on needs of our own.

Compassion Fatigue

When a coach overidentifies with their client's pain or situation they may start to find themselves becoming more reluctant to truly engage with their clients. They may find themselves pulling back emotionally and fighting the urge to connect more closely. Hearing another story of difficulty, we may react by diminishing the very coaching presence that is essential to helping our client to work through their challenges.

As we move forward with co-creating a Wellness Plan with our client we engage in strategic coaching with them to address barriers, but our job is not to provide solutions. Compassion fatigue, I believe, can also come from the sense of powerlessness that we may feel when we can't provide the magic solution for our clients that will make their lives better.

As the coach experiences such fatigue they may find their ability to concentrate and really listen to their clients becoming reduced. It may show up physically with difficulty sleeping, a drop in our immune response, headaches, digestive issues, and more. Our ability to be compassionate may be worn a little thin.

An ICF published article by Niamh Gaffney (Gaffney, 2018) defines compassion fatigue as "…a combination of physical, emotional and spiritual depletion associated with caring for people in significant emotional pain and physical distress." The word depletion is perfect in this description. Our well feels as though it has gone dry, or soon will. It may feel like our very soul is being drained. The way out of compassion fatigue is the same as preventing it.

From Depletion to Replenishment

If compassion fatigue is about feeling depleted, then prevention and recovery is about replenishment. Fatigue comes from the expenditure of energy: physically, emotionally, and spiritually. Coaches must ask themselves what they are consciously doing to restore their own energy supplies. Once again, we are talking about the coach's own wellness foundation.

We often think of wellness in terms of exercise and participation in all kinds of wellness activities. To what degree are these activities an expenditure of energy, and to what degree do they provide an energy return and replenishment? While a workout resulting in a good-tired feeling may fatigue us physically, it may invigorate us mentally, emotionally, and even spiritually. Once again it is a matter of balance. Are we engaging in mind/body activities that replenish our energy on multiple levels? Mindfulness practices, meditation, tai chi, xi gong, yoga, all share the intent of this kind of replenishment.

Our wellness foundation is not just about working out and eating well. What we are looking for here is replenishment on the levels at which we are being depleted—more the emotional, mental, and spiritual. Refilling our well on these levels is more about getting our needs met in these areas. Compassion fatigue can generate feelings of isolation, powerlessness, and feeling overwhelmed. Are we connecting with meaningful friendships to combat that isolation? Are we expressing ourselves creatively and feeling competent in other areas of our lives? Are we consciously engaging in device-free time (without cell phones, tablets, etc.), in connection with the natural world, simplifying our lives? Do we feel like we are truly in charge of our own lives? These questions address the three basic human needs (autonomy, competence, and relatedness) that Deci and Ryan talk about in self-determination theory (Deci, 2000).

When we come back to our own center and feel like our needs are getting met, when we feel safe and secure, energized, and in balance, we can extend the heart of compassion to our clients and not fear intimacy. We can be the ally they need.

Masterful Moment

What do you do to replenish your energy?
How often do you do so?

Have you ever had a client you found exhausting?
What was different about that client or that time period for you?

Do you have a place where you can recharge your energy?

Self-Disclosure

We're working with our coaching client and something they bring up reminds us of a relevant experience in our own lives. Perhaps we feel empathy and can relate. Do we share our own experience with the client? Self-disclosure is a powerful part of human communication and a conscious technique that has been studied in therapy, counseling, and coaching since the mid 60s. Yet, it is a topic that leaves most coaching students once again in a quandary. Let's take a look at the pros and cons, how to avoid missteps, and how to make use of self-disclosure effectively.

Our Need to Self-Disclose

To self-disclose is an expression of our need to connect with others, a way to give some of ourselves to the world, and often contains the hope of receiving some of that connection back. We express our psychological boundaries in the way we self-disclose. Contrast an upper-class British person who has been schooled to self-disclose very little, and to do it carefully, with an American teenager on Facebook telling the world about their most intimate moments with little self-censoring. The whole social networking phenomenon is all about self-disclosure.

Our Fear of Self-Disclosing

Simultaneously we often have many fears about self-disclosure. Self-disclosure makes us vulnerable. Our vulnerability, when displayed to people we can't trust, can open us to attack or being taken advantage of. It can result in a loss of face. Cultural groups (ethnic, class, etc.) that are more concerned about this loss of face may very consciously teach their members to reveal less about themselves, or to reveal only to certain people in certain circumstances. Certainly, we must recognize cultural differences when it comes to self-disclosure, and respect them in our clients. It is well-known that some ethnic groups find psychotherapy or counseling very challenging because they have been instilled with a strong admonition to only speak of personal matters with family members.

Jourard's Pioneering Work

Humanistic psychologist Sidney Jourard, initiated some of the earliest studies on self-disclosure. His idea of a fully functioning human being was someone who had at least one person in their lives with whom they could talk to about anything. Without that, he contended, our psychological health would suffer and our efforts to grow would be held back. Jourard's book *The Transparent Self* (Jourard, 1964) was actually a best-seller during the personal growth movement of the late 1960s. In his book *Disclosing Man to Himself* (Jourard, 1968), definitely a title of the times, he shared work he had done on self-disclosure in counseling groups.

Trust, Self-disclosure, and Groups

Jourard studied the relationship between self-disclosure and trust by studying counseling groups. Counseling group members were identified as having disclosed about themselves (information and emotions) in one of three ways over the course of the group experience: 1. self-disclosed very little, 2. self-disclosed a lot and early in the group, or 3. self-disclosed gradually over the course of the group. The level of trust that the group members felt towards each other was then measured. Surprisingly the group that trusted the least was not group one, but rather group two. Those who shared too much about themselves too fast were trusted the least. The gradual self-disclosers were trusted the most. This lines up with the personal experience most of us have with self-disclosure in our daily lives. People who reveal themselves deeply and rapidly often repel us. This is because self-disclosure often implies reciprocity. The expectation is for you to match the self-disclosure level of the other person. Though we may want to self-disclose to a degree in our coaching, it has to be to the benefit of the client.

Types of Self-Disclosure in Coaching

Self-disclosure takes on primarily three faces in the coaching relationship.

- Transparency in the present—sharing awareness
- Historical stories—similar content or theme
- Personal—biographical information

Transparency in the present moment refers to when the coach reveals their own reaction/response to what is occurring in the session. This is not just an observation of the client, but rather a self-observation of the coach's own feelings. *"I'm really touched by what you just said about your family." "Wow! That sounds so difficult! I know how hard that is for me too." "Let me check in with you a moment. I'm aware of some tension in our conversation ever since I asked about your partner's reaction to you starting to take time to go walking.*

What's going on for you?" The coach has to be very conscious about their choice to share in this way and be extremely careful to not convey judgment.

Transparency also means choice. The effective coach is always deciding what to share and what to hold. Our first awareness of either something internal for us, or something that we are perceiving about what is happening in the coaching relationship, may benefit from further experience. Wait and see if your reaction is validated by more evidence. For example, perhaps you feel rebuffed by your client when you suggest a tool for them to try out. Instead of mentioning it, you wait and see if anything similar happens again in the session. Meanwhile you check in and ask yourself about your own sensitivity to what felt like a rejection. Is it more about you, or is there something going on between you and your client?

Sharing observations about your client is different from self-disclosure. Clients benefit greatly from our keen observations about their language, patterns, and behavior. Self-disclosure happens when we are sharing our own responses and owning them as ours.

Historical stories—sharing similar stories from their life—are probably the most common instances of self-disclosure by a coach. These stories may help convey that the coach can relate more closely to the client's experience. It may be a story that is similar in content ("Yes, I've also experienced running a marathon.") or in theme ("You know, I had to muster my courage in a way sort of like you did, when I confronted my supervisor when I worked at a counseling center."). The key in sharing history is to quickly tie it back to the client's story and shift the spotlight back to them.

Coaches choose to share certain biographical information with their clients to help build the coaching alliance. The coach who comes across as secretive about whether they have ever had children, are in a relationship with a partner, etc., may possibly be trusted less. The challenge here is to maintain good professional boundaries while also being willing to relate to the client as an ally, an authentic human being, not an impersonal and distant professional.

Purposes of Self-Disclosure in Coaching

When we self-disclose in coaching we model behavior. By sharing more openly we give our clients permission to do so as well. We come across as less defensive, less guarded and let the client know it's okay for them to do so also.

Self-disclosure also can increase trust in the coaching relationship. It helps build the alliance by making the coach more real, more human. There is less of a top-down relationship and more of a side-by-side way of relating that communicates an intention that "we're working on this together." This balances the power in the relationship and empowers the client more.

As coaches self-disclose effectively it helps the client develop new perspectives. Seeing how someone else experienced a similar situation, but perhaps handled it differently, can open up some new possibility thinking. All of this can, at times, instill hope and encouragement.

The coach's self-disclosure can also help with the client's own self-acceptance as they realize they are not the only one. They may be reassured that their own reaction was not that unusual and that other people who've been through something similar have felt the same way.

An Evidence-Based Conscious Intentional Technique

Professional opinion and recommendations vary a great deal about self-disclosure. Gavin has compiled an extensive literature review regarding self-disclosure in wellness coaching well worth reading (Gavin, 2005).

In research on the client perceptions, some studies show that clients may perceive a self-disclosing coach as more caring than one who discloses little. Other studies show that coaches who disclose too much are seen as lacking in discretion and being untrustworthy or even preoccupied and in need of help themselves. Coaches who disclose too little are not trusted, and those who disclose too much are thought to be incompetent.

Self-Disclosure: How Much and When? How to Use It?

The coach needs to employ self-disclosure as a purposeful strategy. In other words we have to be very conscious of what our intention is in using self-disclosure. Your use of self-disclosure should have a rationale that enhances the coaching process that helps forward the action, maintain the momentum, or deepen the exploration. Self-disclosure needs to be relevant to the client. Always ask yourself, "Will this benefit my client?"

Make your self-disclosure brief, to the point of the discussion, and relevant to the client. Always, always tie it back to the client's experience. If this is not done immediately after the self-disclosure, some clients for whom this is a hot button will quickly feel like the coach is making it about themselves and feel discounted.

An effective way to self-disclose is to:

- Recognize and acknowledge the client's experience (do this verbally).

- Share your own relevant experience.

- Tie it back to the client's story.

- Ask a powerful question that connects the two (the client's story and yours). The question should help the client move forward with their own process.

- When a client shares something about themselves, acknowledge their experience, reflect feelings, and show that you really are with them and "get it" by using good listening skills. THEN, self-disclose if you believe it will enhance the process.

- You may decide to share your rationale for telling your story and ask if it created any new awareness about their own story.

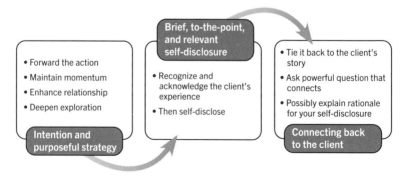

FIGURE 8—SELF-DISCLOSURE

How NOT to Use Self-Disclosure in Coaching

We want to avoid self-disclosure that is:

- Poorly timed—not acknowledging the client's unique experience first.
- Self-serving—ego-driven, where the focus shifts to the coach, not the client.
- Overused. Too much, too frequent self-disclosure leads to distrust and even a perception of lack of competence.
- Underused. Comes across as uncaring, impersonal.
- About persuasion. We never want to use self-disclosure to urge, convince, or persuade a certain course of action (pushing the coach's own agenda, favorite solution, product, etc.)

In an excellent article by Shackleton and Gillie (Shackleton, 2010), the authors address the question of how a coach can possibly determine if the coach's emotional reaction is a genuine response to the client or if it is the coach's own stuff.

> *Sometimes it is obvious, as when a client reminds you of someone else, or brings material which evokes a strong reaction reactivating a past event or relationship of your own, or touches on a strong value that you hold. Here it is probably more appropriate to refrain from disclosing, reflect further, and take your reaction to supervision* (Shackleton, 2010).

The authors then go on to warn the coach about unknowingly shaping the agenda with a client by pushing in the direction of your interest or expertise. A wellness coach could easily do this by relating how their own experience is relevant to the client when it is really more about the coach's own issues.

Self-Monitoring and Self-Disclosure

When coaches are solid in their way of self-disclosing—following the method described above for effective self-disclosure—they can relax into the coaching conversation knowing that it usually helps more than hinders. However, we don't know what we don't know. That's why self-monitoring by frequently recording sessions (with complete client permission) and reviewing them is important. Supervision for the independent coach means connecting with a great mentor coach and periodically getting those blind spots examined. Mentor coaching is especially critical for the neophyte coach but will never lose its value as you attain more experience.

Using self-disclosure in coaching can help open doors or close them. The coaching conversation is different than a simple friend-to-friend chat. It's different than meeting folks at a party. The coaching conversation is a professional exchange of energy and ideas, of planning and possibility thinking. It is purposeful, conscious, and intentional, yet natural and entirely human. Self-disclosure (to be in this trusted space together and shared for the purpose of growth and increased health and wellness) means expressing who we truly are, but doing so with a keen awareness of choice and responsibility.

Self-Deception

What happens outside of our awareness in the coaching relationship may or may not have an effect upon that relationship. The problem, of course, is that we don't know what we don't know.

The Arbinger Institute (Arbinger Institute, 2010) defines self-deception simply as "Not knowing and resisting the possibility that one has a problem." They believe that "Most conflicts are perpetuated by self-deception. So are most failures in communication. And most breakdowns in trust and accountability." The manager who thinks she is doing a great job while all the people who report to her can't stand working for her, or the person who really believes they hold no prejudices as they operate on blatant principles of inequality, would be just a couple of examples.

Deceiving ourselves, by definition, is not intentional. We slip into certain thought patterns and behavior without realizing it. The challenge to our own self-vigilance is to pick up on the emergence of such dynamics as collusion and projection.

One great weapon for fighting self-deception in our coaching is to record our sessions on a regular basis and go over them, observing from three different angles:

1. Listen to how well you are observing your client. Are you picking up on changes in tone of voice, energy levels, shifts in topic? Are you working with your client's emotions, or are you avoiding them? Are you noticing all you can and are you using it in the session by sharing observations with your client so the two of you can process them?

2. Notice what was going on for you, the coach. As you listen to recordings of your sessions you will find that your memory of the experience is stimulated, and you will be better able to recall your thoughts and emotions from that time. This process is used in counselor supervision and is known as Interpersonal Process Recall, or IPR (Cashwell, 1994). Ask yourself if you felt any uneasiness, mixed emotions, or had any other unusual observations.

3. Observe the coaching relationship itself. Notice what is transpiring between you and your client. Notice not just the communication, but the connection. Are you two still working in concert with each other, or straying into different directions? Are you missing subtle requests from the client for a change in topic, for more reassurance, or other needs?

Another even more courageous step that effective coaches take on a regular basis is to subject the coaching to ongoing evaluation. Engage your client every few weeks in a safe and frank conversation about how satisfied the client is with the coaching. Are they seeing progress? Are they pleased with the level of support, accountability, and action planning? See what needs to be changed. If all seems good, see what can become even better.

The real antidote to self-deception, however, lies in awareness and in what the Arbinger Institute's authors call "getting out of the box." This means being willing to look at ourselves and to see. Our mental and emotional blinders cut out our peripheral awareness of ourselves and the world around us, limiting our view of what's right in front of us, to our current perception of what is.

Collusion in the Coaching Relationship

The term collusion can have a variety of meanings, and a search done on "coaching and collusion" will yield an array of articles that seem to mostly add to the confusion. While politics or murder mysteries usually portray collusion as two parties conspiring to evil ends, the collusion we're talking about in coaching is more subconscious, more unintended, than conscious or deliberate.

> *Collusion occurs when a coach somehow merges with their client's view of themselves and the world instead of helping their client explore it.*

We might say that collusion is going along with our client to the point where there is little distinction between the role and function of the coach and the thoughts and behavior of the client. The disheartened client complains that the task they are taking on is so difficult and the coach quickly agrees. That might not sound like much but when a coach responds this way again and again to their client, we see a pattern that is not empowering the client but rather is contributing to their disempowerment. It is helping the client to stay stuck. The coach has drifted from their objective stance of compassionate detachment. The coach unknowingly strays from the belief that their client is naturally creative, resourceful, and whole to somehow become enmeshed with their client's beliefs about themselves and their situation. It is a breach of the clear boundaries that allow compassionate detachment to take place.

"Oh, that's okay. I know it's hard to keep track of all of this." "Yes, it really is hard to monitor your diet all the time." The coach's unique perspective meshes with the client's and a valuable coaching tool is lost. The client no longer benefits from the point of view of someone other than himself or herself. The coach buys the client's story about themselves and fails to help the client discover how they no longer need to be a prisoner of that story. Accountability may become softened and coaching is no longer about possibility thinking.

Motivation for Collusion

So how does a coach slip into collusion with their client? There are a number of motivations that can play into a coach's own self-deception.

Happening outside the coach's awareness, collusion can be motivated by a desire to protect the client. There is a confusion between empathy and sympathy. The coach feels sorry for the client and their plight and may extend great caring and kindness, but also wants to shelter their client from how tough life can be. A client begins to become emotional talking about their body image and the coach rescues them by shifting to how most people their age and gender have issues with body image. The client is whisked away from processing their feelings and encouraged to get intellectual about the subject driving their emotion.

We collude with a client's illness, not their wellness.

Collusion can also occur when the coach over-identifies with their client and their experience. The middle-aged male coach with the midriff bulge is quick to discount the importance of their middle-aged male client's desire to lose their belly fat. The single-mom coach is quick to agree with their client that their parenting stresses make self-care almost impossible. The coach may become quite tolerant of their client's resistance to change because they resist similar changes in their own life. The coach may also self-disclose about their own similar experience but in a way that simply reinforces the client's existing point of view and does not cause them to examine it.

A coach who wants their client to like them may alter their way of interacting. They may strive to keep everything positive to the point where they are not allowing their client to process their fears, worries, etc.

Even more serious collusion may occur when the coach shares a wound similar to their client and it has become a blind spot. The coach may have not done their own emotional healing work in this area and blindly colludes with any client who has experienced something similar to them.

Results of Collusion

When a coach colludes with their client the most harmful result is a lack of progress by the client. They are stuck and the coach's interaction with them is aiding the "stuckness" instead of spurring forward momentum.

The coach and client go around and round in a combination of storytelling, commiserating, and endless attempts to fix the problem.

With the loss or weakening of coaching structure and coaching mindset, progress also slows. In wellness coaching, the result is little or no change in lifestyle behavior and health consequences that may mount.

Projection and the Self-Vigilant Coach

Another aspect of self-deception for the coach to be aware of is the human tendency to project onto others emotions that are actually our own. A classic defense mechanism, psychological projection is when we attribute to others feelings of our own that we find unacceptable. We find it hard to own these feelings and instead we project them on to other people. The most common example is when we have unwanted feelings of anger and instead see hostile and aggressive qualities in the behavior and affect of others.

We often attempt to understand others by asking ourselves how would I feel/what would I do, if I was experiencing that? We put ourselves in their situation, and at times rather than go into a place of empathic understanding, we project our own feelings, imaginings, conclusions, solutions onto the other person. We know what they ought to do!

Projection comes in when we begin to react to our client as though they are much like someone else, perhaps amplifying qualities that belong not to them, but to the source of our projection. Could the client who seems to bother us in ways that we find hard to explain be the unfortunate recipient of our projection? Do they remind us of someone else, a personal relationship from our past, or perhaps even a former client who struggled with the same issues? Do we see them struggling with a similar health challenge, relationship issue, or family of origin issue as we have? Are we bringing our own unfinished emotional business or our own prejudices into the coaching relationship?

When we are on the receiving end of our client's projections, how do we handle it? A client who treats us as the expert may cause us to take on too much of that role, or to overcompensate by being so informal and friendly that we now come across as a buddy or pal instead of a professional coach. The client who projects a parental role onto us may bring out our need to protect and shelter them. We make our assumptions without even realizing them. We slip into feeling that we know best for our client and slip out of the coaching mindset. This is where a continual process of self-monitoring pays off. Let's look at some ways to minimize projection and collusion as well.

THE SELF-VIGILANT COACH GUIDELINES FOR MINIMIZING COLLUSION AND PROJECTION

- Set clear boundaries and expectations for the coaching relationship as you create the coaching alliance.

- Draw a clear distinction between coaching and therapy. This includes operating from a coaching mindset, not an analytical, diagnostic mindset in our relationship with our client.

- Set clear professional boundaries. Stick to the coaching process. Stay professional, remain a coach.

- Convey clearly to your client what is okay and what is not okay in the way coaching works and in the coaching relationship.

- Have clear agreements, not expectations. Your client is not here to live up to your expectations.

- Have coaching conversations with your client about the coaching's effectiveness as well as the client's progress. Get and give feedback.

- Be very clear about the distinction between sympathy and empathy.

- Coach with a sense of self-monitoring. Check in with your own affective and bodily sensations and determine what they are telling you.

- Look carefully at client progress versus stuckness.

- Look for patterns in your coaching process with this particular client or similar clients. Collusive behavior repeats itself.

- Don't be afraid to challenge your client. Examine your own reluctance to do so when this comes up.

- Be vigilant for parental feelings that arise when you believe that you know what is best for your client.

- Reflect upon the client who brings out unusual feelings in you that are hard to explain or understand. Listen to recordings (with client permission) and examine your responses to your client.

- Seek out mentoring/supervision to explore puzzling client relationships that your intuition is telling you don't feel right.

- Do your own work! Your own journey of personal growth and gaining self-awareness is ongoing. Growth as a human being is growth as a coach.

Can a Coaching Client Be Resistive?

What do we mean by saying a wellness coaching client is being resistive? Usually this term is used in treatment settings to describe patients who don't comply with treatment or adhere to a treatment plan. To be resistive, we must be resisting something external that is being foisted upon us. If coaching is a client-centered process where self-determined goals are being pursued by a willing client, with the coach's assistance, how can there be resistance? Think about it. If reluctance to participate or engage appears, we might first self-reflect and examine to see if we have strayed from a coach approach into a treatment approach. Has our coaching become so directive that we are attached to a certain course of action by our client? Have we left the arena of coaching and slipped into being a consultant or treatment provider instead? Our client is not eating the steel-cut oatmeal or kale smoothies we have suggested. They still haven't ordered the how-to-be-well book that we recommended. Is this resistance, conflict, or simply something to discuss in the coaching conversation?

Resistance and Self-Efficacy

I've encountered health professionals who have made statements such as "These people don't want to be healthy!" This usually comes from a frustrated health professional who has seen little progress by their patients in succeeding at lasting lifestyle improvement. Sometimes it may be an indicator of burnout on the part of the health professional. The reality is, of course, everyone wants to be healthy and well. What we are labeling as resistance may, in reality, be an exhibition of very low self-efficacy (the degree of confidence a person has that change will be beneficial to them and that they are capable of succeeding at change).

We see low self-efficacy in clients who come to wellness coaching carrying with them a long history of failed attempts at successfully making changes and making them last. These failure experiences can lead to a state of demoralization. The client becomes so discouraged that they begin to believe that change may not be possible, or that the price to be paid (energy, effort, inconvenience, or actual expenses) is just too great. The thought of attempting, yet again, to make changes brings up the painful memory of their past failures. Recalling those failures may generate feelings of not just disappointment, but embarrassment, shame, guilt, and self-blame.

Our client's failure experiences may have led them to conclude that successful lifestyle change is just not possible for them. They begin to attribute their failure to inherent faults that they can do nothing about. Having tried to summon enough willpower to be successful, yet failed, they conclude that somehow, they just weren't issued enough willpower when it was being handed out. Perhaps they blame their difficulties on their family body type and genetic make-up or other factors outside of their control.

Coaching to build self-efficacy may be a far more logical initial strategy then plunging into goal setting and action planning.

Look at our discussion of Albert Bandura's ways of building self-efficacy in Chapter Six.

Resistance and Readiness for Change

People in pre-contemplation are often labeled as being uncooperative, resistant, unmotivated, or not ready for behavior change programs. However, our research showed us that it was the health professionals who were not ready for the pre-contemplators (Prochaska and Prochaska, 2016).

The work of James Prochaska that yielded the transtheoretical model of change (TTM), or the stages of change model, has shown us the value of viewing change as usually happening as a process, not an event. We will cover how this important theory relates to coaching in Chapter Eight. In their 2016 book, *Changing to Thrive* (Prochaska and Prochaska, 2016), James and Janice Prochaska drive home the fact that most behavioral change programs (weight loss, smoking cessation, etc.) are action-based. The patient or client is expected to be ready to take action on the required behaviors, or they are sometimes labeled as resistive and told to return to the program when they are ready. The Prochaskas' research shows that only 20% of people are ready to take action on changing any particular behavior. The other 80% are not. This vast majority are in the earlier stages of pre-contemplation, contemplation, or preparation.

Rather than view the not-ready client as resistive, the effective coach meets their client where the client is. Yes, it may be medically urgent for a stroke patient to stop smoking, but if they are not ready to take that action, our job is to help them get ready. We do that by coaching them through the stages of change, at their own rate, as we'll see in the upcoming chapter.

Coaching with Difficult Clients: When Conflict Arises

Coaching isn't always easy, and frankly, not all clients are either. Every client brings their unique personality to the coaching relationship. They bring their current experience of the world with them and with that, their own reaction to it. Fortunately, the vast majority of clients see coaching as a positive opportunity, one without the stigma of therapy. What makes a client *difficult* is either their reluctance to be in the coaching process or their own interpersonal traits.

The Incentivized Client and the Forced Referral

The use of incentives is an increasingly common strategy to drive engagement in corporate wellness programs, and, within those, wellness coaching services. Employees are offered rewards or discounts for participation in wellness programs, or for their effective performance on their own wellness goals within those programs. Incentives may take the form of cash rewards, such as being paid large sums to take a health risk assessment. They may also be in the form of time off from work, or some sort of prizes. A more common tactic is to require participation in some aspect of a wellness program (perhaps even wellness coaching) in order to receive a 10-20% discount on the employee's health insurance premium. With the extreme cost of health insurance in America, this type of incentive pushes many employees towards joining a wellness program they would not typically utilize and may not believe they need.

The use of incentives is a topic of much debate in the field of health promotion with critics arguing that incentives don't work in the long run. All too often employees meet the requirements to receive the incentive and then they drop out of the wellness program. In his book, *Drive: The Surprising Truth About What Motivates Us* (Pink, 2011), author Daniel Pink cites extensive psychological research showing that external rewards are not effective at changing complex behavior. Pink, and other critics of incentives, argue that wellness programs need to do a better job of promoting intrinsic motivation. Incentive critics propose that wellness programs focus on creating a culture of wellness within organizations that make it easier for employees to be well.

For the wellness coach, the result is that we often see incentivized clients coming through our door who really don't want to be there. Such clients can arrive feeling resentful at having to submit to some process they see as unnecessary and an intrusion on their private lives, to say nothing of an addition to their already busy schedule. Wellness coaches sometimes receive the brunt of such client's hostility.

In a similar fashion, your wellness coaching client may be there under pressure from a supervisor, a physician, or even a loved one, who thinks that they need to see a coach. The client may not see things the same way for a variety of reasons. The result at times is similar to the incentivized client—anger, resentment, and seeing coaching as an unneeded intrusion.

Coaching the Incentivized Client and the Forced Referral

In such situations, the coach's principal challenge is to transform the perception of the coaching relationship from enemy to ally. This starts with the coach's own challenge to not take what may feel like their client's attack personally. Before we even express empathic understanding of the other person, we have to feel it ourselves. When the coach can literally put themselves in their client's place and imagine what it is like for them to be there for coaching when they truly don't want to be, we can begin to see our client with compassion. Our client is angry with the system, not with us as a person. They may express that anger towards us because we are the concrete representative of that system, but it truly is not personal. Here are some step-by-step suggestions for meeting with the forced coaching client.

WORKING WITH THE FORCED COACHING CLIENT

- Be aware of your own initial reaction. Your client may have caught you off guard with their hostility.

- Realize how truly safe you are. Distinguish between this situation and past situations where you have felt fearful or in danger.

- Take your client seriously and convey that you are doing so with a face of intent listening. Trying to be nice may be misinterpreted as being dismissive or even condescending. Match your client's energy.

- Don't be offended by rough language. Remember it's not about you!

- F.A.V.E., First Acknowledge, Validate, and Empathize (see Chapter Four). First acknowledge your client's situation. "Sounds like this incentive program gave you what feels like no choice but to be here for coaching." Validate that they have a right to feel the way they feel. "You've got every right to feel resentful about having to be here." Empathize with your client. "It must be really frustrating to have to take time out to do something you don't value." Catch your tendency to judge.

- Then offer an alliance. "You certainly want to get that incentive (or please the person forcing the referral). I'm here to help you get it! Let's work together to get you the results you want and to do our best to make your time here worthwhile."

- If your client is inappropriate terminate the session. Calmly explain that you will not work with someone who cannot treat you with respect.

Coaching with Difficult Clients: Aikido Moves

It is your responsibility to protect the person who is attacking you. If you are unfairly accused of something, you can protect your accuser by looking at him with compassion. You try to understand why he unfairly accused you. Then you withdraw your venom from your response to him.

Terry Dobson, *It's a Lot Like Dancing: An Aikido Journey*

The martial art of Aikido originated in Japan in the early 20th Century. Rather than an attack-oriented martial art, Aikido employs turning movements that redirect the attacker's momentum, often combined with various throws and joint locks. The goal is to defend oneself while not intentionally harming the opponent. Observing an Aikido master demonstrating how Aikido works, you will see whirling, fluid movements that blend with the attacker and through subtle redirection send them flying away from the master.

Its relevance to coaching comes from the work of Terry Dobson, author of *Aikido in Everyday Life* (Dobson, 1993), and Tom Crum, author of *The Magic of Conflict* (Crum, 1998). In their work we see how the principles of Aikido apply to interpersonal conflict.

In their book, *Crucial Conversations* (Patterson, Grenny, McMillan, Switzler, 2011), the authors point out how frequently when people deal with conflict, they either go toward silence or violence. The person either clams up and withdraws or elevates the aggression. Likewise, when we encounter conflict it sometimes feels like a physical attack coming at us. Someone is hurling demands or provocations, perhaps even stooping to insults, and it does feel like an attack. This is where the Aikido approach that Dobson and Crum advocate works better than counter attacking, or allowing ourselves to take it on the chin and be hurt.

Expect nothing. Be prepared for anything!

Permit me to introduce a simplified method for dealing with conflict and then elaborate on each part, showing how we can apply it in coaching and in everyday life.

MEETING CONFLICT WITH AN AIKIDO ABC APPROACH

- Acknowledge and meet what is brought to you.
- Acknowledge that your client's frustration, anger, and/or resentment, etc., is real.
- Blend—without agreeing with them, hear them out.
- Compassion—express empathy and genuine understanding.
- Center yourself.
- Deflect all negativity brought to you.
- Energy—recognize and honor the energy brought by the other person.
- Follow the energy. Go where the energy is most.

Acknowledge and meet what is brought to you. Accept that your client is feeling the way they feel and is expressing it. Don't try to deny it to yourself, or to them. Acknowledge that the conflict appears real and is not to be dismissed or minimized. It is like accepting the fact that the physical opponent is throwing a punch at you—it's real!

Acknowledge that your client's frustration, anger, and/or resentment, etc., is real. Make statements acknowledging how genuine it is for them. Paraphrase what they are saying and make sure you are hearing them accurately by asking if you are understanding them correctly so far.

Blend without necessarily agreeing with them, hear them out. Instead of digging in and taking an oppositional stance, imagine turning your body and line up with your opponent looking at the world from the same angle they are. Question your own locked-in viewpoint and consider adopting a new point of view. You don't have to agree with your client to encourage them to tell you more about their point of view. Tell me more about that.

Compassion. Express empathy and genuine understanding. As you begin to understand your client's concerns, express real empathic understanding. In a sincere tone make genuine statements. "Wow! That must be incredibly frustrating (disappointing, painful, etc.) for you." Inquire in a compassionate way to find out more so that you may deepen your understanding and to allow your client to feel heard and understood.

Center yourself. The more centered you are the easier it is to engage in the process of working with conflict. (See Chapter Three.) It begins with living a lifestyle that allows you to be more centered in your life. Doing so will allow you to react appropriately. It also means centering yourself physically during the conflict. Sit up straight with your feet flat on the floor or stand up straight with your weight evenly distributed. Be aware of your breathing and deepen it consciously.

Deflect all negativity brought to you. Step aside and let it fly by. Don't take it personally! It's not about you.

Energy. Recognize and honor the energy brought by the other person. Don't be afraid of passion. Match their energy (but not their violence).

Follow the energy. Go where the energy is most invested. Talk about what they are most passionate about. Don't try to persuade or dissuade. Notice when energy is out of proportion. That usually indicates underlying issues are fueling the fire.

Following this approach may not result in a complete resolution of conflict, but it will most likely shift the dialogue from confrontation to, we would hope, collaboration. Offer to work with your client to continue pursuing resolution. Even when resolution is not possible, you have established that you are an ally, not the enemy!

> **Masterful Moment**
>
> How comfortable are you with working through conflict? Do you avoid it as much as possible?
>
> What feelings arise when you are confronted with a client who appears "resistive"?
>
> Can you empathize with your difficult client?

Courageous Coaching

As we seek to resolve our own quandary of closeness with our clients we must remember that when we are trusting the coaching process, we are able to stay centered enough to connect with our client regardless of what they bring to the coaching session. From that balanced place we are able to be with our client as they face their own fears and challenges. We are able to stand beside them during those times because we are not taking on our client's burden for them or taking it home with us. Respecting our client's own strength, we don't have to deplete our own. By becoming aware of and setting aside our own issues and prejudices we are able to be the ally our client needs on their wellness journey.

I never said it would be easy. I only said it would be worth it.

— **Mae West**

This chapter showed us how the being aspect of coaching isn't always easy. We looked at the question of how to provide the compassion our clients need yet be detached enough to serve ourselves and the coaching relationship well. The vital topics of self-disclosure, collusion, and projection were examined as well. Finally, we explored how to coach clients who appear resistive and difficult.

Chapter Six — Advanced Coaching Skills And Methods — Motivation and Awareness, will introduce Part Three of our book: What to

Do. We will take a deep dive into the vital topic of motivation, how to mobilize it, and the relevance of meaning and purpose. We will examine two key theories of motivation: Self-Determination Theory and Social Cognitive Theory. We will then round out the chapter with a look at how we can help our clients to increase awareness.

REFFERENCES

The Arbinger Institute. (2010). *Leadership and Self-Deception: Getting out of the Box.* Hawking Books.

Cashwell, C. (1994). *Interpersonal Process Recall.* ERIC Digest, American Counseling Association.

Crum, T. (1998). *The Magic of Conflict: Turning a Life of Work into a Work of Art.* Touchstone.

Deci, E. A. (2000). Self-Determination Theory and the Facilitation of Intrinsic Motivation, Social Development and Well-Being. American psychologist.

Dobson, T. (1993). *Aikido in Everyday Life: Giving in to Get Your Way.* North Atlantic Books.

Gaffney, N. (2018, March 2). *Are You Tired of Coaching?* Retrieved from Coaching World - a publication of the ICF: https://coachfederation.org/blog/are-you-tired-of-coaching

Gavin, J. (2005). *Lifestyle Fitness Coaching.* Human Kinetics.

Jourard, S. (1964). *The Transparent Self.* Van Nostrand.

Jourard, S. (1968). *Disclosing Man To Himself.* Van Nostrand.

Patterson, K. G. (2011). *Crucial Conversations Tools for Talking When Stakes Are High, Second Edition.* McGraw Hill Education.

Pink, D. (2011). *Drive: The Surprising Truth About What Motivates Us.* Riverhead Books.

Prochaska, J. O. & Prochaska M. J. (2016). *Changing to Thrive.* Hazelden Publishing.

Shackleton, M. &. (2010). The Use of Self and Self Disclosure in Coaching.pdf. *AoEC Conference 2010.* Marjorie Shackleton and Marion Gillie.

PART THREE
What to Do

Chapter 6—Advanced Coaching Skills and Methods

CHAPTER SIX

Advanced Coaching Skills and Methods

The craft of masterful coaching is a combination of *being* and *doing* performed at a high level. As we have seen in the previous chapters the foundation for all techniques of coaching is the coach's way of being with their client. The coaching mindset cannot be emphasized enough. Our job is to facilitate the client's work, not to do it for them. Our work is to catalyze the growth of our client and help them to thrive.

Motivation for Lifestyle Improvement

You'll see it when you believe it.

—**Wayne Dyer**

Much of the coach approach was founded upon the theories of self-actualization and human potential that Abraham Maslow advocated. Coaching operates on the basic tenet that people are inherently motivated to actualize their potential, to be their best and to thrive. Our clients are inherently motivated to maximize their abilities and seek fulfillment. However, as Maslow further notes, the part of us seeking self-actualization can be easily diminished and discouraged by some of life's harsh realities. It is the job of the wellness coach to nurture the part of our client that wants to grow and to act as a catalyst for that noble purpose. As we hold our clients to be "naturally creative, resourceful and whole" (Kimsey-House, 2018) we are embracing a view that sees our clients naturally striving to be well. The motivation to be healthy and well is there. It is our job to help our clients clear the way to be in touch with their self-actualizing, health-enhancing nature.

Human motivation is a complex topic with many theories and the lifetime work of many psychological scholars. For the coach, the first question may simply be: Is it my job to motivate anyone? I believe it was during my first year after my master's degree in counseling, when working at a residential adolescent treatment center, that I concluded, "I can't motivate anyone to do anything. I can invite. I can support."

An approach that the coach may benefit from is to realize that your best work happens when you help a person discover the motivation that they have inside of them. Motivation for lasting lifestyle change begins within.

The fields of wellness, public health, and medicine have a long history of attempting to motivate through fear. Pictures of diseased lungs and tracheotomy patients seem to have had little success in reducing smoking rates. Avoiding illness is a noble goal, but a negative one. Why not seek health instead?

Our clients are often puzzled by a lack of success in their efforts to start living a healthy lifestyle, or keep such efforts going. They blame it on either a lack of motivation to get started, or that their motivation fades as old habits reassert their rule. "I just don't seem to have the motivation to really make changes." Your work as a wellness coach is, in part, to help your clients find their own sources of motivation and then to harness that energy to an effective methodology for change.

Coaches often help their clients examine and re-examine whatever sources of motivation they have mentioned. They help their clients revisit their desire to change and what drives it. They look at fear-based motivations such as not wanting to have an illness get worse, or not wanting to develop the maladies that have been prevalent in their family. They look at the love-based motivators like caring enough about one's self, or wanting to be there for their grandchildren as they grow up. They explore the intrinsic motivators found in such things as the joy of dancing, swimming, tasting delicious and nutritious food, etc.

Perhaps, not seeing progress at change, the client concludes that these motivators just aren't sufficient. The coach and client may then search for additional motivators, without seeing how these motivators spark change.

Mobilizing Motivation

Your client may have enough motivation. They may in fact have listed three, four, or more reasons they want to change. Motivation is like the fuel for a vehicle to run on. The problem might not be the fuel, but the lack of an actual vehicle! The vehicle is a methodology, a structure, and a process that facilitates change. To get where they need and want to go, the client needs both a vehicle to carry them and the fuel to put in it. How do we mobilize motivation? By providing our client with the methodology they need.

— — —

Case Study

A mentee of mine was recently coaching a middle-aged woman who complained about a lack of motivation holding her back. As we began listening to the recording of their last session, we heard the coach helping the client to describe at least four strong motivators that had propelled her into seeking coaching and beginning to act. She realized that when her children were younger playing with them had provided her with more activity and energy. Now her energy was low, and she wanted to reclaim that. She talked about her grandchildren and wanting to be a very active part of their lives. The client was concerned about her advancing age, not wanting to lose the health she had. She didn't want to become a burden to anyone. She went on to list at least two more motivators.

As the client described her lack of success at change, her conclusion was that she was just lacking motivation. She described coming home from work tired and just fixing a quick (though not necessarily healthy) meal and watching television in the evening. "I just don't have the motivation I need!" the client lamented. She intended to be more active and intended to eat better. All she had for a plan were intentions.

Doing a great job of coaching, my mentee gently confronted his client and recited the substantial list of motivators that she did, in fact, have. He questioned whether it was a lack of motivation, or something else that was missing. The gentle confrontation paid off with the client reconnecting with her sources of motivation and recommitting to the coaching process.

— — —

Setting Up the Needed Structure

In co-creating the coaching alliance, part of what an effective coach does is to explain, in a succinct fashion, exactly how coaching works, how it is structured, and what the benefits are. The client-centered nature of coaching is conveyed with reassurance that the client remains the one in the driver's seat.

Part of the coach's job is to facilitate the client's use of the coaching structure. The coach does this by showing the client how advantageous it can be to operate with a solid plan, to track one's progress at making changes, etc. The coach provides tools that make these processes easier. Mobile apps for tracking can be recommended and then, importantly, integrated into the coaching accountability.

The Power of Vision as a Motivator

What can be the ultimate motivation for a client is the vision of themselves living their best life possible. Such a motivator pulls the client forward in a positive way, fortifying their efforts at making the steps needed to actualize the outcome they want to see. To set up such a vision the coaching process begins with helping the client to take stock of their wellness, of their health and well-being. With a more complete picture of where they are presently, we ask where do they want to be. That is, we help them create a Well-Life Vision that epitomizes the healthy life they want to live. There is a gap between where the person is now (their current level of wellness) and where they want to be (the outcome they want to see). What has to change in their way of living for them to bridge that gap and attain their Well Life Vision becomes their Wellness Plan. (For a complete description of how to coach for the creation of a Well Life Vision and a fully integrated Wellness Plan, see Chapter 8 of *Wellness Coaching for Lasting Lifestyle Change, 2nd Ed.*).

When a client is clear about their Well Life Vision it becomes a continual driver of motivation. When a client is faced with the choice of acting in the interest of their health and wellness or making choices that will continue to hold them back, bringing the Well Life Vision to mind can act as a *tipping point*, spurring them on to make the extra effort towards progress.

Motivation is what fuels change. When it is present, a methodology, a structure, is what the client needs to mobilize it. By providing our client with the vehicle, we help them to get where they want to go.

The Motivational Importance of Meaning and Purpose

The French phrase *raison d'etre*—reason to be—may be the bottom line for motivation. In Chapter One we explored how relevant meaning and purpose are to health and wellness. We concluded that the research referenced showed great success in improved health because being in touch with one's values and having a greater sense of purpose provided a foundation of motivation upon which to build. In fact, a reason for being may provide a reason for doing.

Coaching with Intrinsic Motivation

Clients come to wellness coaching with a variety of motivations for change. Fear-based motivation often is the catalyst for initiating efforts at lifestyle improvement. Witnessing someone they identify with (like a similarly aged friend or relative) go through a heart attack or seeing their own blood lipid levels and blood sugar levels rise to dangerous levels may get someone started on their own journey to better health. The drawback of fear-based motivation is, however, that it often does not last.

As coach and client partner to co-create the client's Wellness Plan, intrinsic motivation can be maximized by the selection of Action Steps that are in alignment with the client's values and interests. A goal of becoming more active can take many different paths. Some clients immediately think it means either working out at a fitness facility or becoming a runner. While those may be exciting options for some, many clients will shudder at the thought of each of these strategies. What will be an activity that the client will enjoy while they are doing it? Will they find it fun? Is it something that aligns with their interest? Your client may be gregarious and find a dance class much more engaging. You may have an outdoors-oriented client who would rather work on finding a friend to go hiking with frequently.

Helping your client to discover the intrinsic rewards in the actions they are taking is another way that coaches can help build intrinsic motivation. When your client reports that they went out on a walk three times last week as agreed in their commitments to action, seize the opportunity to do more than just say "very good" or "okay." Inquire. Ask your client to tell you more about their walks. Where did they go? What did they see? What did it feel like when they were out there walking? What did they enjoy about it?

When you ask a client to elaborate about their experience, they remember it, and in some sense, relive it. They recall what it was like, and in their imagination re-experience it. Emphasizing the positive reinforces the action. As our walking client recounts taking a public walking path, they may recall waterfowl they saw on a pond, sunflowers in full bloom, or the beauty of a snowy landscape. When the event was not so esthetically pleasing, or may have even been done under trying circumstances, such as a rainy day, the coach can acknowledge the strength of character that showed up in the client's determination of complete the task.

Help your client discover the reinforcing intrinsic rewards in what they have done by noticing. Guide them to notice more through their senses, taking note of not only visual cues, but also sounds, tastes, and physical sensations. Encourage mindfulness. Ask your client who has started strength training if they are beginning to enjoy the feeling of accomplishment at getting stronger. Explore for bonus benefits as well. Is that strength training client noticing that they can get up out of a chair much more easily now? Are they experiencing better sleep now that they are walking five times a week? What else is showing up?

As clients become more aware of the intrinsic rewards in the action steps they are taking, the reinforcing value of these actions becomes locked in and positive habits become formed. Seeing the motivational connection between the steps they are taking and their sources of motivation is key. Such a client might be able to say, *"I'm walking three times a week, which I enjoy, to increase my activity level. This will help me attain and maintain a healthy weight so that I can be fit and strong enough to play with my grandchildren for years to come."*

The Volitional and the Imperative

When our wellness coaching clients take on the tasks of lifestyle improvement, are they doing so because they *want* to, or because they feel they must, or should? They have been told that it is imperative that they stop tobacco use after their stroke. They have been told that it is imperative that they lose weight to manage their diabetes. Yet, do they want to? Or, rather, do they feel that they can? What allows our client to choose to make these needed lifestyle changes? Yes, self-efficacy is central here, but what else is at play?

There can be a strange interplay between the volitional and the imperative. What supplies our client with the motivation to again and again engage in their lifestyle improvement actions? They know they should, but what happens that allows them to own their choice, to embrace it enough to stay with these new behaviors long enough to establish them as habits? How can the locus of control shift from external to internal, from an external imperative to an internal imperative that is embraced?

We certainly want our clients to be engaging in their wellness because they genuinely want to. Acting out of their own volition will produce better performance than if they are just doing so from sheer compliance. Yet, how can our client choose to execute these wellness tasks because of a reason that seems positively imperative? Instead of operating on a fear-based imperative — stop smoking or die — how can we help our client to reframe the imperative into something positive?

A *positive imperative* can tie back to one's values and sense of meaning and purpose. It can connect with what they love in life. "I want to be a great example for my grandchildren and be around to help them grow into wonderful human beings." "I want to be healthy enough to continue to be of service to others in need." Have coaching conversations that explore your client's motivation and help them to discover a positive imperative for their wellness.

Integrating Behavioral Change Theory

In theory there is no difference between theory and practice.
In practice there is.

— **Yogi Berra**

Discerning which behavioral change theories to use in our coaching can be a daunting task. Theory is fascinating, and it also can lead us into the abstract world closer to pure science. Perhaps our mantra for discriminating theory is to apply our own version of the inimitable song qualifier developed by the teen television show of the 1950s and 60s—*American Bandstand*. "Does it have a good beat, and can you dance to it?" That is, can we apply the theory to our coaching in a direct and sensible way that allows us to guide the work that we do? It is so easy to remain theoretical when practicality is required.

When we rise to a more masterful level of practice with our coaching, I believe that theory becomes background, not front and center. As a counseling graduate student, I became not just enamored with theories of psychotherapy, I became an ardent investigator. I was fortunate to be exposed academically to not just one theory but to many. What I found myself doing in practice was synthesizing the congruent aspects of these different approaches. As I worked with more and more clients, I found theory receding into the background because I "knew" just what to do. The Coaches Training Institute (CTI) refers to this as getting to the point in your coaching where it is in the bones. How did I know? I had studied theory and combined it with experience in direct service.

Theory is essential. When it is integrated into who you are as a coach, it allows you to think on your feet. You don't sit there and think "Let's see. I guess I should proceed by applying some social cognitive theory here." However, because you've integrated the important teachings of Social Cognitive Theory, you might, with little thought, remember to inquire more about social factors affecting your client's health choices, or pursue more ways to build self-efficacy. Because behavioral change theories have been extensively researched, coaches can operate from more of an informed, evidence-based approach.

As wellness coach training has evolved, there has been a greater emphasis on theory, research, and creating the solid evidential base for the field. This is a wonderful and necessary step in the evolution of this discipline. However, we should remember that coaching is not psychotherapy, and while it draws heavily upon the work of the field of psychology, it is not a sub-domain. The depth and level of education for a coach versus a psychologist is vastly different and should remain that way. In practicality, it is not necessary for coaches to emulate practicing mental health professionals. So, with this word of caution, let's examine how coaches can rise to a more masterful level of coaching by learning more about relevant motivational theory.

Rather than attempt to provide a smorgasbord review of behavioral change theory, in this chapter let us focus on two highly relevant and useful theoretical contributions from behavioral science.

Relevant Theory
Self-Determination Theory and Motivation in Coaching

Don't ask how you can motivate others.
Ask how you can create the conditions within which
others will motivate themselves.

— Edward L. Deci

The life work of psychologists Edward Deci and Richard Ryan has yielded a theory of human motivation that not only fully supports the coach approach but also adds valuable tools of understanding. In complete alignment with the tenets of humanistic psychology (Maslow, 2014), Self-Determination Theory (SDT) views human beings as constantly striving towards actualizing their potential, seeking out ways to foster their growth and development. It is also very much in alignment with the client-centered (or person-centered) approach of Carl Rogers (Rogers, 2004). The congruence with SDT is apparent when we see the way coaches trained in the ICF core competencies and the coaching foundations laid out in sources such as *Co-Active Coaching* (Kimsey-House, 2018) work with their clients.

A core contribution of SDT is the way it demonstrates how it is the type of motivation, not the quantity that is key to success with behavioral change. According to Self-Determination Theory there are two types of motivation, *controlled motivation* and *autonomous motivation*. SDT presents a motivational spectrum with *amotivation*, or total indifference at one end and *intrinsic* and *autonomous motivation*, doing something for its own inherent satisfaction, at the opposite end. In between these two extremes lies *extrinsic motivation* with its own motivational spectrum from the most *externalized (controlled)* to the most *internalized (becoming autonomous)* types of motivation.

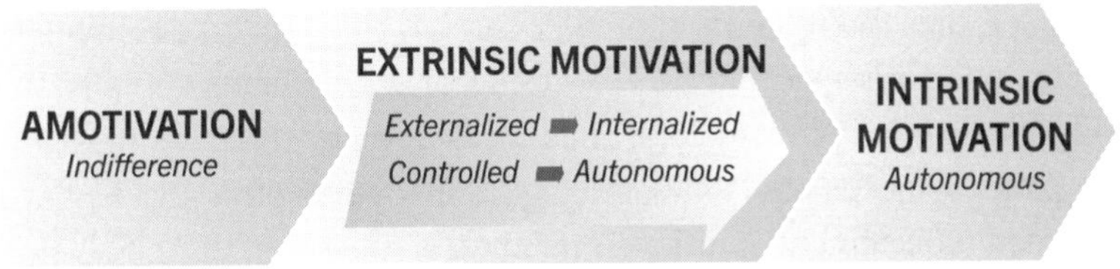

FIGURE 9—MOTIVATIONAL SPECTRUM

A client is viewed as potentially having different types of motivation related to different behaviors, like what we have seen in the transtheoretical model of change. Your client may be in the action stage when it comes to improving their nutrition, but in the contemplation stage regarding beginning an exercise program. Likewise, in the SDT model, your client may feel controlled motivation from an extrinsic source (e.g., pressure from physician and spouse) to begin exercising, and yet possess autonomous intrinsic motivation to improve their nutrition because of a lifelong fascination with and enjoyment of healthy eating.

Coaches certainly encounter clients who are indifferent to making changes in some areas of their lives. This would be referred to as amotivation, or simply lacking motivation. SDT looks at the process of motivation as part of the behavior change process, rather than as a prerequisite for coaching. The client does not have to be ready for coaching; rather, it is the coach's function to help the client get in touch with the motivation they need for change and to resolve ambivalence Again, it is our job to meet our client where they are (Spence, 2011).

Controlled Motivation

All too frequently the wellness coach encounters clients who are feeling the pressure of controlled motivation. This is the carrot and stick approach. It means doing something to get a reward or to avoid punishment. It is characterized by feeling seduced (towards a reward) or coerced (to avoid a negative consequence). Either way there is a perception of being pressured, obligated, or even forced. A perfect example is the coaching client coming to fulfill a requirement for a wellness program incentive plan. The client feels forced into coaching for the reward of a 10-20% discount on their health insurance premium (and to avoid the implied penalty of missing this discount). Deci has emphasized that this type of approach can have negative consequences for both performance and well-being. Deci and Ryan also noticed that individuals coming from controlled motivation tend to take the shortest path to the desired outcome. They often complete the wellness program requirement and then immediately quit.

Autonomous Motivation

Autonomous motivation has two aspects. The first is interest and enjoyment. If these two are present, so is motivation because *I don't have to be convinced to do what I love doing*. The second type centers on deeply held values and beliefs. Behaviors that are in sync with values and beliefs are coherent with one's sense of self. According to Deci, the research demonstrates that when behavior comes from autonomous motivation people are more creative and better at problem solving. When confronted with challenges or obstacles they are more able to think outside the box. Overall, performance is better especially around hands-on learning and people feel better about themselves. "When people's goal-directed behavior is autonomous rather than controlled, the correlates and consequences are more positive in terms of the quality of their behavior as well as their health and well-being" (Deci E, 2000).

Autonomous behavior is about choice. Deci, in an informative video interview (Deci, 2017), points out that it is not the same as independence. A person can be experiencing autonomous motivation (operating out of their own volition) when they choose to seek out a walking group. Autonomous motivation can drive both individualistic and collectivistic behaviors.

SDT also acknowledges that there is often a process experienced by people whereby their motivation may progress from Controlled External Motivation to eventually become a choice that they fully embrace—Autonomous Intrinsic Motivation. What may begin as a requirement of the program (see a wellness coach to get an incentive)—external controlled motivation—may move to compliance with the program (continue to see the coach out of an introjected sense that they should do so). However, if the coach is effective at creating a true coaching alliance with their client, helping them to see the benefits that they may gain by continuing coaching, the motivation shifts. Through a sense of identification, it now becomes autonomous motivation—client is truly choosing to be involved in coaching. Finally, as the client experiences the benefits of coaching and enjoys it, they have fully integrated the process and are experiencing autonomous intrinsic motivation to engage genuinely in the coaching process.

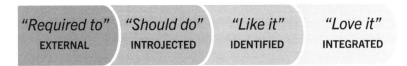

FIGURE 10—FORMS OF EXTRINSIC REGULATION

The Three Innate Psychological Needs

At the motivational heart of self-determination theory is the underlying assumption that there is an inherent human need for fulfillment and self-actualization through personal growth:

1. Development and mastery (competence)

2. Connectedness, (relatedness)

3. Experience of behavior as self-determined and congruent with one's sense of self (autonomy)

These three needs are considered universal and essential for well-being. Whatever supports the positive experience of competence, relatedness, and autonomy promotes choice, willingness and volition, interest, full engagement, enjoyment, and perceived value—the inherent qualities of intrinsic motivation. It also leads to higher quality performance, persistence, and creativity.

The degree that these needs are supported or compromised and thwarted has a significant impact on the individual and the individual's social context (the physical and social setting in which people live and work and the institutions with which they interact). If all three needs are satisfied, "People will develop and function effectively and experience wellness, and if not...people will more likely evidence ill-being and non-optimal functioning" (Ryan R, 2019).

We believe that all human beings have a set of basic psychological needs. The needs that we feel are important are the need for competence. That is to say to feel confident

and effective in relation to whatever it is you're doing.
Second, to feel relatedness, that is to say to feel cared for by
others, to care for others, to feel like you belong in various
groups that are important to you. And the third need is
autonomy… Human need is something that must get satisfied
for optimal wellness and optimal performance.
If they don't get the need satisfied, then there will be negative
psychological consequences that follow.

— **Deci, 2017**

Coaching in Support of Autonomy

People need to feel they are operating their lives by their own choice. Supporting the client's need for autonomy is considered one of the primary tasks of a coach. The client-centered nature of coaching supports client autonomy throughout the coaching process. Coaching operates on mutual agreements between client and coach. Agendas are co-created in a partnering, with the client always in the lead. In health and wellness coaching this is especially true as client-generated wellness goals have more inherent buy-in — that is, more motivational connection. The coaching cornerstone stance that the client is "naturally creative, resourceful, and whole" (NCRW) fosters autonomy as the coach works to evoke the inner wisdom of the client. Rather than operating from an expert point of view, the coach provides support for the client's own decision making, even though they assist in the process.

Coaching in Support of Competence

This NCRW stance also supports the other critical human need, according to SDT, of seeking to achieve competence. Again, in line with the tenets of humanistic psychology and the more recent developments in positive psychology, clients are treated as though they are indeed capable and possessing great potential. The strengths-based, positive psychology nature of coaching emphasizes acknowledging and building upon the client's attributes and qualities they already possess. A key here is acknowledgment. Clients often minimize or fail to recognize their strengths and achievements. If their self-efficacy is already low, having been brought down by previous failure experiences, they may tend to overlook what they are accomplishing, or to downplay it. The active listening skill of acknowledgment needs to be used by the coach whenever it can be genuinely utilized.

As client and coach work on self-determined goals and break those goals down into doable action steps, the client will enjoy more and more successful experiences. As they do so, they begin to feel more competent at improving their lifestyle, which naturally builds their feelings of self-efficacy. By co-creating the Wellness Plan, the client takes more ownership of their success. This ownership can be far more potent than experiencing a prescribed wellness program in which they are a passive participant.

Coaching in Support of Relatedness

The heart of coaching is the coaching relationship itself. Creating that alliance supplies the client with a trusted resource for support that can be relied upon unconditionally. As the coach exhibits the qualities of the great coaching presence, supplying the facilitative conditions of coaching, the client feels accepted, acknowledged, and cared for. Often our clients lack relationships in their lives where they experience adequate empathic understanding and are free from judgment.

> *It is important to note that whilst a coachee may have close relationships outside coaching, s/he may not consistently feel heard, understood, valued and/or genuinely supported within those relationships. If not, they are unlikely to feel strongly and positively connected to others and in an attempt to satisfy this basic need, may attempt to connect by acting in accordance with the preferences of others, rather than one's own.*
>
> — Spence, 2011

For the client, it is not only refreshing to relate to someone who provides unconditional positive regard and validates their experience and feelings; it may free the client up to explore their lives with new openness and independence. As Spence mentions above, they may have been holding themselves back from making some of the lifestyle changes they need to make because the fear of losing connection, to some degree, with others. Perhaps with the support of the coach, the client may be willing to take such risks to live in a healthier way.

Coaching for Connectedness to Meet Relatedness Needs

Masterful coaches have long recognized the importance and power of *coaching for connectedness*. We realize that coaching is a very brief moment in someone's life and that lasting lifestyle improvement often hinges upon finding the support of others for the changes clients need to make. As we help our clients choose action steps in their Wellness Plan we continually ask, "Who else can support you in doing this?" Building in strategies to seek out and gain support for wellness goals and the action steps needed to achieve them is often critical to success.

Of course, not all our clients enjoy lives rich in connectedness at home, work, and in their communities. As we partner with our clients to co-create the Wellness Plan, we may want to include developing more connectedness as an area of focus to be consciously worked on. Part of that process may be exploring ways in which the client holds themselves back from reaching out and making more interpersonal connections in their lives. As clients feel empowered by the autonomous nature of choice in the coaching process, they may be more willing to increase their connectedness.

As one's sense of autonomy increases, so does the likelihood they will make decisions to engage in interesting activities, to exercise capacities, and pursue connectedness in social groups.

— **Richard Ryan**

Supporting More Self-Determined Living

In summary, the work of Deci and Ryan shows us that part of our journey towards greater wellness is about becoming more internally motivated, fueled by getting more of our needs met. While we might observe a well-trained and experienced coach inherently demonstrating Self-Determination Theory in action, they may have never read a word on the subject. The congruency is there. However, functioning as good theory should, SDT can provide the coach with greater awareness of the *nature* of motivation, not only the quantity. It can show us the importance of grounding our coaching in process and structure that acknowledges the needs of our clients for *competence*, *autonomy*, and *relatedness*.

Masterful Moment

Look at the way you coach right now. Does it inherently include addressing the three innate psychological needs that SDT speaks of?

If not, how can you integrate meeting those needs into the way you coach? See how you can make this a natural part of your coaching.

Relevant Theory
Self-Efficacy and the Work of Albert Bandura— Lessons for Wellness Coaches

Self-efficacy or belief in one's ability to perform determines whether behavior will be initiated, how much effort will be expended, and whether the effort will be sustained.

People with high assurance in their capabilities approach difficult tasks as challenges to be mastered rather than as threats to be avoided.

— Albert Bandura

Albert Bandura

From ancient philosophers to Sigmund Freud and down to today's latest psychological research, people have been attempting to understand what drives human behavior. If you were to pose the idea that what we do as human beings is a result of what we think and how we interact with our environment, you would get few arguments. Yet such a theory is a relatively recent development in the study of psychology. Social psychologist Albert Bandura was primary among the people who have helped us validate the idea that our behavior is an interplay between what we observe in the world around us, how we self-reflect about it, and how we decide (cognitively) to go forward with action.

With the publication of *Social Foundations of Thought and Action: A Social Cognitive Theory*, Bandura (1986) advanced a view of human functioning that accords a central role to cognitive, vicarious, self-regulatory, and self-reflective processes in human adaptation and change. People are viewed as self-organizing, proactive, self-reflecting, and self-regulating rather than as reactive organisms shaped and shepherded by environmental forces or driven by concealed inner impulses (Pajares, 2002).

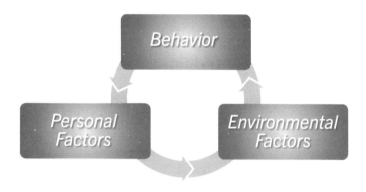

FIGURE 11—MODEL OF RECIPROCAL DETERMINISM, Bandura

Because social cognitive theory sees our behavior as part of a reciprocal, continually interacting circle, our coaching efforts can be directed at the personal, environmental, and behavioral factors.

For the wellness professional who works with people to help them improve their lifestyle behavior, this is an easy theory to identify. We see our clients continuously facing inner and outer barriers that challenge their attempts at behavioral change. Internal barriers include the personal factors that Bandura talks about: cognitive, affective, and biological events. More simply put, how our thoughts and belief systems limit us; how our emotions override our logic in self-defeating ways; and how our emotional-biological connection all influence our efforts at change. Outer barriers include the environmental factors that add stress and/or support to our lives.

Bandura's work shows us that both internal and external factors drive behavior. There is no single factor, such as our cognitive processing, that exclusively determines behavior. Personal factors include cognition, but also emotion and biological events. Think of the coaching client challenged with a medical condition. Their medical compliance/adherence behavior will be influenced by a reciprocal interaction of their thoughts about their condition and the needed adherent behaviors. ("I don't stand a chance with this diabetes. Why should I even bother checking my sugar levels?") Perhaps these thoughts are exacerbated by the fatigue they are presently feeling as their blood sugar levels dip (biological event). Their fears and feeling of hopelessness combine with these thoughts and physical sensations to result in the person failing to use their glucometer and check their blood sugar levels. Environmental factors such as the price of test strips for their glucometer, a lack of social support from family members, friends, or co-workers may also be in the mix, adding to the triadic effect. Because social cognitive theory sees our behavior as part of a reciprocal, continually interacting circle, our coaching efforts can be directed at all of the personal, environmental, and behavioral factors.

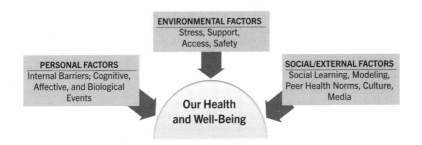

FIGURE 12—SOCIAL COGNITIVE HEALTH MODEL

We learn from others and the world around us. To truly comprehend what factors determine our health and well-being we must acknowledge physiological drivers (genetic predisposition, exposure, etc.), as well as the three influencers illustrated above. We can benefit from acknowledging the personal factors (internal barriers, cognition, affect, and biological events), the environmental factors (stress, support, access, safety, etc.), and the more social/external factors (social learning, modeling, peer health norms, culture, media). Bandura's work on social learning and modeling has shown us our tendency to adopt the behaviors we see exhibited around us. This can work in our favor when we help our clients to discover positive and successful lifestyle improvement examples in people with whom they identify. Bandura sees this as another way to raise self-efficacy and labels this as vicarious experience. The work of Robert and Judd Allen has shown us the influential power of peer health norms (Allen, 2019). The research by James Sallis and others working with the Active Living Research organization (Sallis, 2019) has shown us how health improves when communities become more activity-friendly. In the field of health promotion there is a vast movement to influence the entire culture of workplaces to be more health-generative instead of destructive.

Almost 30 years ago, my family and I made the fortuitous decision to move to Fort Collins, Colorado. This community is a perfect illustration of a place where it is easier to be well. Situated where the Great Plains end at the base of the Rocky Mountain foothills, Fort Collins is a very outdoor activity-oriented town. There is easy access to endless miles of hiking, and over 30 miles of dedicated bike trails and over 285 miles of bicycle lanes. There is plentiful access to healthy food. Another key factor is that most everyone I know is physically active through hiking, biking, dancing, skiing, and other activities. One is surrounded by encouragement to be well. The result, looking at one measure, is that the Gallup Poll found our community to be the leanest in the entire United States. Many communities are not so fortunate and present a whole host of environmental and social barriers to one's wellness. Effective wellness coaches are continually exploring with their clients how the steps they take to be well are going to be either supported or discouraged by the client's environment.

Part of the reciprocity of Bandura's model is that people are not viewed as passive recipients of the effects of their environment, but that they have the capacity to affect their environment. Beliefs and values can be translated into actions that can shape the environment. Fort Collins did not become a wellness mecca by chance. City planners made deliberate decisions to value bike trails over other projects. The people attracted to moving there were bringing with them values around being outdoors oriented and physically active as well as valuing whole and healthy foods.

Part of the empowerment of coaching is helping people to realize that they can advocate for their own health and wellbeing in many ways. A client can get the support they need from their coach, strategizing and rehearsing in an appointment to speak to their supervisor about more humane work hours and expectations. A family can begin an organic garden on a rooftop to improve access to healthy vegetables. In Detroit, Michigan, where the downturn of heavy industry led to widespread poverty and urban decline, there is a vigorous community garden program being enthusiastically embraced. In coaching, people learn that they can affect their environment.

> Bandura provided a view of human behavior in which the beliefs that people have about themselves are critical elements in the exercise of control and personal agency. Thus, individuals are viewed both as products and as producers of their own environments and of their social systems. Because human lives are not lived in isolation, Bandura expanded the conception of human agency to include collective agency. People work together on shared beliefs about their capabilities and common aspirations to better their lives. This conceptual extension makes the theory applicable to human adaptation and change in collectivistically-oriented societies as well as individualistically oriented ones (Pajares, 2002).

More masterful coaches recognize that what derails the best-laid Wellness Plans are usually these inner and outer barriers. Central to the coach approach is the contention that human beings are accepted in coaching as being "naturally creative, resourceful and whole" (Kimsey-House, 2018). They have the ability, with the right support, to positively impact their world and their own lives.

> Social cognitive theory is rooted in a view of human agency in which individuals are agents proactively engaged in their own development and can make things happen by their actions. Key to this sense of agency is the fact that, among other personal factors, individuals possess self-beliefs that enable them to exercise a measure of control over their thoughts, feelings, and actions, that what people think, believe, and feel affects how they behave (Bandura).

What wellness coaches observe is that there is often significant disparity regarding the degree to which their clients believe that the efforts they make to improve their health and well-being will be effective. Do they believe that they can affect their health, and to what degree? For the wellness coach and client, this is the very essence of "self-efficacy."

> Of all the thoughts that affect human functioning, and standing at the very core of social cognitive theory, are *self-efficacy* beliefs, people's judgments of their capabilities to organize and execute courses of action required to attain designated types of performances (Bandura).

> Self-efficacy beliefs provide the foundation for human motivation, well-being, and personal accomplishment. This is because unless people believe that their actions can produce the outcomes they desire, they have little incentive to act or to persevere in the face of difficulties. Much empirical evidence now supports Bandura's contention that self-efficacy beliefs touch virtually every aspect of people's lives—whether they think productively, self-debilitatingly, pessimistically or optimistically; how well they motivate themselves and persevere in the face of adversities; their vulnerability to stress and depression, and the life choices they make (Pajares, 2002).

Many clients arrive at wellness coaching after experiencing failures that negatively impacted their self-efficacy. Discouraged by perhaps numerous attempts to quit smoking, manage stress, or attain and then maintain a healthy weight, their belief in their own ability to succeed at lasting lifestyle improvement is damaged. Yet, as Bandura has shown us, this belief needs to be strengthened for the person to garner the motivation to change and the tenacity to succeed.

> *All that we are is the result of what we have thought; it is founded on our thoughts; it is made up of our thoughts. A man's life is the direct result of his thoughts... We are what we think. All that we are arises with our thoughts. With our thoughts we make the world.*
>
> **— Gautama Siddhartha (Buddha)**

Though he is not quoted as saying so, the essence of Bandura's work would agree with the old saying that we create our own reality. "Most human motivation is cognitively generated," Bandura argues. We anticipate our actions with forethought and figure our chances of success primarily based upon our past experience in this arena. This calculation forms beliefs about what we can and cannot do. We set goals and form plans to realize the outcomes we desire. The way we set those goals is largely determined by perception of our experience and our level of self-efficacy. This, combined with our current thinking, yields our performance in attempting to reach our desired outcome.

Efficacy—The Belief That Change Is Possible

Many of the clients who come to wellness coaching are more than just discouraged; their belief in their ability to affect their health has dropped to an exceptionally low point. They have tried and failed and tried and failed. There is not much energy left for another attempt. In their book *Changing to Thrive* (Prochaska, 2016), James and Janice Prochaska speak of demoralization as one of the dynamics that keeps people stuck in the stage of pre-contemplation. Such clients attribute their lack of hope to their shortcomings, believing that they lack sufficient willpower and strength of character.

> *Self-belief does not necessarily ensure success, but self-disbelief assuredly spawns failure.*
>
> **—A. Bandura**

The vital question for the wellness coaching client becomes, "To what degree do I believe I can affect my own health? Will the actions that I take produce the results I want when it comes to losing weight, quitting smoking, finally managing stress in my life better, etc.?" Bandura reminds us that the efficacy belief system is not a singular and pervasive trait, but instead differs from one realm of functioning to another. The same person who cannot seem to kick the tobacco habit may be extremely efficacious at operating a small business and managing employees. Self-efficacy regarding lifestyle improvement rests on a scale, varying from low to high; it is not a dichotomous concept. A history of unsuccessful attempts at lasting improvement damages self-efficacy. The person may cope with this by minimization and denial, or by a passive acceptance of powerlessness.

> *Reality is not so much what happens to us; rather, it is how we think about those events that create the reality we experience. In a very real sense, this means that we each create the reality in which we live.*
>
> — Dr. Albert Ellis

This also applies to our capabilities as well. We may be quite capable of pursuing successful change in an area of our life, possessing all the skills and knowledge required. However, it is our self-beliefs about our capacity to make this change that will more likely determine what change is actually attempted. Bandura states, "People's level of motivation, affective states, and actions are based more on what they believe than on what is objectively true" (Bandura, 1977).

We must also view self-efficacy as a social construct. Shared group beliefs about health behavior create a certain level of collective efficacy. A peer group (friends or co-workers), family, ethnic group, or such may hold certain beliefs about the utility of engaging in certain wellness-oriented activities. While one group, for example, might embrace practicing yoga for stress management and fitness, another may reject it because they do not identify with it, or see it as the practice of a foreign culture. Thus, a potentially viable resource for them might be eliminated. As a coach we must work with our clients in a way that respects their belief systems yet helps them to examine how it is working for them or against them and help them find workable alternatives.

The Coach Approach to Enhancing Self-Efficacy

How does a person overcome a history of failure in lifestyle improvement? If self-efficacy has been reduced by past events, processed as failures by the person, or even worse, as evidence of their own personal shortcomings, how can coaching help them succeed?

Causal Structure

Perception of past experience affects self-efficacy. This, in turn, affects expectations and the level where we set personal goals. Filtered through our thinking, or as Bandura puts it, our analytic strategies, this combination of personal goals and thinking affects performance and outcome.

This view of causal structure begins with the client having a history of failure at weight loss (for example) and low self-efficacy and belief about succeeding at another attempt. Based upon this past experience they set personal goals that are ineffective. Then, attempting to achieve these goals, they use strategies influenced by a lack of confidence, discouragement, and self-doubt, and, as a result, their performance, or outcome, suffers.

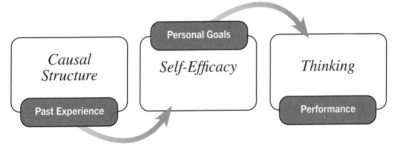

FIGURE 13—CAUSAL STRUCTURE OF CHANGE BASED ON PAST EXPERIENCE

A Coach Approach Difference

Let us say I now have a wellness coach helping me with the process of change. To begin with, I speak to my coach about my past experience, and they help me reframe my experience less negatively. I get empathy and support, even acknowledgment for how challenging weight loss has been for me, but I don't get sympathy. My coach helps me discover what in my experience was effective. What did work that can be used again?

My coach also works with me to improve my self-efficacy and helps me build my feelings of greater self-esteem, self-confidence, and helps me recognize and acknowledge my strengths that I can use in the change process. My coach is using the positive psychology approach that is inherent in coaching. Together my coach and I co-create a better set of personal goals that are optimistic yet realistic. Through the coaching I discover more of the motivation that I have for improving my life, including losing weight. The coaching helps me see the motivational link between what action I am taking and how it will help me reach my greater desired outcome of living my healthiest, best life. This motivation helps me produce more significant effort, push through barriers, and, with my coach's help, strategize both internal and external barriers. The result is improved performance.

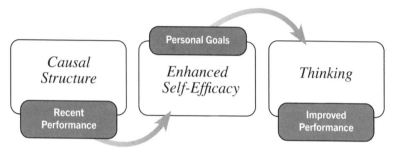

FIGURE 14—CAUSAL STRUCTURE OF CHANGE BASED ON RECENT PERFORMANCE

Now, when I look at my recent performance, I am encouraged by even a minimal level of progress. I now begin the causal structure of the change process again and this time I begin by basing it on my recent performance, not past performance. This helps push a higher level of self-efficacy within me. I set even better personal goals. My thinking, my analytic strategies, are more positive and effective, and these yield even better performance. We are now on a positive circle of action and success that we can repeat, instead of a vicious circle of defeat.

Through effective wellness coaching, we can help the person to shift their efficacy beliefs and enhance the probability of success.

The Coach:

- Uses a positive psychology approach—acknowledging and appreciating what the client has done to be successful.

- Helps the client re-frame their experience.

- Enhances self-efficacy, self-esteem, and self-confidence through the coaching process.

- Co-creates positive, optimistic, and yet realistic goals.

- Establishes a motivational link between actions taken and lifestyle improvement desired.

- Helps generate greater motivation and productive coaching strategies to help the client push beyond internal and external barriers.

- Helps the client see improved performance.

The client's improved performance becomes a new base for continued success.

How to Build Self-Efficacy

Most wellness professionals are already familiar with the term self-efficacy and set improved self-efficacy as a desired outcome in virtually all of their wellness programming. Wellness coaches seek to help clients have greater belief in their ability, capacity, and confidence in positively affecting their health and improving their lifestyles. The question is, "How?"

Fortunately, effective wellness coaching methodologies have built into them the very factors that Bandura has found successful.

Bandura identified four sources of information that affect our self-efficacy:

- Mastery experiences—self-mastery
- Vicarious experiences—role modeling
- Verbal persuasion—social persuasion
- Physiological cues

Let's look at how wellness coaches can help clients improve self-efficacy by working with these four factors.

Mastery Experiences

Mastery experiences are the strongest and most effective source of building self-efficacy. An effective coach helps their client recognize and acknowledge themselves for even the smallest accomplishment. Many clients are notoriously poor at giving themselves credit for what they do accomplish. Coaching can help them reframe this.

The coach helps their client avoid repeating self-defeating strategies used in the past and helps them devise more effective experiments for change. As clients put in place a Wellness Plan that sets out manageable goals and specific (easy) action steps that are in alignment with the client's readiness for change (Prochaska, 2016) the probability of success is much greater. As the client experiences mastery it is self-reinforcing, and self-efficacy beliefs elevate.

Vicarious Experiences—Role Modeling

A cornerstone of social psychology is that we all learn from one another, and that this influences our behavior. Much of Bandura's work has been around modeling, whether it was the famous BoBo Doll Experiment (Bandura A. R., 1961), or filming people crossing the street against a traffic light just because a well-dressed man carrying a briefcase did so. When we see someone who is successful at a specific behavior we are more likely to try it ourselves. Thus, the omnipresence of fad diets and all the fitness trends we witness. Television and the internet expose us to even more models to imitate. Self-efficacy, then, can be affected by observing what others experience.

People who observe a model perform successfully in a challenging situation are more likely to develop an expectation that they can acquire the same skill (Alderman, 1999). Coaches can encourage clients to find models that will both encourage them and, perhaps, show them the strategies and skills they need to be successful like their models.

What we know about effective models is that they need to be people we feel positive about and to whom we can relate. Most fitness and wellness magazines, for example, forget this, and continuously hold up exceptional examples for us to follow. We may find it extremely hard to identify with celebrities or a seventy-five-year-old ultra-marathoner who was an All-American track star in college. Models who are seen as having similar attributes (age, gender, ethnicity, etc.) as we do and who have struggled imperfectly, but persevered and succeeded at a similar task, are the most effective.

Verbal Persuasion—Social Persuasion

The messages we get from others can have a profoundly positive or negative effect on our efficacy expectations. When one receives encouragement that "you can do it," our belief in our capacity for change increases. For these positive verbal statements to be effective, though, they must be believable and conveyed by someone the person sees as trustworthy.

The term persuasion may be a bit misleading for the coach. The reality is that we really cannot persuade someone to be well. It is not a convincing sales pitch that works, but instead the "I believe you can do it; I believe in you" statements that a coach sincerely makes go beyond simple cheerleading.

At the heart of good coaching is what we call coaching for connectedness. A key to successful and lasting lifestyle improvement is coaching with the client to help them consciously develop a system of support that will help them attain and maintain the changes they seek. This social support is a central part of Bandura's message. When clients find walking buddies, connect with social groups with positive peer health norms, or learn how to ask for the support they need, they are much more likely to succeed.

Physiological Cues

Individuals sometimes judge their capability to perform a task by their own physical or emotional experience as they face it or perform it. They doubt their ability, possibly fear the consequences of failure, etc. They may experience anxiousness, increased heart rate, sweating, and so on. When clients are aware of these symptoms, or are experiencing pain, fatigue, nausea, or other effects of their chronic illness or medical treatments, self-doubt and fear can be triggered. Their self-efficacy plunges down further and affects performance.

Bandura contends that individuals have the capacity for self-regulation. We can affect our physiological states through our awareness, our thought processes, and techniques of breathing and relaxation. Wellness coaches can help their clients to become aware of these patterns of anxiousness and teach them to seek out methods for self-management. Coaching takes it further by helping clients establish accountability around practicing these self-management techniques. Positive mental rehearsal can reduce anticipatory anxiety and increase confidence in one's capacity for positive performance. The coach and client can rehearse in role-play for an upcoming event for the same purposes.

Bandura's work with social cognitive theory helps us see ways to be more effective working with our clients. It validates the coach approach. There is congruity between what coaches do and what this theory advises.

Applying Theory Through Advanced Coaching Methods

Once grounded in evidence-based theory, especially around motivation, the coach must hone their craft to bring specific skills to a higher level. Helping our clients to increase awareness of their wellness, their thought patterns, their lifestyle behavior and its consequences can be achieved through skillful coaching.

> *And I believe that this is the great thing to understand: that awareness per se—by and of itself—can be curative.*
>
> **—Frederick S. Perls**

Awareness

So much of awareness is about noticing. It is tuning in to the vast array of information being taken in through our senses, and the way we cognitively process it all. It is the integration of all that information coming on different pathways and arriving at conclusions about what is really happening. In coaching, your three-fold challenge is to be able to move fluidly between your awareness of yourself, awareness of your client, and awareness of what is going on between the two of you. You tune in to your bodily sensations, your perceptions of your affect, while simultaneously keenly observing your client in all that they say and do, noticing nonverbal as well as verbal behavior. To complicate the task, you must periodically step back and tune in to the dynamics of your interaction with your client in the context of the broader coaching relationship. This is where you tap into your third person observer and take a look over your own shoulder.

The more masterful coach is gliding between three levels of awareness throughout the coaching session:

- Awareness of self
- Awareness of our client
- Awareness of the coaching relationship

Awareness of Self

Begin tuning into your awareness of yourself before the coaching session even begins. Take some time before the upcoming session to stop whatever else you are doing, to shift your posture, perhaps stand up, and breathe deeply. Scan over your body quickly and notice how you feel. Stretch, roll your shoulders, and do whatever feels right and it will help you feel more grounded physically. Take note of your own mental/emotional state. Are you feeling grounded and centered, or do you notice how stressed, anxious, or worried you are? Are you ready to really make full contact with the client you will be coaching in just a few minutes? Ask yourself what you need to do to become more present.

Once in the coaching session, continue inventory of your physical awareness as well as your awareness of your thoughts and emotions. Are you noticing that you are triggered by something your client has just said? Did your client just bring up a topic that relates to some tender, unfinished emotional business of your own? The more you are in touch with your own thoughts and feelings and can name them, the more likely you are to remain connected to your client.

Much of what we refer to as the coaching skill of using intuition emerges from a combination of our observations of the client and our contact with our own body wisdom. What shows up as an intuitive hit often begins with this subtle and almost subconscious awareness.

Awareness of Our Client

Our challenge in keenly observing our client is to watch and listen as though looking through a tightly focused lens, with the microphone turned up to maximum sensitivity. Yet, we still must refrain from analysis and interpretation. Judgment dulls awareness. Judgment is like a set of blinders, like those used on the eyes of a horse drawing a carriage, eliminating peripheral vision. It narrows our field of view, and potentially vital information is missed. Notice! But don't judge.

There is so much to notice. If you have the benefit of a live, in-person session with your client (as opposed to only telephonic), keenly observe their body language and nonverbal behavior. A session using real time video can also yield more visual information for you. Notice your client's posture and any shifts that take place, changes in facial expression (again don't rush to interpret), and repetitive movements (possibly reflecting anxiety). The usefulness of this and other observations is twofold. You can file the observations away until you see more behavior that forms a pattern. You can also feed observations back to the client. Simply say, "Are you aware that…." This is particularly helpful when you can tie it to the content of what the client is talking about. "Are you aware that you began to frown when you started talking about getting your partner's cooperation with meal planning?" Then patiently wait as you allow your client to work with that feedback and respond.

Also, take note of your client's appearance. Again, without judgment, look for patterns. Is your client managing their hygiene and clothing in an improved way as coaching has gone on, or has it deteriorated? As some Swami somewhere once said, "As without, so within." How we express ourselves through our appearance is sometimes very telling.

For in-person sessions and in telephonic sessions as well, pay close attention to all of the variations in vocal behavior that take place. Carefully observe your client's speech for shifts in rapidity, tone, and volume. How does it tie into what they are saying? The way someone says something is a far more significant part of communication than just what they have said. Is there a trace of sarcasm or cynicism in their voice? Did their volume descend quickly when they started to express a sense of hopelessness? Again, feed it back to your client when you believe it will be of value. Your job here is to help them increase their awareness, to help them make contact with what is going on for them. Often such feedback fills in a blind spot and leads to a significant insight.

Get to know your client's style of expressing themselves. You may learn that your quiet, somewhat introverted client has an incredible reservoir of strength behind that calm exterior. Personalities and even ethnic differences show up in our ways of expressing ourselves. Misunderstandings can often be avoided by not rushing to an interpretation of our client's intentions or feelings when they express themselves in a way we are not accustomed to. One of my best friends was a boisterous and highly opinionated man who was the son of parents from the Caribbean; one Dominican and one Puerto Rican. It was quite common for people to mistake his tremendous passion when conversing about politics, music, or practically any topic as an expression of anger. When confronted about being angry, he would laugh.

Awareness of the Coaching Relationship

As the coach is tracking their awareness of self and awareness of their client, there needs to be consciousness of the coaching relationship and its unfolding dynamics. Hopefully, the coach has worked to develop a strong alliance with their client built upon trust. Part of that is done by conveying to the client that it is safe to talk about the coaching process itself and to adopt an attitude of continuous improvement. The hope is that difficulties can be avoided by honest interchange about what is happening in the coaching process. If the client is feeling pushed by the coach towards a particular line of action, we want the client to bring this to the coach's attention and work it out. Is coaching structure working to enhance both the efficiency of coaching and the coaching relationship? Is the way accountability is being used both effective and satisfactory to the client? All too often, though, breakdowns in the coaching alliance are suffered in silence by the client or missed by the coach.

To avoid setbacks in the coaching alliance, pay attention to the flow of communication. Is the coaching conversation easy? Is it punctuated with humor and lightness, or is it dead serious or even grim? Is the conversation reciprocal and mutual, or does one party dominate? Clients can take over the conversation and end up getting little value from the coach's few contributions. Coaches can also feel like they are carrying the burden of maintaining the conversation as their client sits and passively just responds to questions.

To address what the coach suspects is a breakdown in the coaching alliance, courageous coaching is required. This is the proverbial "talking about the elephant in the living room." It is time to process the process. Bring your concerns to the client in a way that engages them, looking at the coaching alliance and how to improve it together. Inquire about their satisfaction with how coaching is working. Are they receiving the value that they had hoped? Begin by sharing your observations in a very blame-free way. Again, it is about increasing awareness—in this case for you and your client—of what is happening. Engage your client in a mutual task of how to improve the coaching process. Don't just tell them what you think needs to happen. Be open to their ideas. Seek their perspective. Remember one of Steven Covey's Seven Habits of Highly Effective People: "Seek first to understand, then to be understood" (Covey, 2013).

Coaching for Greater Client Awareness

Coaching puts its faith in the client's internal wisdom, but also realizes that the job of the coach is to help to evoke it. Bringing forth that wisdom is primarily about increasing awareness. We trust that increased awareness will allow our client to integrate greater knowledge, allowing them to make efficacious decisions about living. Coaching is grounded in a theory that people are inherently moving towards actualization of their potential in life-enhancing ways. We often say that people are "doing the best they can, given their level of awareness." If we are aware of more, we can make even better decisions. Trust your client.

When we think of health and wellness behavior, we know that some awareness can grow through effective health education. Learning about the importance of minimizing highly refined carbohydrates in the diet of a person challenged by diabetes may be crucial to their health. Sometimes, increased awareness through increased information is sufficient. Do not overlook the value of great health education.

Increased Awareness Through Mindfulness

> Mindfulness is...*the awareness that arises from paying attention, on purpose, in the present moment, and non-judgmentally.*
>
> —**Jon Kabat-Zinn,** *Full Catastrophe Living*

As clients become more consciously aware of their behavior, they can gather more information and make better choices. The client who ruins their caloric intake goal for the day by unconscious evening snacking may benefit from learning how to eat more mindfully. Coaches can help their clients to do this by first presenting mindful eating as a learning option for the client. Once the client sees the value in this new approach and buys into trying it, then the experiment can begin.

An experiment in mindful eating might begin with the client keeping a log of what they were aware of when they noticed their desire to snack arising. Was it real hunger, stomach growling, etc., or were they feeling bored, lonely, frustrated, or some other feeling? What were their circumstances: watching television, on a break at work, just finishing an upsetting phone call, or receiving a disconcerting text? Their old pattern was to notice the desire and then to react by snacking. Now, they are urged to notice the desire and see what else they see before deciding whether food is really what they want. More can be learned about mindful eating by exploring the "Am I Hungry" mindful eating program (May, 2019).

A great deal of our lifestyle is a collection of habitual behaviors that we perform without a lot of consciousness. Coaching with our clients with this mindful process of conscious noticing can help them become aware of habits that they may want to work on changing.

Awareness of Behavior

A great deal of insight can be gained by noticing. Coaching offers the client a chance to explore the patterns of their behavior and see how they are working for their health and wellness or against it. A place to begin is with increasing awareness of what the client is doing to enhance their health and wellness. The coach approach helps the client to realize the positive things they are already doing to live a healthier lifestyle. As you and your client explore their current lifestyle, be sure to take every opportunity to use the coaching skill of acknowledgment. Bring their attention to their attitude and behavior and how it is working to maintain or improve their health and wellbeing.

As the exploration continues, clients will bring up things about their lifestyle that they know they want to change. Those goals can be integrated into their Wellness Plan. The additional value that coaching brings is to help the client to examine how their current lifestyle behaviors work against them living the healthy life they desire.

When you notice a self-defeating pattern bring the client's awareness to it gently. If you come across accusatory or judgmental, be prepared for resistance. Instead, share with your client your neutral observation. "I hear you saying that you enjoy time alone, but I also hear you saying that the only time you eat healthily is with friends." At that point, don't follow up with a question. Just listen. See what your client does with the shared observation. If the client proceeds with exploration of that observation, great! Go with the client to explore it more. If they hesitate, then ask if they would find value in pursuing it. As you explore, think of your task as simply helping your client to increase awareness of their current behavior, to enhance understanding. As you use your active listening skills (paraphrase, request for clarification, etc.) and pursue this line of inquiry with powerful questions, hopefully your client will gain some insights. Once they do, you can then move on to forwarding the action and see what the client wants to change.

Awareness of Feeling

We speak of being "in touch with" or "out of touch with" our feelings. Feelings are present. The question is: how much contact do we have with them? At times feelings are overwhelming and we swim in a sea of emotion. At other times we employ various psychological defense mechanisms to distance ourselves from our feelings. Sometimes we are so caught up in our cognition that feelings elude us.

While coaching sometimes is pursued as a type of intellectual exercise in goal setting, the reality is that for real and lasting progress to take place, the emotional realm must be brought into our awareness. Emotions are affecting our decisions every day. Decisions such as how to pursue our lifestyle through a myriad of health behavior choices are made on an emotional, not just logical, level. If this is so, then we had better give our feelings their due (Lerner, 2015).

An important value of coaching is helping our clients make full contact with their feelings. If we believe in the capacity of our clients to be "naturally creative, resourceful, and whole," then we begin with faith that they can handle being in touch with their emotions. We will explore the whole area of process coaching—how to coach with emotions—in detail in Chapter Nine. For now, let's look at how we can help our clients to become more aware of their affective side.

Use the coaching skill of reflection of feeling. Unless the coach has a counseling background, this is probably their most underutilized coaching skill. When we reflect feeling, the first thing it does is to convey to the client that emotions are within the scope of coaching and okay to talk about. We cease to merely engage in intellectual exploration and begin to include the whole person.

Reflecting feelings helps the client check in with their emotions and determine what they are feeling. When we give our clients our best take on what emotion we are observing, we seek their validation that we perceive accurately. "It sounds like tracking your exercise has become very frustrating." "I hear some real disappointment in your voice right now." Doing so helps our client sample the feeling we are reflecting, and if on target, to make more contact with that emotion. "Yes! I am disappointed that the walking group didn't work out. I'm afraid I'll never make progress getting out walking."

Sometimes instead of reflecting feeling, we need ask, "What are you aware of right now?" This often works even better than asking, "What are you feeling right now?" or "How does that make you feel?" You are simply bringing their attention to their emotions in a very non-directive and non-demanding way. This can be especially effective when a client, for example, goes through an exhaustive list of all the items on their stressful to-do list. Instead of addressing what's on the list, ask, "So! Hearing yourself go through that list, what are you aware of right now?" That turns the conversation to what is most important—how the client feels about their list. Now they are in contact with their feeling of overwhelm, exhaustion, resentment, or whatever the real issue is.

The client-centered coach approach is apparent here when we help our client to make contact with their emotion and then leave it up to them to direct the work on it. We do not interpret the meaning of the emotion or speculate about its importance.

Masterful Moment

When we begin an expedition of awareness with our client, we have no idea where we will be going. It is the land of our client's awareness of their own experience that we are journeying in, not ours. To accompany our client, to facilitate their exploration we must be centered, grounded, courageous, and confident that we can always come back to the present moment. In fact, it is within the present moment, the here and now, where awareness resides.

All else is memory and imagination.

This chapter shifted into Part Three of our book: What to Do. We took a deep dive into the vital topic of motivation, how to mobilize it, and the relevance of meaning and purpose. We introduced two key theories of motivation that are critical for the coach to understand: self-determination theory and social cognitive theory. We then rounded out the chapter with a look at how we can help our clients to increase awareness.

Our next chapter, Advanced Coaching Skills and Methods — The Craft of Coaching Skills, will bring us into the concrete skills of what to do in wellness coaching. We will show how the skills of listening are not about active listening skills. They are about how to listen and what to listen for. We will examine each active listening skill and look at how we can respond more masterfully to what we are hearing. The use of questions will be explored showing how we can employ them effectively in our coaching.

We will also see how language plays a central role in coaching and explore how the way the client and the coach talk impact the coaching process. The essential coaching skill of reframing will be demonstrated and the value of using metaphors will be presented. Lastly, we will discuss laser coaching and show how to coach efficiently when we may or may not have all the time we would like with our client.

REFERENCES

Alderman, M. (1999). *Motivation for achievement: possibilities for teaching and learning.* Lawrence Erlbaum Associates.

Allen, J. (2019). Home page. Human Resources Institute. Healthy Culture.com: http://www.healthyculture.com/schedule_presentation.html

Bandura, A., Ross, D., & Ross, S. A. (1961). Transmission of aggression through imitation of aggressive models. *The Journal of Abnormal and Social Psychology, 63*(3), 575–582. https://doi.org/10.1037/h0045925

Bandura, A. (1986). *Social foundations of thought and action: A social cognitive theory.* Prentice Hall.

Bandura, A. (1997). *Self-efficacy: The exercise of control.* Freeman.

Brewer, J. (2018). The craving mind: From cigarettes to smartphones to love – why we get hooked and how we can break bad habits (Reprint Ed.). Yale University Press.

Covey, S. (2013). *The 7 habits of highly effective people: Powerful lessons in personal change* (Anniversary Ed.). Simon & Schuster.

Deci, E. (2017). *Self-determination theory*. Retrieved January 4, 2019, from Youtube. com. https://www.youtube.com/watch?v=m6fm1gt5YAM

Kimsey-House, K. K., Kimsey-House, H., Sandhal, P., & Whiteworth, L.(2018) *Co-active coaching: The proven framework for transformative conversations at work and in life* (4th Ed.). Nicholas Brealey.

Lerner, J. L. (2015). Emotion and decision making. *Annual review of psychology*, 66(33),1-33.

Maslow, A. (1998). *Toward a psychology of being. (3rd Ed.).* Sublime.

May, M. (2019, January 4). Homepage. *Am I hungry? Eat mindfully, live vibrantly.* https://amihungry.com

Pajares, F. (2002). Overview of social cognitive theory and self-efficacy. *University of Kentucky.* http://www.uky.edu/~eushe2/Pajares/eff.html

Pink, D. (2011). *Drive: The surprising truth about what motivates us.* Riverhead Books.

Prochaska, J. O. & Prochaska, M. J. (2016). *Changing to thrive: Using the stages of change to overcome the topthreats to your health and happiness.* Hazelden Publishing.

Rogers, C. (2004). *On becoming a person: A therapist's view of psychotherapy.* Constable & Robinson Ltd.

Ryan, R. M. (2000). Self-determination theory and the facilitation of intrinsic motivation, social development and well-being. *American Pschologist*, 55(1), 229.

Ryan, R. M. (2017). *Self-determination theory: Basic psychological needs in motivation, development, and wellness.* Springer.

Ryan, R. M. (2019, January 4). Self-determination theory. *Self-determination theory.* http://selfdeterminationtheory.org/theory/

Sallis, J. (2019, January 4). Homepage. *Active living research.* https://activelivingresearch.org

Spence, G. B. (2011). Coaching with self-determination theory in mind: Using theory to advance evidence-based coaching practice. *International journal of evidence-based coaching and mentoring.* 9(2), 37-55.

PART THREE

What to Do

Chapter 7—Advanced Coaching Skills and Methods— The Craft of Coaching Skills

Advanced Coaching Skills and Methods—The Craft of Coaching Skills

Deep Listening: "I can hear tears"

What is it that allows masterful coaches to become aware of things that most people miss in a conversation? How do they tune in to their client in such a way that the coaching conversation becomes rich, productive, and even enlightening?

In a class discussion about listening, one of my Real Balance students, who demonstrated she was an already accomplished coach, shared with us the poignant statement, "I can hear tears." She was referring to coaching over the phone where the visual nonverbal cues are absent. She was picking up on both the client's subtle vocal cues and the context of the conversation. At such a tender moment, a client may make an effort to be as silent as possible. The vocal cues such as a voice that breaks in tone or stammers are not there for the coach to perceive during such a silence. The context can undoubtedly tip the coach off that it would be natural for a client to cry upon sharing a painful experience or talking about a profound loss. Yet people react to experience and emotion in many different ways, from hysteria to stoicism. How does a more masterful coach *hear* tears that silently run down the cheek?

The powers of observation of the more masterful coach are as keen and sharp as a razor. They don't miss much. They notice. They are mindfulness in action. They also don't allow judgment to interfere and throw their subsequent observations in a prejudiced direction, blinding them to the full picture of what is unfolding. They stay on pace with their client instead of ahead of them. These practices allow them to stay in the present and in touch with all of their senses. They are not rushing ahead with their imagined conclusions about where the dialogue is going. By maintaining a coaching mindset, they are able to facilitate the client's work instead of attempting to do the work for their client. By not engaging in the *headwork* (analyzing, deducing, imagining, problem solving, continually thinking of the next question to ask, etc.) they can be *present* with their client and hear more. This way of being, combined with providing the facilitative conditions of coaching discussed in Chapter Four, is the very essence of *coaching presence*.

Observing by Scanning

One aspect of effective observation is what I call *scanning*. If you ever take a nature walk with a trained naturalist, or perhaps the type of experienced hunter who is keenly in touch with the natural world, you realize that they are constantly scanning the landscape as they move through it. I remember reading Barry Lopez's award-winning book *Artic Dreams* (Lopez, 1986). He spoke of his time with the Inuit people of the far north who were out on a hunting expedition. They walked over the tundra all day, slowly, silently. Then, at night around a campfire, they spoke of all the things they had seen. Lopez, one of America's greatest nature writers who has developed intense powers of observation himself, was amazed at what these indigenous people had picked up on, down to minute details of the land and its creatures. The Inuits had been scanning both the horizon, where they were walking, and everything in between. They had been scanning visually, looking for movement, shifts, changes, anything out of order in shape or color. They had been scanning auditorily, hearing birdsong, wind, twigs snapping. They had been scanning olfactorily, smelling the scent of whatever flowers, animals, carrion, or people might be in the region. They had been doing all of this effortlessly. It was simply how they hunted.

Just like our friends in Lopez's book, we, as coaches, want to be noticing shifts, changes, anything out of the ordinary with our clients. While the Inuit hunter might spot the movement of a ptarmigan in a bush, we may notice the shift in our client's tone of voice, in their posture, in the speed with which they are now talking. When we listen beyond words, beyond content, we hear more. The verbal content is important. It's like the landscape itself; it is the context of the conversation. Yet, what's important is what is happening on that landscape. What movement is there in the bushes, so to speak? What is the client thinking and feeling regarding the content about which they are speaking?

The novice coach, new to the coaching landscape, may focus mostly on the content of their client's communication. Yet they progress in their coaching so much more when they realize that the client is not just speaking to them about a subject, they are communicating! It's not just what they say, it's how they are saying it. The content might sound like "I've walked only two times this week." All the while the client is attempting to convey to their coach that they are becoming very worried that they will never get their lung capacity back after their acute heart failure if they don't exercise more often. Did the coach see the frightened bird that just froze on the tree branch, or were they lost looking at the trees? What is the client communicating?

What Are We Listening For?

Just like the skilled naturalist, or the Inuit people that Lopez observed, the more masterful coach has learned what to look for in our coaching landscape. The novice coach may travel the same landscape and not notice half of what the more masterful coach will pick up on. They have learned how to read the signs, to distinguish a track from a mere depression in the soil. To deepen your listening ability, what can you tune in to? Within the content of what is being said and beyond the content, what will help our coaching be more productive?

The Coach's Listening Day-Pack

As we develop greater skills, we begin to notice so much that is going on that we can't possibly comment on all of it during the coaching session. We will be constantly choosing what to respond to in the moment and what to stash away in what we might call our *listening day-pack* for future use in the coaching process. Hold on to those observations and perceptions. Write them down in your notes after the session is over.

Listening for "The Big Five"

In their excellent book, *Becoming a Professional Life Coach*, Pat Williams and Diane Menendez (Williams, 2015), explore five critical elements for coaches to tune into with their listening. My take on *The Big Five* is a little different. Allow me to share the value I see in each.

1. Focus. Your client begins by connecting with you, telling their story, and explaining what brought them to coaching. Either directly, or indirectly, they begin to center in on what they want to get out of the coaching experience, what they want to accomplish, realize, and learn. Their goals emerge, perhaps in terms that require clarification. Listen within the content for what the client wants. Listen for aspects of the beginnings of their *well life vision* as it begins to appear. If we are beginning on a journey together, what is the destination they are imagining?

Often clients arrive for coaching with ambiguous goals, or a shopping list of all of the things they want to change to live a better life. For them clarity is their ally. Listen for specifics that the client mentions. What aspects of their goals seem most often referred to? What qualities do they hope to have present in the changes they want to see? Listen for how their values show up in the coaching conversation, or perhaps inquire more about what they value. How are their values reflected in their goals? Listen for the hopes, dreams, fears, and concerns the client is expressing.

When we use a developed wellness coaching process, we begin with helping our clients to take stock of their wellness through a thorough self-assessment process. By doing this before we nail down the Wellness Plan, the client can gain a more holistic picture of themselves and co-create with the coach better goals to work on. During this process listen for desires, hopes, and themes in the process that help the client to winnow down their goals to ones that are feasible and will serve them well.

Alternatively, some clients arrive for wellness coaching stating a very simple and direct goal. "I want to lose XX lbs." They seem to have the *focus* part down. They may even seem hyper-focused. With such a client listen for ways you can help them expand their peripheral vision. As you inquire more about their past efforts at change, listen for what worked and what did not. Listen for the barriers to change that occurred before and inquire about their concerns that such barriers may arise again. If you are able to help such a client see the benefits of beginning with a more holistic self-assessment, they may discover keys to success that were missing in the narrow approach they tried before.

2. Mindset/Attitude. Few of our clients come through the door of coaching wearing sweatshirts that say *Optimist* or *Pessimist*. The mindset that our clients approach life with is slowly, but inevitably revealed as they speak and engage in the coaching process. Williams and Menendez (Williams, 2015) share six ways through which clients eventually reveal their mindset:

1. The ways they characteristically approach people and relationships.

2. The ways they define success and themselves in relation to people, events, and circumstances.

3. Whether they tend to see themselves as actors, participants, or victims.

4. How they draw conclusions about events and experiences.

5. How they think about their ability to create and influence.

6. How they evaluate the importance and value of people, situations, experiences, and results.

Take in your client's mindset without judgment, even if it appears to you to be rather self-defeating. Coaches work with the client they have, not the ideal one they might imagine. You can always challenge your client with the good old "How's that working for you?" question.

Fundamental to wellness coaching is the question of your client's degree of self-efficacy. To what degree do they believe that they can affect change in their life? How confident are they that engaging in this lifestyle improvement effort will be worth it? Listen for the references your client will make about their past experience of success and failure and how it affects their attitudes and beliefs today. Listen for how they speak about becoming discouraged and perhaps demoralized. Listen beyond the words to the tone of voice and all of the affective cues that come through in how they talk about their experience.

Listen for the nature of their *locus of control*. Do they believe that they have agency in life, that they can affect their world through their own will and efforts? Do they believe that most of what determines success and failure in life is external to them? Do they seem to feel overwhelmed by the social and environmental determinants of health? Where do they feel empowered to make change happen, or not? Is this what is keeping them stuck?

3. Skills and Capabilities. As you continue your coaching conversation with your client, listen for attributes that might prove useful on their journey toward a healthier and happier life. As these show up, you may, again, want to put them into your listening daypack and pull them out at an opportune time later on. Considering the nature of the lifestyle improvement process what skills and capabilities would prove useful? This is again implementing coaching's strengths-based, positive psychology approach.

Lifestyle change is a process of changing many daily habits, some lifelong in nature. To do so requires tenacity and consistent persistence. Listen for the presence of these qualities as your client speaks.

Sometimes you may come across skills or capabilities that can be celebrated in the moment instead of saved for later use. When I coached a policewoman and a policeman on weight loss, we were able to encourage them by celebrating the fact that their work had trained them to be incredible, detail-oriented trackers of behavior. This was a key factor in their eventual success.

An Example of Applying Skills and Capabilities Now

When doing a coaching demonstration with a student in one of our webinar classes the student-client spoke of how she had been successfully working on losing weight in order to help with her recent knee replacement. She had been exercising three days a week at a fitness center at 5:30 p.m. on Monday, Wednesday, and Friday as this was very convenient for her to do immediately after work. Then she relayed how "Life happened!" A complex series of events at home and work led to her abandoning her workout routine. I inquired, "Tell me about life happened." The client went on to describe how she had dealt with the chaos. Through some real skills at organization and conflict resolution she had brought order out of that chaos. She was still being affected by the unpredictable nature of the circumstances and hence had not returned to her workout routine. I was hearing attributes here that she could use at once. I immediately acknowledged her skills at organization and how they had served her so well in dealing with how messy life had become. I then challenged her to use those same organizational thinking skills to tackle the problem of getting back to working out regularly enough to help her weight-loss/knee rehabilitation program. She jumped right in with a laser-like analysis of the current situation and began putting order to it. Suddenly she realized that she had been stuck on her workout schedule of Monday/Wednesday/Friday at 5:30 p.m. The light bulb went on and she used the same sense of flexibility that had served her so well in dealing with the home and work problems. She only had to get in three workouts a week, and the exact time to do so could be flexible. It didn't matter when she did the workouts, just so she got them done. Applying her same skill at organization and her capability to be flexible allowed her to return to the regular workouts she needed so badly.

4. Habits, Practices, and Patterns. Habits, practices, and patterns fall into two categories: the ones clients are aware of and those they are not aware of. Wellness is all about changing the habits, practices, and patterns of lifestyle so that they are working for a client's health and well-being and not against it. Many times our clients realize what some of their self-defeating habits are. A classic would be late-night snacking. Our client knows it is a problem and may choose to work on changing it in coaching. What we want to especially be listening for are the habits, practices, and patterns that the client is not aware of.

The coach is positioned perfectly to notice the ways in which their clients are behaving that they might not be conscious of. It is like we are sitting in the car's passenger seat and we can more easily twist around to see the blind spot that the driver cannot. The client's own hopes, desires, dreams, and fears may be blinding them even more to how what they are doing is working against them.

I once coached a single dad who had joint custody of his children. They lived with him half of the time in their home in the country. He came to me for coaching on being more productive with his self-employed business. As he described his lifestyle I heard again and again references to making the half-hour drive into town to accommodate every request his children made. His desire to please his kids was strong and pizza, video games, movies, etc., all added up to many time-consuming trips back and forth. What seemed obvious to me was not something that he could see. Rather than confront him with judgment, I simply urged him to keep a diary of how he was using each hour of his waking day. The numbers did not lie and now the mystery of his lack of time to devote to his own business was solved. Listen for what your client is not *hearing* themselves.

Patterns in Client Language and Behavior

One of the things that can prove most useful to a client is when the coach is able to put together patterns that emerge in the stories the client tells. Barriers and self-defeating behavior tend to repeat. Again, the coach may be able to spot what is going on more easily than the client. Listen for what clusters together. Bring it to your client's attention by using a simple awareness technique. "Are you aware that each time you talk about how challenging it is to take time for self-care, you end up talking about your partner? Would you find value in exploring that?"

5. Follow the Energy. In my previous training and work in Gestalt therapy we were taught the value of becoming acutely aware of our client's energy and especially the shifts in it. As clients speak, their emotional energy may hold steady for long periods of time or go up and down. This is manifested in their feelings and emotions. *Listen* for your client's energy. Do they show excitement (a noticeable increase of speech volume, rapidity, and tone) as they speak about something they feel passionate about? A client might mention something and *light up* talking about an interest they have. We might respond in the moment, bringing their awareness to it, or stash it again in our listening daypack. Perhaps that interest could become part of the client's Wellness Plan.

Do you notice your client's voice slowing down, decreasing in volume and tone as they speak about a particular subject? Once again, bring it to their awareness. "Are you aware of how your voice has shifted since you started talking about the upcoming holidays?" Following the energy means also noticing long stretches that seem devoid of affect. Bringing that observation to our client's attention can help them discover what is going on for them. Are they bored, stuck, or discouraged? How is this low, but steady, level of energy related to the subject they are talking about? How related is it to the coaching relationship? The long-haul process of improving lifestyle can create both discouragement and fatigue. This can show up in the client's voice. Listen for it. Client energy always tells a story. Follow it.

A Deeper Look at Active Listening

What do we do with the new information we are hearing? Once we pick up on the totality of communication from our client, what do we do with it? This is where the ICF core competency of active listening comes in.

The *active listening skills* that we talk about aren't really skills about how to listen more effectively. They are critical skills for how we give evidence to our client that we *are* listening and truly *hearing* them. They are skills that further the coaching conversation. They are how we respond to our client when we take in their communication. This is the *active* part of listening: what the coach says and does.

Let's take a deeper dive into each of the active listening skills.

Active Listening Skills

Restatement—saying back to the client what they have just said in essentially the same words.

Paraphrasing or Reflection—saying back to the client the *essence* of what they have just said, usually in a more condensed way.

Reflection of Feeling—mirroring back to the client more of the feeling that is present and being experienced, rather than the content; getting at the meaning behind the words.

Use of Silence—strategically waiting a moment or two before responding, allowing the client to elaborate in the direction they choose; allowing the story to unfold.

Requesting Clarification—asking for elaboration; allowing the client to continue and deepen their exploration. *Tell me more about…*

Acknowledging—sharing with the client the value of who they are and the validity of their experience, as well as what they did.

Relying on Intuition—using your *gut feeling* and sharing it, offered tentatively.

Summarization—reviewing in a concise way what has been expressed and experienced in the coaching so far, or at the conclusion of the session.

Restatement—Simple Enough

Coaches seldom say back to their client exactly what they have just said. The power here is not what is said, but how it is said. At a tender moment in the coaching conversation a client might say, "I'm so worried about this." The coach may respond by simply saying, "So worried." The coach's tone of voice may convey the compassion the client needs. It may convey that the coach is right there with them, listening deeply. Restatement may be used rarely, but don't pass up its potential strategic effectiveness.

Paraphrasing/Reflection—More Powerful Than You Might Think

In the taxonomy of coaching skills, some approaches speak of paraphrasing as *reflection*. We are reflecting back to the client the *essence* of what they have just said. Paraphrasing does more work than is first apparent.

Paraphrasing has the function of condensing down what is being said in the coaching conversation. Think of it as a distillation. A more masterful coach is able to grasp the essence of what their client is saying quickly and keep the client moving ahead efficiently and productively. We often hear the client responding by saying, "Yes! Exactly! That's what I'm trying to say." The client feels heard, understood and trust grows.

Paraphrasing functions surprisingly well to keep the client on track, focused, and moving forward in their exploration. Observe a coach who utilizes paraphrasing rarely and you will often see a client ramble. Without the benefit of paraphrasing the client keeps elaborating and going off on a tangent rather than sharpening their focus. A strong line of inquiry fails to develop and less is accomplished in the session. Had the coach been hearing what the client was actually saying, reflecting back to them in condensed and essential form, they would have been able to focus in on what the client really wanted and needed to explore and express.

Paraphrasing can also convey to the client that this is a two-way conversation. When a coach remains silent for too long it communicates to the client that the way coaching works is *you talk and I (the coach) listen.* When you, the coach, interject with paraphrasing it communicates that you are an active participant in a coaching conversation! Doing so will allow the coach to assert themselves into the role of a real ally who has input in the process. It will prevent the client from engaging in long reports about what happened and instead engage in more thoughtful exploration.

Examples of Paraphrasing

Client: *My last bloodwork labs caused my doctor to put me on all these new medications. I'm already taking too many meds!*

Coach: *So now you're challenged by even more meds to take.*

Client: *Yeah! Some are twice a day with food, others are once a day with or without food. I can't keep track of all of this!*

Coach: *You don't think you can keep up with all these new and different instructions.*

Client: *My sleep pattern is really poor. I'm only getting six hours at the most, sometimes only four or five a night. And I'm coming to work tired at the beginning of the day.*

Coach: *So you're very concerned about the amount of sleep you're getting and the effect it's having on you.*

Client: *I sure am. I'm just not as sharp on the job. I miss putting appointments on my calendar and then blow a potential contract.*

Coach: *You're seeing some tough consequences.*

As you can see in these examples, paraphrasing, like all active listening skills, is best used in combination with other skills. In these examples a coach would want to pursue the feeling that is accompanying these statements by the client and do so by using our next active listening skill—reflection of feeling.

Reflection of Feeling—Taking It to the Next Level

Progressing on your journey to coaching mastery requires developing ease with the use of reflection of feeling. Often when the feeling level of interaction is not accepted, acknowledged, and explored, all of the goal setting and action steps seem never to get traction. Helping clients explore their feelings and work with them is often referred to as *process coaching*.

> **Process coaching** focuses on the internal experience, on what is happening in the moment. The goal of process coaching is to enhance the ability of clients to be aware of the moment and to name it…Sometimes the most important change happens at the internal level and may even be necessary before external change can take place (Kinsey-House, 2011).

My observation is that this critical skill is one coaches may underutilize the most. (That is, unless they have a counseling background where they may even over-utilize it!)

What coaches are overlooking by not using reflection of feeling is the power of simply feeding back to the client their estimation of what feeling is present in what the client is saying and experiencing. The place to start is by naming it. Do your best to identify what the feeling is: worry, fear, concern, overwhelm (yes, that's a feeling), delight, joy, anxiousness, hopefulness, etc. Then, without interpretation simply offer it to the client for them to validate, refute, or clarify. "Well, I'm not really angry. More like resentful."

Your job, once again, is to facilitate your client's work. By bringing their awareness to the feeling being expressed it allows them to bring attention to it, make greater contact with it, and then do their own work.

There are times our clients are reaching out to us with their expression of emotion. They are essentially saying, "I feel this way, please understand!" Staying focused on the content we can miss what is actually being communicated.

We can use phrases like *"Sounds like..."; "You seem to be..."; "What I hear is..."* to reflect feeling back to our clients. We can also put it in question form, checking out if our attempt at identifying their feeling is accurate. *"Are you feeling frightened right now?"* We can also simply use an awareness technique to bring their attention to an expression of a feeling without identifying it ourselves. *"Are you aware of the shift in your tone of voice as you say that?" "Are you aware of your clenched fists?" "Are you aware of how tight your voice became talking about that?"*

> ### Masterful Moment
> Periodically examine recordings of your own coaching. If you notice that you are seldom using reflection of feeling do some self-vigilant inquiry with yourself. Are you steering away from feelings that you find uncomfortable? Are you feeling less confident working with the emotional side of coaching?

Use of Silence: When Less Is More

The standard joke here is "Don't use this skill too much!" Yet, strategic use of silence can deepen the coaching process. Coaches often feel uncomfortable with silence, sometimes thinking that it reflects poorly upon them. They can feel responsible for keeping the coaching conversation moving. When we consciously choose to remain quiet and still, we are creating space for our client to do more of their work. We are keeping them in the lead and giving them time to think, feel, and react.

When a client makes a particularly powerful statement, "I'm so stressed out by this job! My supervisor is constantly pushing me." it is the perfect time to literally or figuratively bite your tongue and see what happens next. The silence allows the client to remain in touch with their own thoughts and feelings and gives them the opportunity to continue with the expression that is needed, or to collect their thoughts. At times like this I have been surprised by the direction the client takes. When I hear a statement like the one above, I could easily think, "The client is going to talk about their conflict with their supervisor now." I would then be shocked to hear them continue with something like: "Yeah, my spouse is fed up with me working at this company. They're giving me a really hard time about finding something else for work." Now, the conversation is really about the relationship with their spouse. We would never have known that if we had pursued our own line of thought and asked about the work supervisor.

We as coaches want to develop a patient balance between active engagement and calm silence. Even a coach with a high-energy personality, if more accomplished in their skills, will consciously choose when to be quiet and to be even more effective. There are truly times when less is more.

To realize when the use of silence might be effective the coach has to be centered themselves. If you find it difficult to utilize silence in your coaching, you can ask yourself, "What's going on for me right now that is causing me to push the pace of this conversation? What do I have to do to be more grounded and centered in my coaching?"

Requesting Clarification

The more masterful coach realizes that coaching is most productive when the client is actively exploring, learning, and gaining insight about themselves. To encourage that exploration we often request clarification from the client about what they are saying. "Tell me more about…" type phrases can help the client to elaborate and gain greater clarity. The coach may gain greater clarity as well but what we really want is for the client to explore further. Clients often fall into the practice of coming to coaching and merely reporting about what they have done to work on improving their lifestyle. That is acceptable, but when they actually use their experience as a jumping off place for exploration, more learning takes place.

Another use of the skill of requesting clarification is to further the development of *intrinsic motivation*. When a client reports in on an accomplished action step that they had committed to ("I walked four times last week."), the coach can take advantage of the opportunity to enhance intrinsic motivation. "So, tell me about one of those walks that you particularly enjoyed."

Request for clarification is also much more neutral than a question. Your client has to answer your question in the direction the question points. Request for clarification allows them to answer any way they want. Coaches sometimes ask many questions in a row, to the exclusion of all of the other active listening skills. Substituting request for clarification can break that cycle and enrich the coaching conversation.

Acknowledging—Positivity in Action

Effective coaches seize the opportunity to acknowledge every bit of success their clients achieve. The acknowledgment has to be genuine and heartfelt. Nothing goes over worse than insincere, phony cheerleading. There are so many things that a more masterful coach can pick up on and acknowledge.

Acknowledge:

- What your client did. The action taken, the behavior they performed.

- What aspect of your client's character showed up (was exhibited) that allowed them to perform the action.

- What your client knows. Their knowledge about how to live a healthy lifestyle, how much they know about their health challenge, what they know about successful behavior change or positive thinking.

- What your client has already done to improve their lifestyle. What they have done before they began coaching.

- What your client has done successfully in the past. Their previous successes (if temporary) on lifestyle improvement.

- The resources and assets they have that will help make change easier.

- Values, beliefs, and attitudes that are strengths that will aid them in being successful at lifestyle improvement.

- Every bit of success!

Our clients often fail to recognize what they have accomplished, what they already know, or what strengths they have. Their past failed experiences make them vulnerable to self-criticism and often blind them to what they are doing well. Faced with the perceived enormity of their challenges they often don't give themselves credit for their progress, only for the final achievement of their goal.

When hampered by low self-efficacy, demoralization, and discouragement, our clients often cannot see the accomplishments they are making in their progress towards their goals. It is our job as coaches to see these accomplishments and qualities, and acknowledge them. When we do, we help our clients to notice their progress and accept it more. It builds motivation and encouragement.

When I have observed coaches who are good at effective and frequent acknowledgment, I see sessions that move along with a steady and productive pace driven by positive emotion. Their clients are responding positively, and it seems to stimulate them to realize more about what they are doing and how they are doing it. The pace often picks up, gaining momentum, and the coach is then simply *tapping the top of the tire*. Have you ever watched a child playing with an old auto or truck tire? Or, perhaps can you remember doing so yourself as a kid? The hard part is lifting the tire and pushing it to get started. Then as the tire starts to roll, all the child has to do is gleefully run alongside and tap the top of the tire to keep the momentum going.

Encouraging Self-Acknowledgment—Coaching Experiment

To encourage your client to increase their ability to notice what they are doing that deserves acknowledgment, suggest to them this experiment.

- Each day for at least a week or two, write down three things to acknowledge themselves for. A key is to write it down, not just think about it.

- It can be something that they actually did and accomplished: "I acknowledge myself for getting eight hours of sleep last night." "I acknowledge myself for keeping track of my calories on my phone app today."

- Or, it can be acknowledging themselves for some aspect of their character that showed up that allowed them to accomplish something, feel good about themselves, or act in accordance with their values. "I acknowledge myself for having the courage to ask my boss for some flex time so I can pick my child up after school." "I acknowledge myself for caring enough to take the time to work on the environmental petition that is important to me and our community." "I acknowledge myself for caring enough about myself to make an appointment with my dermatologist."

Relying on Intuition—That Gut Feeling

Our intuition can serve us well. So, what is that *gut feeling* that we get at times that guides us to make a leap in the conversation? An intuitive feeling seems to arise spontaneously. It is more of an awareness that comes to us in ways we don't completely understand but can be surprising in its wisdom. We certainly can't bring it forth on demand.

We may be coaching a person who is exploring a particular topic when we have a realization that what the person is really talking about, or is trying to get to, is something that hasn't been spoken about yet. When we tentatively offer our *hunch* to them, for them to accept or reject, we are often surprised at how frequently we are on target. Our client may be talking about their stressful situation at work. They may be going into detail about the demanding nature of their work both mentally and physically. As the client speaks, we get that internal awareness that brings forth our idea that perhaps they are concerned about how their health challenges might limit them as they get older, increasingly interfering with their ability to do their work. When we share our gut feeling with them, they light up and vigorously validate what we have offered. Now we are coaching around what they are deeply concerned about, not just the daily tasks at work.

It's important to differentiate the emergence of intuition from a conclusion we might reach from an analytic process. We are not using deductive reasoning, analyzing the client's story, and seeing connections or drawing conclusions. Sharp minds will do this anyway at lightning speed. The question is what do we do with it? We might store our information for later, or we might consciously choose to be a bit directive and offer the client the consideration of our hypothesis, but don't mistake this for intuition.

So how does intuition arise? There may be many theories about it, but my notion is that what we experience as intuition is the collective awareness that has resulted from a combination of:

- The context of our coaching with the person.
- The history of what we have already talked about.
- The input from all of our senses (visual, auditory, etc.) based upon our observation of the client.
- The client's affect, their behavior, and our body wisdom (our internal bodily reactions to what is going on in the coaching).
- A little extrasensory perception may be at play here too.

I contend that the synthesis of all of this information somehow shows up as an awareness within us that leads us to draw a conclusive hypothesis about what is going on for our client at a deeper level.

However it comes to us, the key question is how do we make use of it? Our intuitive hunch must be humbly offered to our client with the utmost tentativeness. "So, let me know if I'm on target here..." "Tell me if I'm off base here, but I get the feeling that..." This allows the client to accept, reject, or take our offering and clarify it further. "Well, that's kind of it, but it's really more like this..."

The danger in offering our gut feeling is that it may instead be our own projection. We are continually trying to understand others by imagining what we would think, feel, or do in the same circumstances. What we do with what our client is saying may not at all be where our client is headed. Our own needs, wants, prejudices, or perceptions may be getting in the way. In light of this, we offer our intuition very humbly.

The upside is that when it clicks, the coaching conversation leaps ahead into productive territory at once. Trust your gut.

Summarization—More Than Just a Recap

Coaches are often taught the value of providing the client with a concise summary of the session as time is winding down. This summary helps refresh the learning that has taken place and can clarify what agreements were made for the next steps. Some coaches approach this from a client-centered style where they quiz the client about what they have learned; sometimes asking what the *take-aways* were for the client. At times the process of summarizing the session yields new insights as the coach and client consider the session as a whole. This can lead to even more fruitful discussions.

The other use of summarization can be as a periodic refresher throughout the session. Shorter, even more concise summaries can help the client to stay focused while staying in touch with the larger theme they are exploring. Think of such summaries as *paraphrasing on steroids*. Often the summary sets up the perfect opportunity for a great question. It brings the coaching conversation to, "What's next?"; "Where do we go from here?"

Summarization may allow for a shift in question form more like:

- Okay. So, what would be an entirely different way of looking at this same situation?

- What different perspective can you take on this?

- Alright, so what would be the view your partner would have about this?

Such *perspective coaching* can be very valuable.

Think of summarization as a technique to provide you, the coach, with an opportunity to increase your involvement in the coaching conversation. You can use the break to:

- Share an observation.

- Ask a powerful question.

- Ask permission to explore more deeply into a sensitive area.

- Check in with the client and ask if this line of inquiry is being productive for them.

- Interrupt a client's long monologue and return it to a dialogue with you (a very useful technique that we will expound upon later in this chapter).

Types and Depth of Reflections—Motivational Interviewing

- The motivational interviewing approach to behavior change has developed an entirely different way of approaching active listening skills. They take the term reflection and break it down to cover a number of active listening skills. What might be called paraphrasing and restatment, reflection of feeling, use of intuition, and summarization are all referred to as reflection. Reflections are then categorized in terms of their depth and more specific purposes, varying from simple to complex.

- Simple reflection—repeat—this is simply repeating back to the person, or slightly rephrasing what they have said. We might also include the simplest form as a Restatement.
  Client: *I need to know more about how to eat better.*
  Coach: *You need to know more about how to eat better.*

- Simple reflection—rephrase—(paraphrasing) saying back to the client the essence of what they have just said slightly altered.
  Client: *I really want to improve the way I eat.*
  Coach: *A better way to eat is really important to you.*

- Complex reflections add meaning and emphasis to what our client has said. MI practitioners sometimes "Make a guess about the unspoken content or what might come next" (Miller, 2013). We will explore, in depth, more MI Reflection categories in Chapter Nine.

The Power of Active Listening

The coaching demonstrations, and the coaching sessions I've reviewed that have impressed me the most with their true and effortless power, have been the ones where there was a *balance* between active listening skills and the effective use of questions and more directive techniques. There is great wisdom in the client-centered approach that coaching was founded upon. If we coach as though we truly embrace the Coaching Cornerstone *"People are naturally creative, resourceful and whole"* (Kimsey-House, 2018) then we will be fine with keeping them in the lead. Think of the Active Listening Skills, along with questions, as an artist's pallet. Paint with lots of different colors!

> ### Masterful Moment
>
> The more accomplished coach is like a musician who can reach all of the notes at their disposal. Are you allowing yourself to make use of the full range of active listening skills? Are you finding yourself playing the same notes over and over again? Examine your coaching and see what *sounds* are missing. Are you seldom using Reflection of Feeling, or Acknowledgment? It is important to get a true reading on your facility with active listening skills.

The Fine Art of Coaching Questions

Everything we know has its origins in questions.
Questions, we might say, are the principal intellectual
instruments available to human beings.

— Neil Postman

Observe a masterful coach and you will see and hear questions that sound like they come from a true ally. Strategically placed in the conversation, they seem to bridge thoughts together and build a line of inquiry that yields a positive result. Such a coach laces together these questions with a balance of Active Listening Skills and empathic understanding. The client experiences these questions as gifts that open doors to new perspectives, connect with new awareness and insight.

When the coach first meets their client, they are building the coaching alliance as they are hearing the client's story and becoming informed about many aspects of the client's life. Clarifying questions help the coach understand more about their client than just the information filled out in a welcome packet. At this point, many of the questions, we might say, are for the coach. My client may share with me details about their family, their health challenges and such, yielding no great insight for them, but providing me with much greater understanding of their life. If I operate from a consultant mindset (treatment, education, etc.), I may continue to ask more and more questions for me so that I can function as a good consultant—analyze the situation, determine and convey recommendations. If I have made the shift to the coaching mindset, my questioning becomes far different. Now I am using questions to help my client to explore and assess themselves. Now I am composing questions for them to ask themselves. I think of my challenge as "What is a great question that I could offer to my client right now that would help them gain greater insight, understanding, etc.?"

When the coach becomes a question composer, their style of coaching shifts entirely. They have moved beyond information gathering and instead are functioning as a coaching ally, helping their client to do the work. We might say that this is ultimately a client-centered way of questioning. Coaches do provide information from time to time, but here we are equipping the client with ways to inquire of themselves. Through effective questioning, we seek to help our clients to:

- Increase awareness.
- Explore more deeply.
- Connect with emotion.
- See patterns and connections.
- Generate possibilities.
- Consider new possibilities.
- Gain insight.
- Become infected with curiosity.
- Provoke new thinking.
- Encourage self-reflection.
- Clarify values.
- Connect with deeper meaning.
- Discover and challenge assumptions.
- Generate energy and forward momentum.

A Taxonomy of Coaching Questions

Several years ago, I rediscovered the pyramid model of Bloom's Taxonomy, and immediately realized its potential for teaching coaching students about the various forms of and uses for questions. As I shared this in coach training classes, students found themselves surprised by and fascinated with its usefulness.

"Bloom's Taxonomy was created by Benjamin Bloom in 1956, published as a kind of classification of learning outcomes and objectives that have, in the more than half-century since, been used for everything from framing digital tasks and evaluating apps to writing questions and assessments" (Heick, 2018).

What I found was that in the midst of this classification system is a process that we follow whenever we explore and take our thinking to higher and higher levels. In fact, it is very similar to the process that we use in coaching. While I would not advocate coaching in some kind of strictly sequential manner using this model, it can expand the thinking of the coach and help them see the myriad uses questions can serve.

The pyramid model works well because the lower levels are foundational, with higher levels building upon them.

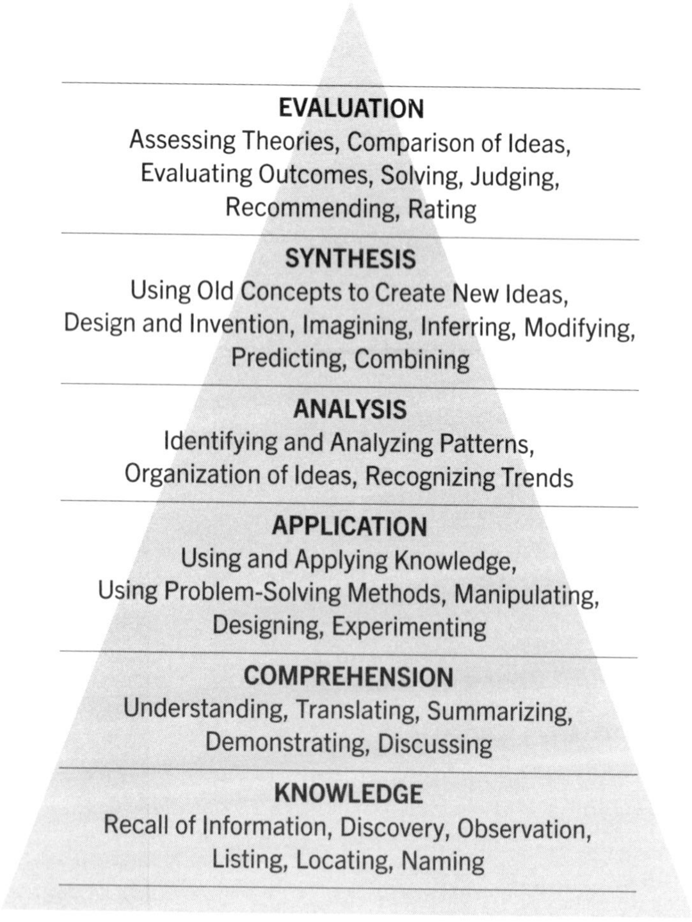

EVALUATION
Assessing Theories, Comparison of Ideas,
Evaluating Outcomes, Solving, Judging,
Recommending, Rating

SYNTHESIS
Using Old Concepts to Create New Ideas,
Design and Invention, Imagining, Inferring, Modifying,
Predicting, Combining

ANALYSIS
Identifying and Analyzing Patterns,
Organization of Ideas, Recognizing Trends

APPLICATION
Using and Applying Knowledge,
Using Problem-Solving Methods, Manipulating,
Designing, Experimenting

COMPREHENSION
Understanding, Translating, Summarizing,
Demonstrating, Discussing

KNOWLEDGE
Recall of Information, Discovery, Observation,
Listing, Locating, Naming

FIGURE 15—BLOOM'S TAXONOMY, Benjamin Bloom

We begin with the knowledge level:

- What does your client know about their health and well-being?
- How aware are they of health challenges, medical conditions, treatments, medications, resources, sources of support?
- Questions here expand client awareness of how their behavior, attitudes, and beliefs are affecting their wellness.
- This level can involve tracking behavior and developing realizations about current functioning.
- This level is about noticing, mindfulness, gathering information.

Next is the comprehension level:

- How much does our client understand about their current health and well-being?
- Questions here are helping the client to process what they noticed at the earlier level.
- Questions get at the essential meaning and implications of the client's lifestyle.
- Questions help the client to organize, compare, contrast, and interpret what they are realizing about themselves.

Now we take what we have learned and put it into application.

- At this level we are using our accumulated knowledge and awareness to develop experiments—action steps.
- Questions here help the client to design action steps that are in alignment with their values, interests, motivation, and level of readiness for change on that particular behavior.
- These questions go into strategic thinking, helping our client to create experiments that take into account barriers.
- Questions at this level explore sources of support for the changes the client is contemplating.

Next, we examine our application work by using analysis.

- Here we use questions to identify and analyze the patterns that emerge as our lifestyle experiments are conducted.
- What are we noticing about the application of lifestyle improvement efforts?
- What kinds of trends are we seeing?
- How consistent or inconsistent are our client's wellness efforts?
- What is supporting change, and what is challenging it?

We then take what we have learned from our analysis and bring all of our information and realizations together in a process of synthesis, which is also referred to as creation in newer models.

- Now questions help the client to explore possibilities, consider alternative solutions, and compose new strategies.
- Questions help the client to compile their information, combine ideas, imagine what could be, see new perspectives now that we have come this far.
- We get into predicting, estimating, theorizing about where we can go from here.

Finally, we examine what our efforts have produced and engage in evaluation.

- Did we get, or are we getting, the outcomes we wanted to see?
- Here our questions examine and assess actions and strategies, and judge their effectiveness.
- We honestly rate the efforts made and explore what worked well, and what still needs to be improved.
- Questions here might challenge a client's own assessment of their success if it appears that they are being too hard on themselves.

While I doubt that I have ever or would ever coach with some image of Bloom's Taxonomy floating in my mind, knowing more about it seems to stretch our own knowledge about the wide range of questions the coach has available. Again, knowing theory allows us to think on our feet.

A Balance of Questions and Active Listening Skills

It is not uncommon for beginning coaches to rely heavily on questions. Sometimes when a line of inquiry becomes productive, it is like the coach becomes like a hunting dog on a fresh scent and pursues it with more and more questions. This is especially true when the coach is operating from a "What's wrong and how can we fix it?" mindset. Problem solving becomes paramount and everything else about coaching is swept aside as answers are hotly pursued. The coach seems to forget about providing empathy, building the coaching alliance, or using any of their active listening skills. Opportunities for acknowledgment are missed. Feelings go un-reflected. The coach is actually operating under a great deal of pressure as they feel completely responsible for maintaining the momentum of the conversation by coming up with yet another powerful question.

Active listening skills, as we've already seen, provide many benefits to our coaching. When we fail to use them in adequate balance with effective questions, we miss out on much of the power of coaching. A good balance of active listening skills and effective questions:

- Helps clients feel heard and understood.
- Helps clients to stay focused and on track.
- Reduces rambling and going off subject.
- Reduces defensiveness caused by the prosecutorial effect that too many questions can have.
- Keeps responsibility for the coaching conversation back on the client.
- Allows the coach to seize the opportunities for empathic understanding and acknowledgment that arise.
- Stimulates thinking and participation in the coaching process as the client understands they are not just in the role of answering questions.
- Keeps more of a two-way complete coaching conversation going.

> *Call them forward to learn, improve and grow,*
> *rather than to just get something sorted out.*

—Michael Bungay Stanier

Some Favorite Questions with Commentary

How will you know when you're being successful?

As clients are co-creating action steps with their coach, the question immediately arises: how to track these steps towards lifestyle improvement. At times clients resist the laborious-sounding task of tracking (writing things down, logging them on an app). This straight-forward question always seems to help them realize that, yes, tracking in some form will be needed to get the job done.

What are three things you could do here?

Your client is struggling to figure out the single, right thing to do to make progress, overcome a barrier, etc. They are stumped. When we relieve the pressure by having them consider three options the fear of selecting the wrong answer seems to evaporate. Knowing that they will not have to commit to doing the one thing they come up with, three new ideas emerge with greater ease.

How will you know that you know enough?

A terrific question for the forever-preparing client! I have had clients who get stuck at the preparation level of change. They keep on doing their research, identifying options, finding out more and more, but never pulling the trigger. This question jolts people into considering how they are holding themselves back and often leads to our next favorite question.

What are you afraid would happen if you did that?

When clients tread water, when they hesitate on pursuing a course of action, it is often more about fear of the consequences that might come as a result. Exploring fears is vital to helping our clients evaluate what to do next. Are they operating on the cliché that FEAR = False Evidence Appearing Real? Or, are they being realistically and legitimately cautious? Will there be serious push-back from others? Will they endure criticism or ridicule? Are they once again afraid that failure will result? Asking this question can open up an essential dialogue.

When have you been successful doing this before?

Most of our clients have had at least some success at lifestyle improvement in their past attempts. They were often doing all of the right things to lose weight, stop smoking, etc., but the success did not last. There can be many reasons why they may have failed, but using this question here can yield two things: 1. It builds the client's self-efficacy to recall past successes; 2. What worked before may work even better today with the support of coaching.

Questions—The Dark Side

For all the supreme utility of effective use of questions in coaching, there are definitely some ways of asking questions that can work against the coaching process. Most of these coaching errors are outside of the coach's awareness, or may even be done out of good intentions, but the result is a lack of progress at best.

Coaches may use leading questions to nudge a client toward a certain conclusion. Wellness coaches often have their own favorite ways to be well and sometimes, without even realizing it, use leading questions to help their client see the benefits of yoga or kale smoothies. We may push certain methods or even products because we really believe they will be helpful. Using questions in this way may be considered a type of covert suggestion. The self-vigilant coach has to guard against this. By analyzing our coaching recordings, we can spot the use of leading questions and change it. This makes us more transparent in our coaching. If a suggestion seems valuable, a coach may ask permission and offer their suggestion for the client to directly accept, reject, or consider.

Questions also start working against the coaching process when the coach has slipped away from a coaching mindset. If we revert back to our consultative, treatment-oriented, or educational mindset it will quickly show up in our use of questions. The questions head in the direction of determining diagnosis, prescribing the way forward, or helping the coach determine a solution rather than co-creating one with our client.

Effective coaches have been taught to ask permission to pursue a line of inquiry into sensitive areas. I love to ask, "Would it be of value to you to…?" I always ask this when the topic of intimate relationships, finances, or personal mental health history of any kind comes up in the coaching conversation. Clients feel honored and respected that we ask. It builds the coaching alliance. The key is to truly convey that they have complete freedom to set a boundary and say no.

The Miracle of Miracle Questions

The ultimately stuck client sometimes seems to need a miracle. They appear faced with an unsolvable problem, a barrier so great that they just can't think of any way over, under, around, or through it. The client who cannot think of a way to fit exercise at all into their life, or the one who feels held back from living the life they really want to live. Such clients are often saying to themselves, "If it wasn't for this great barrier, then I'd be able to be healthy and well." Or, more specifically they might be saying, "If it wasn't for this overdemanding job, being married to this person, having this chronic illness,"… and more.

Steve de Shazer's work in *Solution Focused Therapy* is one of the most brilliant contributions of coaching. He states that the way through a barrier is to describe the outcome the client wants to see. In other words, describe the client's goals. This is what de Shazer called "the miracle question."

The Miracle Question

What if overnight a miracle happened, and your problem was solved? You were asleep. It doesn't matter how it was solved. It was a miracle. Once you wake up in the morning, a) how will you go about discovering that this miracle has happened to you? or, b) how will your best friend know that this miracle happened to you (Gaiswinkler, 2000)?

The coaching conversation that results from questions like these is the real key. The skillful coach will help the client to explore what this brings up for them. What emerges with the barrier eliminated (at least imagining that it is so) brings the client to the other side of the wall, into the future instead of their stuck present experience. Listen, inquire slowly, helping the client to see themselves in this new situation. Some coaches like to use this as a closed-eyes fantasy exercise. Perhaps you will ask your client to take you through a day in the life of themselves in this new situation.

The short-hand version of the miracle question is the "What would it look like?" question. While the full-on miracle question is rarely used in coaching, the "What would it look like?" question is a strategic coaching question that can serve two different purposes:

The coach may be helping the client explore a way forward towards their goals. The "What would it look like?" question can help the client to envision the outcome they want to see and perhaps, with more clarity, now be able to consider more ways to achieve it. Visualizing it makes the goal more real and possible, thus opening up creative thinking.

The other major use of the "What would it look like?" question is with a client experiencing or imagining a dilemma or barrier that is keeping them stuck. This is the client who hasn't been able, despite great effort thinking about it, to find time to eat well, exercise regularly, recreate in a rewarding way, etc. "So, what would it look like if you really could eat healthfully the way that you truly want to?" "What would your ideal exercise pattern look like?" Again, by describing the outcome we want to see and attaining real clarity, we often find that small, step-by-step solutions start to emerge in our thinking. The client response is most often, "Well, I could at least do that right away."

At the end of the day, the questions we ask of ourselves determine the type of people that we will become.

— Leo Babauta

Masterful Moment

As you did with active listening skills, examine your use of questions. Are you using your questioning as a way to facilitate your client's exploration and discovery? Or, are you demonstrating your expertise, your knowledge in a more consultative way of questioning? Do you find yourself trying to think of a really powerful question to ask your client next? That may indicate that you are either still operating from the expert-consultant mindset, or you are not shifting enough between active listening skills and effective use of questions. Trust the coaching process.

Communicating Effectively at a Masterful Level

Effective active listening skills and powerful questions are foundational components of masterful coaching communication. Communication is more than skills and questions, however. When coaches reach a level of some mastery of their craft the communication takes on qualities that go even further. Masterful coaching communication is authentic, direct, honest, and yet kind. It's fun, at times, entertaining, yet very much down to business. The communication is something shared between coach and client with a high level of equality and respect. The coach is encouraging the client to do as they do; to challenge, to question, to explore, to look at the big picture, and at the practicality of small details. There is a mild level of self-vigilance on the part of the coach, always questioning if they are keeping themselves out of the way, always keeping the agenda as the client's. The coach can share observations, their intuitive hits, and provide feedback to their client without being attached to the outcome. The coach has a rationale for what they share, a methodology for how to proceed, and a sensitivity for how everything lands, or is taken in, by the client. Their communication reflects the work of two allies on a shared journey of discovery.

The Sound of Effective Coaching Communication

Masterful coaches notice and make use of the language of their clients. They pick up on key words and phrases and adopt them into the conversation. Taking your coaching to a higher level means paying attention to and learning about our use of language. The linguistics of coaching are valuable to understand and then use to improve our craft.

Refining Coaching Linguistics: Verbal Tics, Placeholders, and Fingerprint Words

Verbal placeholders are empty expressions that we use, often habitually with little awareness. Our client, for example, might use their own placeholders, saying "you know," "I'm just saying," drawing out words like "welllllll…," and speaking in ways that keep the talking stick in their own hand.

I was first shocked into awareness of my favorite placeholder when, as a late teenager, a very astute young woman on a phone call with me said, "Oh my God! You just said 17 'you knows'"! It was an embarrassing encounter with a verbal habit I hadn't even been aware of. As I studied psychology and counseling, tape recordings and videotapes revealed other linguistic repetitions of mine so I could work on jettisoning my reflexive verbal placeholders from my work.

Listen to your recordings to catch your own *verbal tics*. Saying okay, or some equivalent, quickly after one's client speaks is often a way to let the client know that we are tracking with them. When psychologist Allen Ivey taught *Micro-Counseling* skills, he referred to such words, as well as head nods and mmhh-hmms, as "minimal encourages." Such responses by the counselor or coach encourage the client to go on.

The downside of your minimal encourages, especially when it is reflexive, is that it is a very quick signal to the client to keep on talking. The result with the overly talkative client is like a quick squirt of gasoline on an already hot fire. The client continues to hold the floor, often rambles, and the coach has an extremely hard time saying anything. The conversation is no longer a conversation, but a monologue. Respectful interruption is needed, but even that may be hard to do after we have already primed the client to keep talking with our okays.

Listening to your recordings also helps you discover your own *fingerprint* words. A coach may discover that they have pet words that they use over and over again. Again, we do this without even being aware of it. The fingerprints may have a healthcare flavor or may be the trending words of current business-speak. Leveraging, optimize, or cognizant and the like are words that, when used habitually, not only become like identifying fingerprints, they sometimes are unintended turn-offs to our clients.

A very powerful coaching technique is to identify fingerprint words. When we see them used in a context that reflects emotional and/or strategic importance to our client, we feed this back to them to consider. *"Are you aware that each time you speak about taking time for self-care in any way you use the word indulgent?"*

When coaching we will run into someone whose speech is different than ours due to cultural or family differences. Sociolinguistics professor Diana Boxer says that in such situations we usually respond in one of two ways. "We either start to mimic them in some way or distinguish ourselves from their usage" (Boxer, 2014). We need to ask ourselves how natural it feels to speak in ways that are more similar to our client. In coaching we want to always convey that our relationship is one of allies. Clients realize that there may be differences in speech and expression and don't expect or even want us to alter who we are in order to communicate with them. Doing so can be perceived as patronizing or condescending. The client will feel more respect from the coach if the coach remains true to their way of speaking.

Reframing and Perspective

We sometimes say, "Things are not always as they appear." A coach might add, "And, they don't always have to be." We all explore our worlds looking through the lenses that shape our perspective and lead to our conclusions. These lenses are the result of past learning and current circumstances and awareness. Sometimes a new way of looking at things opens up new possibilities. Coaching can help people either polish up those lenses or try on new ones by using the technique of reframing.

Reframing is a way to help someone consider a new perspective on an event that has taken place or is about to, a circumstance of their life, a relationship they are involved in, and more. What would be a new way for your client to look at the same situation? How could shifting perspective change their course of action? An effective reframe can empower a previously stuck and helpless-feeling client to engage in change.

Reframing can help clients to:

- See a personal quality previously seen as a liability as an asset.

- See what they believed was a personal weakness as a strength.

- See a potential problem as an opportunity.

- See the upside of a situation and how they can benefit from it.

In today's world of political spin doctors, we can cynically view reframing as manipulation. Reframing is not about tricking people, convincing, or persuading. It is about offering the consideration of a different perspective.

Probably the best reframes are ones that are client-generated. Instead of feeling as though you, the coach, are responsible for coming to your client's rescue, invite your client to come up with a new lens to try out. The key word here is invite. You cannot force a new perspective on someone not ready to try it out. Your client may be entrenched in their thinking or may even be getting what therapists call secondary gain by holding fast to the current perspective. Secondary gain is when a person somehow benefits from continuing to behave as they do even when it may appear self-defeating. For example, you may come across a client reluctant to practice their physical therapy exercises because they are receiving comforting pity from family members for their painful condition. They may not even be conscious of the reason behind their reluctance to adhere to their treatment program. If you are hit with such resistance, back off without attachment.

Clients, however, are often keen to discover a new way of looking at things. You can help them bring forth a more positive reframe by using invitations such as, *"What would be at least two other ways of looking at this?" "If this went well, what would be an upside to this?" "Tell me what the part of you that really cares about you would say here." "And the upside could be...?"*

Coaches can also provide reframes for their clients to consider. This is where already operating on a positive psychology basis helps. You may have already noted strengths, skills, and capabilities in your client from the coaching up to this point. You can draw upon that and what you have learned about your client's situation, values, beliefs, and attitudes to compose a reframe. You also have the immediate ability to look at your client's situation from a different perspective — yours! This does not mean for you to tell your client the way you would look at it, or how you would handle a situation. Your solution, or perspective, might not work for your client. However, you may be able to see a possible reframe that your client is not able to at this moment.

First empathize, acknowledge the client's perception of their situation and validate their feelings about it. Don't make your client wrong to be feeling the way they feel. Then offer a reframe for them to consider.

> **Client:** *My children are involved in so many baseball and soccer teams that I end up attending all of these games and practices and I can never get in any time for walking.*

Coach: *So, you're telling me that you attend events where you are outdoors with hours of free time.*
Client: *Well, yeah. I'm kind of stuck there with nothing to do. I mean, I love watching them play, but it takes up hours!*
Coach: *Think about this for a moment. You are outdoors with hours of free time. Instead of sitting at these events, what else could you do?*
Client: *Wow! I could walk around the entire field while they play!*

Coaching from a positive psychology approach does not mean we are shoving a pair of rose-colored glasses at our client and minimizing some of life's harsher realities. It hardly works to ask a client *"So! What's the upside of being poor?"* Not everything can be smoothed over by a positive reframe. In Barbara Frederickson's book *Positivity* (Frederickson, 2009), she makes this point with a humorous tale of a woman waking up in the morning and her partner in bed, who is still asleep, rolls over, and unknowingly smacks her on the nose with their arm. The woman quickly reframes this by saying to herself, "Oh, well. At least I have someone to wake up in bed with." She then jumps into the shower and waits for the water to warm up. It never does. Dripping with cold water she dries herself with a towel saying, "Oh, well. At least I live in a place where I do have running water." Reframing is not rationalizing or fooling yourself. It is taking on a new perspective.

Weaknesses as Strengths

Clients are often quite self-critical. They are frustrated by what they perceive as their weaknesses and see them as liabilities, more barriers holding them back from success at improving their lives. Often these same weaknesses in other situations can be strengths. The person who is easily hurt by harsh comments from others criticizes themselves for being too sensitive. In another situation that same sensitivity might be a real asset, allowing them to notice the pain others are experiencing and come to someone's aid. Someone who can at times be so stubborn that they miss opportunities that a more flexible person would benefit from can also be helped to see how in another situation that same stubbornness shows up as having the strength to stand by their convictions and values in trying circumstances.

Coaching Reframing Exercise
Weakness Becomes a Useful Strength

- Invite your client to list three weaknesses that they possess and dislike the most.

- Coach and client have a coaching conversation to discover at least two situations where each weakness could be useful. (If the client gets stuck and can't think of any situations, urge them to think in extremes, even to the point of absurdity.)

- Coach and client process how this could be applied in the client's life.

Shifting Perspective

In order to succeed at implementing their Wellness Plan, clients need to gain the support of others and overcome the obstacles in their way. What often keeps them stuck, or feeling trapped, is their persistence in looking at their situation from only one perspective. This may be the perfect time for your client to get off their point of view and adopt a new viewpoint!

What often leads to an impasse for your clients is seeing an interpersonal conflict or the lack of support from others from only one perspective.

> **Client:** *My supervisor thinks I'm wasting time at work looking at the internet. She doesn't trust me at all! She keeps giving me a hard time.*

> **Coach:** *Sounds like that makes work really tough for you. You've already told me a lot about this situation from your perspective. Go ahead and explain it to me again, only this time from the perspective of your supervisor. Pretend you are her for a moment and tell me about what it's like for her to supervise you.*

A coaching experiment like this can yield some surprising insights. This client might realize the pressure the supervisor is under for production and empathize with her more. The client might acknowledge how challenging they, themselves, are to supervise and become more understanding of their supervisor. The coach may then challenge the client to have a critical conversation with their supervisor now that they are in touch with another perspective on the situation.

The Big Picture

Clients can become stuck and frustrated by getting caught up in the details of situations. They are looking through their magnifying glass and lose perspective on how this situation fits into the larger scheme of things in their life. This is when a skillful coach can spot what is going on and challenge their client to take on a broader perspective. For example, the coach might say:

- Think for a moment about how all of this fits into your whole Wellness Plan.

- So, if you keep doing this for the next five years, how will that play out?

- How important will this be to you next month, next year?

- You've lost ten pounds and that doesn't seem like much when you think of the fifty you want to lose. But, just think. That's the first time in at least five years that you've succeeded in losing ten pounds!

- Right. You weren't able to complete all of the action steps you committed to last week. But, do you realize that you've accomplished 80% of it, and those are steps you've never taken before?

The Use of Metaphors and Analogies in Coaching

Unless you are educated in metaphor, you are not safe to be let loose in the world.

— Robert Frost

A distinguishing feature of more masterful coaching is the skill of using metaphors and analogies. The beauty and utility of a metaphor is that is allows us to understand something outside of our current experience or understanding by associating it with something we are familiar with. I may not know how to convey to someone how exactly I feel about the barrier I face, but when I say "It's like I'm up against a brick wall" they understand.

We use metaphors in daily language much more often than we think. We speak of a weight being lifted from our shoulders, feeling at the end of our rope, drowning in grief, running out of gas, and many more. Metaphors enrich our speech, they evoke imagery, they stimulate creative thinking and can open up new perspectives. Metaphors can help us connect with and give language to the emotions we are experiencing. Extended metaphorical exploration can help us chart a new path forward by expanding our thinking to consider options we were not previously aware of.

In a profoundly useful article, coach Angela Dunbar shows how metaphors can give both the coach and client insight.

> As a tool for coaching, the client's metaphors give you an insight into their unique perception of their situation and their goals. When the client tells you they can "see light at the end of the tunnel," that is what they are experiencing. There is light for them, and they are in a tunnel. They will unconsciously "know" much more about their situation from this metaphoric viewpoint. They are very likely to know in which direction the light is, how far away it is, and where the light comes from. They will know about the structure of the tunnel, how it feels and looks, how narrow the passage, and whereabouts they are in relation to the tunnel.
>
> And more—this is where the power of metaphor comes in. The client will know, on some level, what needs to happen for them to move towards the light and get out of the tunnel. The answer can come in pure metaphor, the person's real perception of their tangible situation will shift as their perception of the metaphor evolves and alters" (Dunbar, 2006).

Metaphors can emerge in the speech of our clients or can be generated by the coach as well. The key is what do we do with them.

The more a coach thinks metaphorically themselves the more they will notice metaphors in the speech of their clients. All metaphors have a function, some more important than others. Listen for the emergence of a metaphor from your client that seems to help the client to express an emotion or communicate the nature and/or importance of that emotion. Listen for metaphors that seem to present a new perspective on what is being discussed. Metaphors are often doing the heavy lifting for a client, helping them express what is otherwise hard to put into words. When such worthy metaphors show up, inquire more about them. Request clarification with a simple "Tell me more about that." "What's that like for you?"

I'm often known to quip, "What's a meta for if you don't use it?" I've been known to take a client metaphor and run with them with it, a metaphor in itself. Extending metaphors with a client is fun, creative work, and often quite productive, leading to greater client insight.

> **Client:** *I'm really feeling stuck. I'm not sure what's the next step to take. It's like I'm stranded on one side of a river.*
>
> **Coach:** *How can you take just one step into the river?"*
>
> **Client:** *I'd like to get across by jumping from one rock to the next. I have taken a few steps already at solving this.*
>
> **Coach:** *Great! So, you're into the river now. You've hopped onto a few rocks. What's next?*
>
> **Client:** *I don't know. I've run out of rocks to step on.*
>
> **Coach:** *How can you build your next rock to step on to?*
>
> **Client:** *Well, I guess I can stay where I am and start digging up stones to pile together and make a place to hop to next.*
>
> **Coach:** *So how can you start gathering those stones in your life right now?*

Such coaching conversations can lead to insight, problem solving, and charting a way forward. Solutions occur to our clients where just asking themselves, "What can I do? What can I do?" seems to be like banging their heads on a wall.

Dunbar's article introduces us to a concept from psychologist David Grove that is critical to our work extending metaphors—clean language. "The language you use is 'clean' because you say nothing to contaminate the client's own perception. You merely direct their attention towards the metaphor, and the shapes and symbols that evolve from it" (Dunbar, 2006). This is important because as you and your client engage in the metaphorical journey together you are both using your own mental imagery. What is essential is that you allow the client to go with their mental imagery, not yours, thus avoiding contamination.

You or your client might strike upon the metaphorical image of a tunnel. My tunnel may look like one created by hammer and pick from solid stone, whereas my client's might be smooth cement. Mine may exude a cool, damp breeze while my client's may emit a hot, dry wind.

As you explore the metaphor with your client be vigilant for subtle ways your language might influence or alter your client's imagery. Don't ask, "How cool is the breeze?" Their tunnel might not be cool and might not even have any air movement at all. A cleaner approach would be, "Is there any air movement? Tell me about the temperature you notice." It is all about the client's own internal perception.

An excellent way to stimulate a metaphor from your client is to use a question from David Grove's work that is a twist on what we often ask. Instead of asking your client, "What's that like?" ask them, "So, that's like what?" "What's that like?" will generate a response describing what they are talking about or the client will go into how they feel about it. When you ask, "That's like what?" you go directly towards a metaphor that describes something similar in the client's experience.

Coaches use metaphors to help their client understand what this new experience called coaching is all about. I frequently explain the role of a coach as being like that of a mountain guide. I might say, "Perhaps taking on this lifestyle challenge is like climbing a truly daunting mountain. You'd be really wise to hire a mountain guide to climb such a mountain with you. I won't climb it for you, but I'll go with you all the way and help you get to the top."

Coaches also generate metaphors when none are forthcoming from the client. Injecting a metaphor into the coaching conversation can enliven it and help a client regain momentum. More masterful coaches just seem to think metaphorically. Metaphors pop into their heads as they visualize what their client is saying. As the client paints a picture of their life, the coach sees the shapes and colors. The skill is then in distinguishing what metaphors to introduce to the coaching conversation. The coach needs a rationale for their use. Is the client in need of a new perspective? Are they struggling to find words for what is going on with them? Or, are they progressing just fine, and I can keep my metaphor to myself?

> **Client:** *I don't know. This new diagnosis has me freaked out. There's so much to know. All of this self-testing, damned finger sticking, keeping track of meds, learning about what to eat and not eat. I'm not used to these diabetes education classes.*
>
> **Coach:** *It's like you're back in high school again.*
>
> **Client:** *Yes! Exactly! I'm feeling like the dumbest kid in the class.*
>
> **Coach:** *Sounds embarrassing for you. You're a full-fledged adult and here you are like a teenager looking at a new textbook.*
>
> **Client:** *Right. And, sometimes I doubt my reading ability! (Laughter.)*
>
> **Coach:** *So, you're the new kid in class. Don't you think everyone else in class was new once too?*
>
> **Client:** *Sure they were. I just feel like the kid who transferred in at mid-year. Guess it's okay that they are a few lessons ahead of me, that's all.*

> *The metaphor is perhaps one of man's most fruitful potentialities. Its efficacy verges on magic, and it seems a tool for creation which God forgot inside one of His creatures when He made him.*
>
> — **Jose Ortega y Gasset**

When you offer your metaphor for your client's situation don't be attached to it. It may not stick. However, you may find that by merely introducing a metaphorical way of looking at things, your client will pick up on the use of metaphor. They may clarify the metaphor you offered or be stimulated to come up with their own. *"No, it's not like I'm up against a wall, it's more like I've painted myself into a corner."* Now you and your client are off to the races!

To develop more of a metaphorical mind, read! Don't just read from work-related sources, read fiction, the higher quality the better. Read poetry. Listen to music searching out poetic lyrics where you find them. Folk music seems to be a rich source for this. Chances are you use metaphors more than you think. Notice it in your review of your coaching recordings. Start to notice how you may already be speaking prose. Notice even the language in movies and on television shows. Also, when you realize that it is not up to you, the coach, to entirely come up with metaphors, and instead work just as often with the metaphors generated by your clients, you may relax into it more and let the metaphors flow like a stream.

> *"Metaphor lives a secret life all around us. We utter about six metaphors a minute. Metaphorical thinking is essential to how we understand ourselves and others, how we communicate, learn, discover and invent. But metaphor is a way of thought before it is a way with words."*
>
> — James Geary

Creativity in Coaching

What allows the more masterful coach to be creative in their craft? Watching a master coach at work is fascinating, not only because they do their work so well, but the fascination comes from knowing that at any moment you might witness something you've never seen before in your field. Suddenly the coach suggests some kind of experiment in the moment for the client and a huge insight is triggered. Out of what seems like thin air the coach brings an idea forward to pursue something you never would have thought of and it pays off. What allows such a coach to work this way? Reaching back to the second chapter of this book you may recall two of George Leonard's steps on the Path to Mastery. *Surrender* and *Pushing the Edge*.

Surrender and Creativity

Surrender to being yourself. The best coaching seems to occur when a coach allows their own personality to come through. Authenticity is not only appreciated by your client it allows you to relax and in doing so allows you more access to your creativity. Learn from others but do it your own way.

Surrender to appearing foolish. Coaching is a relatively safe place to make mistakes, as long as they are not ethical violations. We can usually step back and start all over again with little lost. This freedom to be vulnerable is part of the modeling we want to present for the client. We work at creating a safe, some would say even sacred, space for our coaching to take place in. Remember how safe it is for you, the coach, as well.

This type of freedom allows the coach to create experiments and, as Leonard would say, Push or Play the Edge. We are more willing to try something new. Most of our coaching, by far, will fall within the parameters of well-established and evidence-based practice and theory.

Playing the Edge and Creativity—Creative Experiments

Creativity in coaching comes forth when we work with our client to help them stretch and grow. Inviting them to step outside their comfort zone, but not into their risk zone. We can offer experiments either in the moment, or as homework for our clients to try out. It also helps the coach to offer more experiments like this when they are not attached to the success of the experiment. If we think it's got to work, then we will inhibit our creative process. If we and our client make an agreement to have an experimental attitude—it may succeed or fail, that's why they call it an experiment—we are more likely to generate creative experiments.

Experiments can be experiences that the coach and client co-create in the moment though usually with the coach in the lead. "Would you be willing to stop for a moment, take a couple of deep breaths, and then describe that again?" "Tell me. When you describe all of the challenges you're facing right now, what feelings do you become aware of?" Many in-the-moment experiments are about increasing awareness.

Designing experiments to conduct in the day-to-day life of your client comes more from a place of co-creation. As your client attempts to make progress on their goals, action steps often take on an experimental style. Your client and you come up with ideas and plans, to try out in their everyday life. A client working on increasing connection with others may brainstorm with their coach to come up with new venues for meeting others. A client working on improving sleep may experiment with a whole host of sleep hygiene techniques. Client participation and buy-in is huge in the probable success of experiments, so always *co*-create.

A Word on Using Tools in Coaching

In day-to-day work, great coaches come equipped with tools and use them. The way they use them, however, is what sets the craftsperson apart.

Like the craftsperson, the masterful coach knows all of the tools in their kit and is adept at their use. They know when to use what and when using a tool would interfere in the coaching process. They know what kind of results each tool is capable of bringing forth. They understand how each tool supports the coaching process and is backed up by sound theory. Tools such as strength inventories, rating scales that look at various aspects of one's lifestyle, pie-graph type scales, and more formal tools such as health risk assessments (HRAs) all have their uses.

Perhaps most importantly of all, a masterful coach knows that *the coaching drives the tools; the tools do not drive the coaching*. There are some tools that coaches find value in using with most every client, especially when helping the client begin coaching and engage in self-assessment. There are other tools that require an opportunity for their use. If the need, the opportunity, does not arise, they remain in the tool kit. What we don't want to see are thoughts like these: "I know I've just been using a saw, hammer, and nails on this project, but you know, I've got this great socket wrench set in my toolbox. There's got to be something here I can bolt down and use it!"

Tools require a rationale for their use. If your client requires more insight, a better, more organized way of looking at something, needs to get in touch with their strengths, could benefit from a more holistic perspective, etc., and you've got just the tool for the job, bring it out and offer it. Don't be attached to every tool. Some may sit for a long time in the toolbox. Coaching structure is your friend, but don't make it your master. Using too many tools with a client can make the coaching process laborious and even unpleasant for your client. Clients need to perceive adequate value in everything you do together. We don't want our coaching to have an impersonal feel.

Some tools are best delivered as part of the coaching conversation. The way a skilled coach presents a tool and takes the client through the process of using it can be most productive when it is a blend of the structure of the tool and the processing of what it reveals. Help your client to maximize their learning as they experience using any tool.

Other tools are best delivered as homework assignments (that the client sees the value in doing). Such tools as personal inventories are best completed when the client is home and has the time to go through them thoughtfully. Processing what they learned can take place at the next coaching session.

Time-Limited Coaching—Laser Coaching

Wellness coaches often work in settings where their time with clients is quite limited. Sessions may be as short as 20, 15, or even 10 minutes in length. Many large companies are continually searching for how they can provide meaningful service with the minimum number of sessions and minutes. At other times wellness coaches are meeting with someone for only one session, to go over the results of an HRA (health risk assessment) or perhaps the results of a biometric screening. Some independent coaches discover how challenging it is to go from the 60-minute sessions they were trained on to the 30-minute sessions that more clients prefer. Regardless of the amount of time spent with a client, we want the coaching to be of maximal value. We want our clients to feel like the time they spent in a coaching session was as efficient and productive as possible. Let's look at how what we call laser coaching can work for them.

The Term Laser Coaching

Thomas Leonard (1955-2003), one of the true founders of the life coaching field, was probably the originator of the term laser coaching. His form of laser coaching was quite different from the time-limited coaching that we refer to. Leonard was a brilliant coach who came from a business consulting background and had the ability to take in what a client was saying and quickly cut to the most critical aspects of what the client was dealing with. His insightful observations were usually on target and coaching progress accelerated greatly when Leonard intervened in this way.

> **Laser coaching** defined by Thomas Leonard is a specialized coaching technique and approach that promotes quick alignment, a rapid sense of relief, and a way of quickly unblocking someone who may have felt stuck in their way of thinking for a long time.
>
> Not necessarily a brief time frame but a focus of helping a client become un-stuck around a specific barrier.

We also see business and life coaches offering *laser coaching sessions* that are presented as one-session-only meetings. The idea is to attract clients who are already clear about what they need to talk about but need coaching to help them break through an impasse to greater insight and perhaps spark an action plan to move forward with. Part coaching, part consultation, these one-shot sessions can be helpful for the right client at the right time.

The How-To of Laser Coaching
Move Swiftly but Do Not Hurry

So, what does it mean to move efficiently and swiftly, yet not hurry? That's what the techniques and strategies of laser style coaching are designed to do. Laser coaching is about maximum efficiency no matter how much or how little time we have. Efficient coaching leaves a client feeling like the coaching session was focused and productive, like little if any time was wasted and all served a purpose.

Laser Coaching Mindset

The more masterful coach has learned that when they stick to a coaching mindset they operate more efficiently. A more diagnostic mindset that requires as much detailed information as possible. The client knows the detailed information of their own life. If they are checking in on action steps for accountability that's an important part of coaching. However, if they are simply reporting they are not necessarily working on making progress. When the coach operates from the coaching mindset, they are encouraging the client to explore, to reflect, to learn. They are helping their client to obtain insight about their behavior, not just report it.

The way the coach expresses this coaching mindset is to not ask as many questions about the details but to ask questions that get the client to think about what they have been doing, or not doing. Consequently, the coach and client stay out of the weeds and much time is saved.

Time-Saving Empathy

It seems quite paradoxical, but when the coach takes time to express empathic understanding, it actually saves time. Without empathy, without compassion or acknowledgment of what the client has gone through or is experiencing, the client does not feel heard. When people don't feel heard and understood they either shut down and withdraw, or they keep making an effort to be heard and understood. Meanwhile, the clock keeps ticking.

Clients want their story to be heard and acknowledged. In the foundation session a coach may be wise to let the client express themselves fully while staying actively involved in the coaching conversation by using active listening skills and non-judgmentally expressing empathy. As coaching goes on the more masterful coach helps the client to sort out what is their story, and who they are. Clients can sometimes over-identify with their story. It can be easy to think of one's self only in terms of one's health challenge, or one's situation. Effective coaching honors the client's story and helps them realize that they are not their story.

Even in Laser Coaching, Remain Client-Centered

When coaches feel the pressure of time there is a great temptation to become directive. "Maybe it will save time if I just tell my client how to change their diet." An educative approach looks like it would be quicker and to the point. Can we share information and resources? Certainly. Can we share what other clients of ours have found helpful? Of course. The coach has to ask themselves, however—are they jumping to offering these solutions prematurely, or even pre-emptively, and not giving their client a chance to develop these solutions themselves? Carefully distinguish when to blend education and coaching. Many of your clients are trying out coaching because their experience with learning all of the best ways to be healthy still did not result in success at behavioral change.

Another temptation for saving time is to rush into goal setting. Instead of following a process of adequate exploration, taking stock of one's wellness, and then co-creating an effective Wellness Plan, some coaches move quickly to get goals for change set in place. Some organizations even require their coaches to do this in the very first session. If goals are set prematurely with inadequate attention to the whole coaching process, we may find that the client does not succeed in attaining such goals, so we are back to square one.

Being laser-like in our coaching requires the coach to keep the client in the lead, but to be actively engaged in the coaching conversation. The coach is always monitoring the conversation and trying to determine if forward momentum is being achieved and maintained. The key to the right balance of directive to non-directive coaching is focus. Our challenge is to be directive enough, but to remain client centered.

Structure Is Again Our Friend

When coaches are providing adequate structure, the time used in coaching is much more efficient. You will see that this is one of the key components of a laser style of coaching.

Focus

Paramount in laser coaching is helping our clients to achieve and maintain focus. Are we staying on track? Are we pursuing a line of inquiry efficiently? Are we herding, so to speak, our client away from tangents?

Focus starts with clarity. As we've said before, sometimes clients walk in the door very clear about specific goals they want to achieve. Often though, they are perplexed about their inability to find real success in lifestyle improvement and lack clarity about how to proceed.

A lot of coaching comes down to helping clients answer the questions "What do I want?" and "How do I get it?" Part of a laser-like approach is to cut through the stories about past failures and shift to the present and future. In the process we may help our clients explore how they have held themselves back, etc., but the focus is on where we go from here. Using powerful questions often helps our clients to stay focused on creating this forward momentum.

Clients often feel the need to explain themselves and their past attempts that didn't work out. While a lot can be gained from learning what did and didn't work in the past, a key is for the coach to pick up on a client's attempts to assuage their guilt for past failures. Quickly shifting back to the present is important for not getting bogged down in remorse.

Rabbit holes are an expression often used to describe a conversational journey into unnecessary detail. Clients plunge into these subterranean expeditions for various reasons. For one thing, they often just love to talk about certain topics. Food or exercise are especially great topics for bringing out perseveration on the part of the client, and, all too often on the part of the coach as well. You may be fascinated to know how your client prepares a certain dish they've described, but unless you want to tie up precious time for your own information, don't go there. Hold back on any questions that encourage diving into such rabbit holes.

Is It Actually a Tangent?

Clients do ramble and benefit from the coach noticing their lack of focus and pointing it out to them. However, there are times when there is a method to your client's madness, so to speak. At times clients go into what seems like excessive detail getting to a point they want to make. There really may be a purpose to providing so much information. When you are not sure about where your clients are headed (focal point or rabbit hole), ask, "So, how is what you're telling me now related to what we were just talking about?" "How are you hoping that this information will help us stay on track?" "So Alex, you were just talking about exercise. Is that what you want to stay focused on?" Intervening like this will help your client explain their rationale, get to their point faster, or realize that they are off on a tangent. Just like in our everyday conversations, most people appreciate it when we help them get off of a true tangent.

Problem du Jour

The problem of the day. If coaching lacks structure it is easy to ask the client, "So! What would you like to talk about today?" Such an introduction to a session invites a problem-solving approach and there always seem to be problems to solve. Agreeing upon an agenda for the session right at the start can help both coach and client keep a holistic approach to the coaching process. Thinking that coaching is solving one problem after another is an infinite challenge and keeps a negative focus to the process.

Respectful Interruption

Many of us have been taught to never interrupt someone. To do so is rude. Yet, what does the coach do when confronted by a client who talks endlessly and turns the coaching conversation into a soliloquy?

It is critical that a coach reclaim their part of the conversation. Allowing the client to go on and on may not results in anything insightful or productive on the part of your client. Chances are good that they have a very talkative style and aren't even aware of how much they are speaking. This is where the coach must find a respectful way to interrupt.

"Excuse me. I want to make sure I really understand what you're saying…" Then the coach provides an accurate summarization of what they client has just said. Quickly, the coach follows this with a question, a request for clarification, or some other active listening skill. The summarization softens the interruption. The client usually feels heard and understood when they hear an effective summarization of what they have just said. The break in the action allows the coach to get themselves re-inserted into the conversation. Clients, even talkative ones, appreciate an actively involved coach. They usually feel as though they are getting more value out of the coaching when their coach is an active partner on the journey.

Presentify

Borrowing a term from Gestalt therapy, to presentify is to bring a topic of conversation out of the past and into the present. A sure way to burn time is to journey into the past rehashing what has happened long ago. What may be relevant, though, is how does the past show up in the present? How does past experience affect the client's ability to carry out the change process here and now?

Quicksand—When It's Not About Coaching

A sure way to grind the coaching process to a slow crawl is to delve into issues that are better suited for counseling and therapy. Containing less stigma than therapy, it's not unusual for clients needing more clinical help to seek out coaching instead. Be vigilant about being led into the quicksand of subjects such as family of origin issues, past emotional, physical, or sexual abuse, profound guilt and shame, or dysfunctional intimate relationships. These topics are not only exhausting, they are far better served by working with a licensed mental health professional.

Practical Time Savers

Laser coaching is not just about coaching techniques and style. It's also about very efficient practices that keep the coaching process moving right along and save time.

Laser Coaching Time Saving Tips

- Use a coaching prep form. Have your client fill this out ahead of time and either send it within a day of the appointment or have them bring it with them. You'll know what's coming and your client will be far more prepared and ready to start working faster.

- Tools. Have your client fill out certain tools outside of the coaching appointment. Some tools are better to complete during the coaching session and others are best filled out when the client can take more time at home.

- Share responsibility for clock watching. If your client seems to habitually wait until time is almost up to bring up important issues, urge them to place a time piece (watch, phone, etc.) where they can see it during the session.

- Be firm on time boundaries. Teach your client to use time efficiently by learning that their appointment with a professional coach has professional time limits.

> • Co-create agreements about extending a session beyond the original time limit. Agree to coach for five or ten more minutes when the time is available, but don't keep extending the deal.

Masterful coaches never seem to rush. They aren't pushing or forcing the coaching process. What you observe is efficiency, accuracy, and an economy of action. They understand the importance of being congenial, warm, and friendly, yet they are still all about being down to business. Clients leave their sessions feeling like a lot got done in whatever amount of time they had together.

> *Just be patient. Let the game come to you.*
> *Don't rush. Be quick, but don't hurry.*
>
> **—NBA Hall of Fame member Earl Monroe**

This chapter brought us into the concrete skills of What to Do in wellness coaching. We started the chapter with the realization that the skill of listening is not really about *active listening skills*. It is about how to listen and what to listen for. It is about constantly scanning and noticing on multiple levels as your client communicates with you. We then gave each active listening skill their due and looked at how we respond more masterfully to what we are hearing. The use of questions was then explored showing how we can do so effectively while avoiding the coaching pitfalls that poor use of questions can lead to.

Language plays a central role in coaching, so we explored how the way the client and the coach talk impacts the coaching process. The essential coaching skill of reframing was demonstrated. The value of using metaphors throughout our coaching was also presented. Lastly, we discussed *laser coaching* to show how to coach efficiently when we may or may not have all of the time we would like with our client.

In Chapter Eight we will discuss how to move forward with our client and co-create the momentum that can bring change. We will look at the need for adequate exploration before we launch into goal setting. We will show the distinction between effective exploration and simple reporting of behavior. Then, we will engage in a thorough inquiry into how to use the transtheoretical model of behavior change in the process of coaching.

REFERENCES

Dunbar, A. (2006, February 8). Using metaphors with coaching. *The CleanCollection.* https://www.cleanlanguage.co.uk/AngelaDunbar-using-metaphorswith-coaching.html

Frederickson, B. (2009). *Positivity.* Harmony.

Heick, T. (2018, December 11). What is Bloom's taxonomy? A definition for teachers. *Teachthought.* https://www.teachthought.com/learning/what-isblooms-taxonomy-a-definition-for-teachers/

Lopez, B. (1986). *Artic dreams: Imagination and desire in a northern landscape.* Charles Scribner's Sons.

Malady, M. (2014, September 11). Fingerprint words. *Slate.* https://slate.com/human-interest/2014/09/fingerprint-words-verbal-tics-that-define-us-and-how-they-spread-to-others.html

Shazer, S. (2007). *More than miracles: The state of the art of solution-focused brief therapy* (1st ed.) (Published posthumously.) Routledge.

Williams, P. (2015). *Becoming a professional life coach.* (2nd ed.). W.W. Norton.

PART THREE

What to Do

Chapter 8—Forward Momentum

Forward Momentum

Even a highly skilled coach, well-schooled in theories of behavior change, now faces the challenge of moving forward with their client in their quest for greater health and well-being. Creating progress quickly sounds exciting but let's help our client gain a clear picture of where they are to start. In my previous book, *Wellness Coaching for Lasting Lifestyle Change, 2nd Ed.*, we give a thorough description of the process of helping a client to take stock of their wellness, craft a motivating vision of their best life possible (Well-Life Vision), and co-create a fully integrated Wellness Plan.

In this chapter let's look at the process of adequate exploration more closely. Let's see how a more masterful coach presents the invitation to change and works more deeply with the stages of behavioral change to ensure success as we create forward momentum.

Adequate and Effective Exploration

After establishing the coaching alliance, a masterful coach begins by helping the client to get a thorough picture of their current level of wellness, health, and overall well-being. Instead of rushing into action, the coach and client benefit from a more measured, deliberate, and positive approach to change.

Think of it this way. Your client, with their history of struggles with lifestyle improvement, is embarking with you on what feels to them like a perilous journey. Realistically assessing their current health status and facing their challenges is critical. However, your client also needs to know what they have going for them that will ensure a greater chance of success. They need to thoroughly take inventory of their wellness, their strengths, their assets, and resources before they take on this new challenge of change. This strengths-based coach approach makes use of all the benefits of what we now know of positive psychology. So, to begin our journey, let's help our client take stock of their wellness and adequately explore their strengths and where they are to begin with.

Adequate exploration means coaching your client to look at their life 360 degrees—full circle. For the wellness coach it means getting grounded in your client's current health status, life story, treatments, medications, etc. It starts with getting on the same page with your client by becoming acquainted with all of these aspects of their current situation. As the coach is doing so, however, the process of gaining client information is accompanied by the simultaneous process of building the coaching alliance. The skilled coach is expressing empathy, using all of their active listening skills, helping the client feel heard and understood. They are taking in data but doing so in a very warm and human way. The experience of realizing that their story is being heard and appreciated ignites hope in a process of positive change that might work for them.

As coaching moves beyond that first phase of exploration, the process now focuses on helping our clients to learn more about themselves. Often clients need to fill in gaps in their own wellness knowledge. They may not have had a medical exam with a healthcare provider in years. They may have no idea what their blood pressure, blood lipid levels, or blood sugar levels are. As clients make appointments or otherwise gain such knowledge the key is for the coach to explore with them what effect this new information is having upon them.

Exploration becomes a regular part of ongoing coaching appointments. This is where we help our clients to look at their lives in a more holistic and comprehensive way, gaining insight as they do.

Simple tools of exploration like The Wheel of Life help clients realize how truly holistic wellness is. Taking the time to coach clients around the interconnections of the different areas of their life often pays off in more accurate selection of areas to work on and therefore actually saves time in the long run.

The Power of Story

Our client's story needs to be heard, honored, and understood. Great coaches demonstrate excellent listening skills and show a warm, empathic coaching presence as they hear their client's story. Acknowledgment, validation, and empathy pave the way to both building the relationship and establishing awareness of the client's life as it is today.

At other times the client engages with the coach in a lively conversation that seems as though it should be productive, but never really delivers on that promise. Often, what is going on is that the client is simply conveying what they already know. They are reporting rather than exploring.

Real exploration is when you are exploring new lands, not just taking a walk in your neighborhood. Clients often use a lot of coaching time informing the coach about every tree, bush, and rock in their neighborhood (reporting things they already know). Effective exploration is when we say to the client, "How about going someplace new? Let's go on a journey!" Coaches help people look at the old neighborhood with new eyes, and yes, that is the close-to-home aspect of exploration, developing new perspective on old ground. However, more serious growth usually takes place somewhere less familiar, perhaps even someplace that is more of a stretch.

Some international travelers never stray from the well-worn resort areas, or don't even travel to a country that doesn't speak their own language. Other than many trips to Canada, my first time out of my home country was to dive alone into the heart of Bangkok, Thailand. That adventure stretched me, though not always comfortably, in new ways resulting in growth I never expected. You, the coach, need to become comfortable with being uncomfortable. When you exude more confidence in new territory, your traveling companion client will feel safer and allow themselves to proceed while still perhaps feeling uncomfortable.

> *Life is an adventure, it's not a package tour.*
>
> — **Eckhart Tolle**

The probability of our clients sailing into unchartered waters is vastly improved when they have a traveling companion, and preferably a trusted professional guide. In a way, we might all become better coaches if we fancy ourselves as adventure guides! To do so might mean getting some adventurous miles under our own belts. No need to book that flight to Thailand or the Amazon. Your own exploration is right where you know it is, in the land of your own personal growth. You might not need to jump into years of therapy and confront your shadow side, but simply ask yourself, "What will stretch me?" Your own personal wellness foundation is rooted in your personal growth.

As you work with your client you might ask yourself, "Are we really exploring here?" You might imagine the two of you like the famous explorers in history; Vasco da Gama, Henry Hudson, Daniel Boone, etc. They were all looking for new lands, and, importantly new routes to get to places that they knew existed. Henry Hudson and his crews jammed their way through artic ice again and again searching for the fabled Northwest Passage that would lead them to Cathay (China). They never made it to the Orient, but in the process, they opened up the great land of Canada. Sometimes clients are surprised by what they find. Exploration in coaching helps our clients to discover their own passage, their own route that can lead them to the life they truly want to live.

From Patient to Client

Part of what keeps clients stuck in the neighborhood of their familiar lives is the patient role that they have learned well. As a patient I believe in telling my healthcare provider as much accurate information as I can about my conditions, my current health status, etc., so that they can develop an accurate diagnosis and recommend the best course of treatment. This works great when I am in a professional medical consultation situation. I'm doing my best at reporting in. Coaching, as we know, works differently.

Part of building the coaching alliance is helping our clients learn how to become clients. We can explain how coaching works and ways in which we will be of value to our clients. As we do so we can make a distinction between how the medical consultation works and how things proceed in coaching. After this introduction we will most likely find that we will need to repeatedly coach with the client in such a way as to remind them that we, the coach, don't really need all the details.

Our job is to help the client work with their own situation by facilitating the coaching process with them.

So, what does ineffective and effective coaching exploration sound and look like?

Ineffective Exploration

- Client energy is low, even monotone in voice. On the other hand, client energy is fine, even anxious, speech may even be rapid.
- The same ground gets plowed again and again.
- Tangents and minutia prevail.
- The client tends to stick to favorite topics (e.g., what to eat).
- Drilling down into details never strikes oil (we don't gain insights, only more details).
- The client may be giving the coach what the client thinks the coach wants to hear.
- The coach finds it hard to forward the action.
- May feel like less rewarding hard work.

Effective Exploration

- Client energy is strong and engaged.
- There is a curiosity that the client shows about their own life, behavior, beliefs, etc.
- Stimulates new ideas, insights, connections, potential solutions.
- Challenges the client.
- Asks about the relevance of what is being discussed.
- Asks the client if they are receiving real value out of the current discussion.
- Helps clarify values and beliefs.
- Draws upon what has worked in the past.
- Experiments with new perspectives.

- Can tap into body-wisdom of both the coach and client.
- Includes process coaching where feelings may be explored, and emotions processed.
- Encourages looking into new topics.
- Provides the substance for possibility thinking.

The Sound of Effective Exploration

It often takes some powerful questions to stimulate effective exploration. Here are some questions, requests, and phrases a coach might use to help make exploration more productive.

- "So, is what we're talking about something you're finding of value?"
- "That's one perspective. Now tell me about the same thing, but from a completely different perspective."
- "I understand how important the components of your diet are. Would you find it more productive to continue to explore what you are eating, or is there some other aspect of food and eating that we could benefit from looking at?"
- Summarize and then: "Hearing your long list of all the tasks and activities you are engaged in right now, what are you aware of?"
- "What question are you hoping I will ask you now?"
- "What question are you afraid I might ask you now?"
- "What would be a real stretch for you here?"

Sharing Observations—Saying What Is So

Creating forward momentum is a co-creative process. We want to stimulate our client's thinking with great active listening skills and powerful questions, but we also have something more to contribute. The coach is in a seat that allows for a very different perspective than that of the client who, alone, can only self-examine and self-reflect. So much of the coaching process is about increasing awareness. By sharing what is being observed, the coach can help the client to increase their awareness of themselves, their situation, and more.

After we, as the coach, have done a great job of listening and helping our client to clarify what they are saying, we take what we have been accumulating as observations and fashion a way of sharing that information with our client. We listen and we notice, then we provide feedback to our client by, as the coaching expression goes, saying what is so.

The key here is to keep our observations clean and clear. Clients benefit the most from direct observations that we can substantiate as observable behavior, rather than our own interpretations. As the coaching session goes on you will be noticing many things. You will pick up on patterns in speech, language, emotional expression, and associative patterns. Associative patterns are where the client tends to speak about a particular subject, for example taking time for self-care, and tends to also bring up a topic that is related in some way, such as their relationship with their intimate partner. The conversation may simply start to drift from self-care to talking about the partner with no apparent connection. It may even appear as a shift in topic. However, if you notice a repetitive pattern here and bring the client's awareness to it, the association may trigger some insight. "So, are you aware that three or four times now, when you've been talking about your eating habits you end up talking about the workplace?" Without your own interpretation, simply offer that to your client for them to consider. It may lead to an important insight that can propel coaching forward.

Evoking Discovery and Growth

So how do wellness coaches help their clients move from simply telling their story once again (and experiencing it being appreciated by the coach), to engaging in a process of discovery and growth? How do we help our client to reach down inside themselves and grab ahold of hope and motivation?

Coaches are sometimes confronted with clients who appear as though they do not want to improve their lifestyle even while admitting that such changes would be beneficial, or even critical to their health and well-being. Clients will sometimes make the case for why they cannot change.

Much of our client's argument for why they cannot change comes from a place of low self-efficacy. As we saw in Chapter Six, if one has lost the confidence that all of this wellness effort will be worthwhile and that it can be successful, that low sense of self-efficacy will keep them trapped. Building self-efficacy may be the first order of business.

Beyond that, the effective coach knows that it is often the client's fears that can be trapping them in inaction. Explore with your client what fears are holding them back. *"So, if you do make this change, what are you afraid might happen?"* At this point we often hear our clients talk about the potential they face for rejection, criticism, ridicule, attack, or even punishment. This can come from peers, family, friends, or others. The fear of damaging those relationships may easily outweigh, in your client's mind, the benefits of lifestyle improvement. Never be dismissive about a client's fears. They are very real to them. Acknowledge the effect such fears are having upon your client. Allow them to feel what they feel, then explore further.

Fears are something that can be addressed head-on in coaching. Gently explore them with genuine empathic understanding and help your client to develop some strategies for how to address them. Of particular value is helping your client to realize it when a fear is based upon an assumption. *"So how do you know that to be true?"* As blocks like this are cleared away the client may be more open to consider change now that it seems more possible.

Creating forward momentum in coaching depends not upon the coach's desires, but upon where the client is in terms of the change process. As coaching proceeds the masterful coach begins to form a clearer idea of how ready their client is to move forward. That concept of readiness is explored directly with the client as they have the greatest insight about their own level of readiness. Being an effective ally at this point in the coaching process can be greatly enhanced by a thorough knowledge of the transtheoretical model of behavior change, also known as the stages of change, developed by James Prochaska and his associates (Prochaska J. N., 2016) (Prochaska J. N., 1994).

The Transtheoretical Model of Behavior Change and Wellness Coaching

Few theories of behavior change are as deeply researched and as ubiquitous as the transtheoretical model of behavior change (TTM). Originally coming out of work with tobacco, alcohol, and substance abuse, TTM has found wide application in not only clinical programs, but it is safe to say, most health and wellness programs.

The Development of the Transtheoretical Model

The transtheoretical model is so named because as Dr. Prochaska and his associates developed the model, they integrated the essential principles from several leading theories and therapies including:

Sigmund Freud: Consciousness-Raising. Freud emphasized the importance of the unconscious mind and how it can impact behavior. The goal of psychoanalysis is to make the unconscious conscious.

Fritz Perls: Dramatic relief. Perls developed Gestalt therapy, which emphasized enhanced awareness of sensation, perception, bodily feelings, emotion, and behavior in the present moment.

Rollo May: Self-Liberation. May developed an existentialist psychology that focuses on creativity, love, authenticity, and freedom to discover potential avenues toward transformation, which enables people to live meaningful lives in the face of uncertainty and suffering.

Carl Rogers: Helping relationships. Rogers coined the term "client centered therapy." As a humanistic psychologist Rogers agreed with the main tenets of Abraham Maslow (self-actualization theory), but added that for a person to "grow," they need an environment that provides them with genuineness and acceptance (unconditional positive regard) and empathy.

B. F. Skinner: Reinforcement management. As a behavioral psychologist, Skinner developed the theory of operant conditioning, which postulates that behavior is determined by its consequences, whether negative or positive (reinforcing or punishing) and which make it more or less likely that the behavior will occur again.

Prochaska, et.al, saw behavioral change as a process, not an event. By studying what had worked for people who were successful at managing to achieve change on their own he and his team determined that there were six stages that people typically moved through in their journey.

The Transtheoretical Model: Six Stages of Change

1. Precontemplation: The person is either not aware of the issue (e.g., hypertension) or is aware but may be not willing to even look at changing, sometimes due to being demoralized after having tried and failed. Not ready; not intending to take action in the next six months.

2. Contemplation: The person becomes aware and begins to consider changing, weighing the pros and the cons of change. Getting ready; intending to take action in the next six months.

3. Preparation: The person begins exploring change possibilities (looks for resources, accessibility, affordability, etc.). Ready; ready to take action in the next 30 days.

4. Action: The person initiates and executes the steps necessary for change to take place. Have made the behavior change but for less than six months.

5. Maintenance: The client has established a new behavior and now works on maintaining it. Doing the new health behavior for more than six months.

6. Termination: The new behavior is now integrated into their life. Confident with the change; not tempted to relapse.

Perhaps the very first thing to understand about this model is that it underscores that a person can be at a different stage of change for each different behavior. The overweight, middle-aged smoker who fears weight gain and is firmly in pre-contemplation about quitting tobacco may be more ready to engage in improving their diet (perhaps they are in the preparation or action stages), and more ready to begin an exercise program (again, perhaps preparation or action). They may also have to consider any of these changes by weighing the pros and cons of change in more conversations with their wellness coach (contemplation stage). A common misunderstanding I have observed is the idea that the entire person is either "ready" or "not ready" to change.

At the 2017 Leadership in Healthcare Conference in Boston, Dr. Prochaska presented "Coaching at Every Stage of Change." There he asked the audience, "What is the most important stage of change?" Many responded with "the action stage," while others identified "the preparation stage." Dr. Prochaska surprised much of the audience when he stated that it is the precontemplation stage, because that is the beginning of where change happens.

The Action Model

Too often coaches and others in the helping professions view the action stage as not only the most important stage but see getting their client there as soon as possible as their primary goal. In their 2016 book, *Changing to Thrive* (Prochaska J. O. & Prochaska J. M., 2016), James and Janice Prochaska demonstrate that their research has found for any given behavior, only 20% of people are in the action stage of change—the other 80% are not! They speak about weight loss and smoking cessation programs that screen to determine who among their applicants are in the action stage and only accept those who are. Then, the same programs brag about their high success rates. Our job as coaches is to coach 100% of the people and help the 80% who are not in action to proceed through the stages from precontemplation to contemplation and preparation. The Prochaskas have also found that when a person moves up just one stage, say from precontemplation to contemplation, they double their probability of proceeding to the action stage.

In 1996 I began being trained in life coaching. The field had no concept of readiness for change, and I remember being taught to urge insightful clients into action with the challenge "So! What are you going to do about it?" Even today what is often misunderstood is that the stages of precontemplation, contemplation, and preparation are inherent and important parts of the process of change. Coaches and students often think of the term "ready to change" as meaning the client has arrived at the action stage of readiness. Change does not equal action, per se. Change is a process, not an event. Change equals progressing through the stages of change.

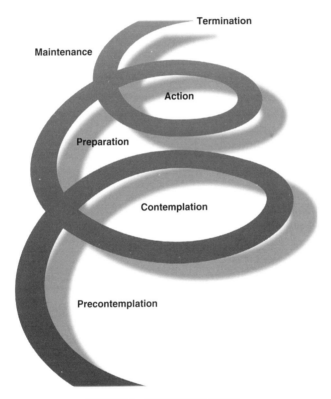

FIGURE 16—STAGES OF CHANGE

The Precontemplation Stage

Imagine that your client has come to you as a referral from their physician or is there because of an employee wellness program incentive that will save them 20% on their health insurance premium. They are not enthused to see you and, despite some serious medical conditions, are not optimistic about coaching helping them to accomplish better health—something they have struggled with for years. They reluctantly tell a story of repeated failure attempts at weight loss, smoking cessation, etc. They would rather not even be talking about trying again to make changes happen. They know that their lifestyle habits are working against their health, but they have no confidence that another wellness program will help, or that they, themselves, would be successful at it.

They have not given up entirely. They do walk their dog every day and have joined friends in participating in a hiking group that gets out every other weekend. They are worried about the effect that secondhand smoke may have on their grandchildren whom they watch two days a week and are seeking more information about using nicotine patches as part of a tobacco cessation program. Yet, they believe that there is no way to change their eating habits and don't even want to discuss this. They have made many attempts at dieting with the classic "yo-yo" effect of weight loss followed by immediate regaining of those pounds. In TTM terms we could help our client to realize that they are in the action stage with becoming more active, and in the preparation stage with smoking cessation. When it comes to improving their diet as part of a weight loss effort, however, they are entrenched in pre-contemplation.

The illustration shows us that every client is a person with a complex set of attitudes, beliefs, behaviors, and experiences. Sometimes our clients are full of contradictions and paradoxes. Sometimes they are angry, frustrated, sad, dejected, or experiencing any combination of emotions. As we apply TTM theory we must remember that this theory acknowledges this complexity, and as we help our clients to become aware of where they are at with the process of change, we must do so with compassion and sensitivity as well. This is especially true with precontemplation.

A common misunderstanding about this stage is the belief that individuals don't want to change. Rather, in precontemplation individuals do not have the intention to change. "There is a big difference between wanting and intending" (Prochaska, J. 0. & Prochaska J. M., 2016).

"People in precontemplation are often labeled as being uncooperative, resistant, unmotivated, or not ready for behavior change programs. However, our research showed us that it was the health profes-

sionals who were not ready for the precontemplators" (Prochaska, J. 0. & Prochaska, J. M., 2016). What is going on for the precontemplator? As I heard a speaker at a lifestyle medicine conference put it, "The dream of better health goes to sleep." The person may have reached a point in life where they stop evaluating how they have been living. Their self-efficacy is usually very low when it comes to changing a particular behavior, or a group of behaviors that might be necessary for improved health and wellbeing. What often gets in the way is what the Prochaskas have identified as The Three Ds.

The Three Ds of Precontemplation

1. Don't know how: This is characterized by a lack of awareness or understanding of how the behavior change may benefit the individual or a lack of awareness of how not improving their lifestyle may bring them harm. The person may benefit from some healthy-living education. The Prochaskas make the point that education is not intended to result in action. It is intended to move someone into contemplation. The client may also not know what to do to begin a process of change. Their attempts at change in the past may have been lacking any real plan, support, or accountability.

2. Demoralization: Often our clients are stuck in uncertainty about their ability to change or they fear failure. This frequently arises from repeated attempts to change that have resulted in failure. They may identify causal attributions or reasons why they can't change. (Not having enough willpower, not having the right genes, low self-efficacy based on repeated failure.) Our client is so discouraged that they don't even want to consider taking on another attempt at change.

3. Defending: Sometimes our clients feel criticized by people in their lives about the way they are living an unhealthy lifestyle. Their tendency may be to defend or protect their current risky behavior. Defensive behavior is in fact most often a way of protecting independence or autonomy. They may do this by:

> a. Turning inward: blaming themselves and/or retreating inward. We may see them withdrawing interpersonally

and dis-attending (tuning out). They may internalize their blame, which leads to lower self-esteem and yet more demoralization.

b. Turning outward: blaming others, outward circumstances, etc. We may see them projecting the blame onto others. "My family won't change the way they eat, so, how can I?" They may displace their own frustration by being angrier and more critical of others.

c. Coaches often hear their clients explaining away risky behaviors. They may rationalize why it is okay for them to maintain the status quo. We sometimes hear intellectualizing, using facts and data to justify bad habits. Everyone seems to know some person who lived to a ripe old age and reveled in exhibiting all of the health-risk behaviors they could.

One of the causal attributions that coaches frequently hear from the client in precontemplation is that they lack motivation. As we saw in Chapter Six, our clients often have plenty of sources of motivation, but have been lacking the vehicle—the behavioral change methodology, the structure that coaching can provide—to put that motivation to work. They have usually participated in action-oriented programs that urged them to start making huge changes in their lives quite suddenly.

The beauty of the TTM approach is that it honors where the person is and helps them gradually progress to where action and success can happen. The Prochaskas direct us to provide hope for our clients. Having a behavioral change ally and the support of that coaching alliance combined with a solid behavioral change process can offer so much more hope than simply trying again to change as our client has before.

By honoring client autonomy, we can avoid bringing out defensiveness in our clients. The last thing a client wants to hear is someone telling them that they are living their lives in the wrong way. There is a story behind every behavior. Our client may have any number of social and environmental determinants of health that make lifestyle improvement very challenging. The key is to help our client frame these factors as just that—challenges—and offer our coaching alliance as a way to co-create strategies to deal with them.

Perhaps another strategy to consider for reducing defensiveness is to move away from the health-risk reduction approach to wellness. Instead focus on building healthy behaviors that the client is attracted to. Help them build on their strengths and engage in experiments that will result in easily achieved success at behavior change. Help them to examine their own belief systems and get in touch with positive sources of motivation.

Masterful Moment
When the more masterful coach hears justifications coming from their client, they are alerted to reflect on how they have been coaching with this person. Have they been saying anything to bring out a defensive posture? Have they been pushing their own agenda of reducing health risks too hard? Are they becoming too directive and not co-creating the conversation with their client?

Creating Forward Momentum — From Precontemplation to Contemplation

In precontemplation our client most likely considers lifestyle improvement ever so briefly, then dismisses it. How do we get our client not to jump into swift action, but to merely give change serious consideration, to contemplate it? TTM offers three primary methods to help coaches tackle this imposing challenge: *raising the pros while reducing the cons of change; dramatic relief; and consciousness raising.*

The First Principle of Progress: Increasing Pros to Move from Precontemplation to Contemplation

Why would anyone begin to change when the reasons against such an endeavor outweigh the perceived benefits that might result? How do we do so without a campaign of persuasion (which most likely will not work)? Have you ever tried to convince someone to be well? Clearly the pros of changing must outweigh the cons, but how do we help our clients to discover this? This is where considerable coaching skill is required.

At the start of precontemplation the cons are high, and the pros are low. This is how our client perceives themselves and their situation. As we begin coaching, we start with an open phase of exploration and encourage the client to engage in a process of self-assessment. By not rushing to set up goals and action steps we avoid pushing the client beyond their stage of readiness. The more coach and client explore together the more apparent the stage of change emerges for each behavior that is being considered for change. The precontemplation stage shows up in our client's language. We hear our client make the case for why they believe they cannot change a particular behavior and/or do not want to. The list of cons is recited sometimes with a sense of helplessness, sometimes defensively. This part of the client's story needs to be met with compassionate understanding, but not collusion. That is, the coach can empathize but not agree with the client that change is so terribly difficult. Reframing it as a challenge can be important here.

The coach proceeds in the coaching conversation not with the goal of stimulating the client into action, but simply to get them thinking — to weigh the pros and cons. We can do so by:

1. Offering education. The Prochaskas do this by providing clients with extensive lists of the benefits of various lifestyle improvements. The wellness coach may offer other resources or help the client to find more information on their own and make those efforts part of the coaching process.

2. Challenging assumptions. James Prochaska is fond of saying that people too often underestimate the benefits and overestimate the costs of change. If our client appears to be operating on an assumption about what would be involved in making changes, it's a perfect time to call out the assumption. Again, a great line for the coach is "So, how do you know that to be true?" This can build into a powerful coaching conversation about re-evaluating their pros and cons.

3. Engaging in *Decisional Balance*. In the context of coaching, this would be a coaching conversation exploring with our client the pros and cons of change. We can help our client to list the advantages and benefits of change that they are aware of. We can help them list the ways in which change may lead to disadvantages or penalties in their life. The

Prochaskas were able to develop brief assessments of six to eight questions to help with this process (Prochaska, J. 0. & Prochaska, J.M., 2016). As they researched decisional balance they came to an important realization. "Although we didn't realize it for some time, we were also discovering that making the decision to change one's behavior for improved health was nowhere near as rational and empirical as we had assumed. Nor was it nearly as conscious" (Prochaska, J. 0. & Prochaska, J.M., 2016).

The Second Principle of Progress: Increasing Your Consciousness

We sometimes hear that *people are doing the best that they can, given their level of awareness*. Perhaps our client has concluded that being stuck in a stage of precontemplation is the best that they can do right now. By helping our client to increase their conscious awareness of themselves, their problems and potential solutions, we can help them to shift out of precontemplation. TTM uses the term *consciousness raising* to describe this process. Consciousness raising can take place a number of ways.

1. Clients are often stuck because they don't know much about how to effectively go forward with a process of change. As coaches we can show them how a developed methodology of change (such as the Wellness Mapping 360° Methodology©) can provide so much more than simple goal setting. The coach can educate the client about the TTM change process. This can reassure the client that it is okay for them to be where they are in the process of change and engender hope for how they can move through the stages of change. Clients are often focused on *what* to change—what to eat, how to get more sleep, etc. Coaching can bring a powerful process to raise awareness of *how* to change. The Prochaskas refer to this as Increasing your Behavior Change IQ.

2. Analyze what is getting in the way. Freud emphasized that consciousness raising works best when resistance is analyzed first. That's what you were doing when you reviewed

your inward and outward defenses and took an honest look at what gets in the way of your self-change efforts (Prochaska, J. 0. & Prochaska, J. M., 2016). In the coaching conversation we ask powerful questions that help our client to explore their internal and external barriers. *What holds you back when you consider making some changes? What are you afraid might happen if you made these changes? When you make an attempt to change, or think about it, what are you aware of? Do you ever feel guilty when you take time for your self-care, or your wellness activities? How do others react when you attempt change?*

3. Explore *Coaching for Greater Client Awareness* in Chapter Six to see how we can use awareness of behavior and feelings as well as mindfulness to support more consciousness raising.

The 3rd Principle of Progress: Use Dramatic Relief to Move from Precontemplation

Drawing upon the work of Fritz Perls in Gestalt therapy, the Prochaskas have found the value of working with emotions for what they call dramatic relief.

When we hold our feelings in, we can get distressed or depressed. However, if we can release difficult emotions like anger or guilt, we also reduce the emotional pressure they contain, and we aren't as tempted to numb them with one or more of the four high-risk behaviors (Prochaska, J. 0. & Prochaska, J. M., 2016).

The four high-risk behaviors are: smoking, alcohol abuse, unhealthy diets, and not enough exercise.

Health and wellness coaching inevitably deals with our client's emotions. Paying attention to the feelings of our client is a key to effective change. As clients experiment with change, as their conscious awareness increases, they get in touch with the affective component of their change process. Insights arise that can lead to release, inspiration, and ultimately more motivation for improving their way of living. Fears can arise when we consider removing the blinders that we have put in place to protect us from change. Helping our clients to process their feelings can lead to the kind of relief that allows them to break out of the hold that their low self-efficacy and demoralization has had on them.

"In TTM, dramatic relief is intended to move you *emotionally* from precontemplation" (Prochaska, J. O. & Prochaska, J. M., 2016). In addition to the processing that can take place in the coaching conversation, the Prochaskas recommend encouraging methods like journaling or keeping a diary. Such a self-reflective process can allow for emotional expression and relief. They also encourage the use of various relaxation techniques to reduce dis-stress.

Honoring the emotional element in the change process allows clients to make powerful connections with motivation and often clears the way for them to move forward.

The Contemplation Stage

All too often coaches see the contemplation stage as a stage to be moved through as quickly as possible on our way to action. Somehow, we believe that just *thinking* about change is not important or may even be a way our client avoids actually changing. In the TTM model, this is where our client is considering the pros and cons of change, and now the pros are strong enough to get them engaged in this process of contemplation. Their intention is to make a change within the next six months.

This is where more exploration takes place in the coaching conversation. The coach helps the client to elaborate about the pros and cons of change. Powerful questions composed by the coach for the client to ask themselves facilitates their client's thinking, helping them gain insight and understanding. As the client discovers more reasons to make a change through this process, forward momentum can increase.

Building the pros of change is important here, but the cons of change are still strong. Often, they show up as what TTM calls the two Ds of contemplation: doubt and delay. "Those in contemplation can be plagued by profound doubt, wondering, 'Is change really worth it?' The rule of thumb for contemplators is: When in doubt, don't act" (Prochaska, J. O. & Prochaska, J. M., 2016). Our client can be stuck here doubting if all of the time and effort, all of the investment in this

Wellness Plan will be worthwhile. When doubt is strong, it leads to delay. Unlike the precontemplator, the contemplator does not abandon considering change, they just keep on considering. They engage more readily in conversation about change, they may begin to look up information about it, research programs, etc., but move ahead with real preparation or action? Not yet.

The forever contemplating client is often what frustrates coaches and healthcare providers. TTM refers to this as chronic contemplation, which they see as one of three forces that hold back our clients. As the Prochaskas put it, it's hard to fail when you're only thinking about change.

The second force TTM finds at play is our client's need for certainty. Afraid of failing (again), our client keeps talking about change, hoping to find a way to completely eliminate all risk and remove all doubt. Clients search for the absolutely perfect solution, helping us understand the seduction of programs that "guarantee success."

TTM has identified a third force that gets in the way of successful change; that of rushing into action before one is adequately prepared. Again, what I call "jumping to solution," or premature goal setting that is often designed to urge our clients into action, is often doomed to failure. Such a setback may keep the client stuck in contemplation or push them back into precontemplation. The desire to rush into action is quite understandable. As we explained earlier, the action model is what dominates our culture and most of our healthcare programs. Smokers are urged to quickly set a quit date within 30 days regardless of readiness. Marketing efforts of weight loss programs promise results in 90 days or less.

The 4th Principle of Progress: Decreasing Cons to Move from Contemplation Towards Preparation

An encouraging result that the Prochaskas discovered is that the cons need to decease by only half as much as the pros need to increase. In the coaching conversation we can ask our clients to examine how their current behavior is working for them and how it is working against them. What do they lose, what do they gain? Perhaps the best approach here is a positive psychology one—building on the client's strengths. Clients often dismiss or ignore the strengths they have that can make lifestyle improvement more possible. How can the changes that are being considered be catalyzed by the person's strengths? Help your client to see the connection and how making change can pay off.

Another method that the Prochaskas use to help move someone from contemplation towards preparation is what they call correct comebacks. This essentially involves a conversation with your client helping them see the upside of change, often backed by healthy living knowledge. While the way the Prochaskas present this in the book is in more of a point-counterpoint method, a coach approach might be to do this using reframing and powerful questions. Instead of supplying the client with information that shows the advantages of change, the coach may ask the client what advantages they might be aware of or could imagine. This is where a "what would it look like" question might be very effective. *So, if you actually did have the time, what would your ideal way of being more active look like?* Perspective coaching can help the client to reframe their view of a situation from impossible to possible.

As your client begins to seriously contemplate change, you may want to challenge them to look up more information about a course of change and how they would benefit from it. Setting up some accountability around that would lead the client into making a commitment to actually taking a step into the preparation stage.

The 5th Principle of Progress: Use Environmental Reevaluation to Move from Contemplation Towards Preparation

Environmental reevaluation is undertaking consideration of how one's lifestyle behavior affects others around them. It is taking into account the effect that one's more risky health behaviors may have on their family, co-workers, friends, and others. The TTM approach is to encourage our client to look at this both cognitively and emotionally.

Many coaching clients find motivation in wanting to be healthier so that they can be a good role model for their children, live long, and be healthy enough to be around to see their grandchildren grow up and be a resource for them. Clients sometimes learn about the 50,000 U.S. deaths each year from second-hand smoke and completely reevaluate their own smoking habits. Coaches can help their clients to contemplate how their lifestyle and the stress it causes does in fact impact those they care about. We can do so by gently asking powerful questions that get them to look at their own behavior through the eyes of others (perspective coaching). We can ask how their food choices for their family affect not only themselves, but everyone else in the household. Clients who may not be moved forward towards change just for themselves will do so for others they love.

One of our coaching students shared how an epiphany about her own health changed everything for her. She had been living a highly stressful life, working hard, and not engaging in much to support her own wellness. She related how she had always believed that the most important thing in the world was her children. And, all too typically, she often sacrificed her own self-care in order to do everything she could for her children. *"Then, one day I realized that my children were not the most important thing in the world! I realized my own health was. If I'm not healthy enough to be there for my children, then they are really in trouble!"*

The Preparation Stage

Once our client is moving beyond the contemplation stage the temptation for both coach and client is to, again, rush into action. There is a purpose to each of the stages and preparation needs to be consciously addressed to ensure that the client approaches action with the information and preparatory steps that they need.

This is where clients often obtain greater clarity (perhaps through your effective coaching) about what they truly want and need. A client may now be clear that they want to improve their sleeping, but they have little idea about how to do this. Our client at this stage may need sleep hygiene information. Their coach may help them research sleep hygiene strategies that have shown to be effective. Another client may be clear that they want to improve nutrition but are overwhelmed with the mountains of information and misinformation available.

Working within the preparation stage, coach and client can develop steps to find out what approach will work best. Building on the coaching alliance can provide support and reassurance to the client who has always hit this spot in the change process before entirely on their own. They can co-create steps that the client takes to prepare more for change. Agreements about looking up research, checking out resources, inquiring about the considered change with friends can all be set up with accountability to ensure follow-through.

Masterful Moment

Client success with lifestyle improvement often hinges upon the support they get from other people in their life. The opposition or support from partners, spouses, family members, co-workers, managers, and others are often the deciding factors for the client's efforts at change. A more masterful coach anticipates this and inquires, "So, if you move ahead with this change, what pushback do you think you will get?" Clients are usually very aware of the challenges they face like this. It is often one of the biggest reasons that they have not already moved forward with change.

One of the best preparation steps a client can take is to set up a crucial conversation with the parties involved and make an accountability agreement with their coach that the appointment to have that conversation has been set. I have seen this pave the way to success many times. Coach and client can even rehearse that anticipated conversation and to help the client to prepare. Well before the client launches their new action plan, critical groundwork can be laid that increases the probability of success.

The Forever-Preparing Client

Just as we've seen the client stuck in chronic contemplation, we can observe clients who stay busy preparing but never take action. They accumulate healthy-eating recipes, look into every school of yoga imaginable, compare and contrast every weight loss program they can find, read incessantly about alternative ways to be well, and scour the internet with its infinite resources. Like the contemplator who is using delay, so too a person in preparation can delay the risk of taking action while appearing (to themselves and others) to be seriously engaged in attempting to change.

A powerful coaching challenge for the forever-preparing client is the question, *"How will you know that you know enough?"*

What else can be holding our preparing client back? TTM points to the Dread of Failing. So many of our clients have tried and failed many times. There is a real fear that another attempt at change will only result in failure, and perhaps not only embarrassment in front of others, but also harsh self-recrimination. There is the memory of how past failures resulted in such painful outcomes. All of this makes pulling the trigger for action much less appealing.

The TTM approach here is very consistent with the Positive Psychology tactic a more masterful coach would take: helping our client reframe their past failure into a learning experience. By examining the previous ineffective attempt, the coach can help the client take on a new perspective. *"What did work at least through part of the change attempt?"* *"What did you learn that did not work so well so that we avoid repeating that again?"*

Our client's trial-and-error approach may have been the best they could come up with on their own, but it took its toll.

> The problem with trial-and-error learning is that it can be highly inefficient and often ineffective — it takes too many trials and too many errors before the desired change is achieved. This can sometimes increase feelings of demoralization to the point that the person hits bottom. The average smoker and drinker experiences too many trials over too many decades, while inflicting too much damage on their minds and bodies and on the lives of others (Prochaska, J. 0. & Prochaska, J. M., 2016).

Together coach and client can engage in what TTM calls "guided learning," which is much more efficient than simple trial-and-error learning. With a more directive coach approach and building upon the tremendous value of having an ally to rely upon in the midst of change, our client can lower their fears and move forward towards action.

The 6th Principle of Progress: Use Self-Reevaluation to Move from Preparation to Action

The road to wellness is paved with self-reflection. The TTM principle of self-reevaluation encourages clients to look backwards at their life and their behavior, and forward towards the life that they really want to have. The Prochaskas emphasize that this is both an emotional and mental reassessment of the self. They recommend that we urge our clients to ask themselves, *"How do I think and feel about myself as a smoker (or drinker, or non-exerciser, or unhealthy eater) and how will I think and feel about myself if I quit my unhealthy behavior"* (Prochaska, J. 0. & Prochaska, J. M., 2016)*?* This process fits in nicely with the work coaches do helping their clients to create a Well Life Vision.

The Action Stage

So far, you've seen how cautious an effective coach is about rushing our clients into to taking action prematurely.

- Was there a thorough period of exploration?
- Were the pros and cons examined to the point where now the pros are exceeding the cons of change?
- Has our client consciously gathered support from those around them for their change efforts?
- Have the coach and client anticipated what may challenge them in the change process?
- Have they co-created some strategies ahead of time to meet those challenges?
- Has our client done their homework researching the practical and logistical aspects of making these changes, and have they taken some small steps?

Surprisingly, the TTM approach may encourage the person not to take action if they realize they are, in fact, not adequately prepared. "Change when you're ready." We may, however, have finally arrived at the time where commitment to action is the way forward. To move ahead with initiating the change process TTM applies the process of Self-Liberation.

The 7th Principle of Progress: Make a Commitment to a Better Life Through Self-Liberation to Move to Action

Borrowing from the existential therapy of Rollo May, the Prochaskas define self-liberation as "…the belief in your ability to change your own behavior and your commitment and recommitment to act on that belief" (Prochaska, J. 0. & Prochaska, J. M., 2016).

This is where our clients talk about getting their willpower up. All too often our clients depend on willpower alone. They hinge their success on what they frame as strength of character. *"When they do this they overtax the willpower they do have and can easily demoralize themselves by ending up feeling powerless"* (Prochaska, J. 0. & Prochaska, J. M., 2016). Upon finding that lifelong habits take more than just willpower to effect change, our clients may become very self-critical.

The Prochaskas are quick to point out that making a commitment is not the same as making a decision. Commitments, they show us, are something that goes beyond evidence or certainty. Perhaps this is the point where our client needs to make a leap of faith. Waiting upon a certain decision may be waiting for something that never comes. All of our work in health and wellness promotion is really about behaving in ways that increase the probability of enhanced health and wellbeing. That's all. "Self-liberation is an acceptance that we need not be absolutely certain about our course of action; we can still commit and recommit to change" ((Prochaska, J. 0. & Prochaska, J. M., 2016).

How can our client strengthen their resolve? A first step is the very act of sharing it with their coach, making it part of a well-designed Wellness Plan. The very act of writing it down makes it more real, more a true commitment. TTM also points out how going public in some way with our commitment to change is another powerful way to strengthen willpower.

By sharing our action plan with others, we deepen our commitment. We may want to coach our client to be very strategic with whom they share this. A coaching conversation about who would be supportive versus critical of their efforts may be yield better results. Your client may want to choose wisely just how public they want to go. Many clients are afraid that the more public they are, the more embarrassment lies ahead with failure. Social media can be a double-edged sword in this regard.

The upside of extending our sharing is gathering unexpected support. While many of our Facebook friends do not really care to see a photo of the healthy meal you just consumed, clients may find an app that allows a group of like-minded people with the same health goals to share such photos is very supportive. According the app maker

MyFitnessPal, their analysis of user data and user surveys found that "MyFitnessPal users who share their daily calorie counts with friends lose two times the weight, on average, as those who don't share. Users who share their food diaries with 10 or more friends lose four times as much weight as the average—an average of 22.75 lbs. during the total time they spend using the app" (Gannes, 2014).

Making changes in one's life inevitably brings some level of stress and distress. The Prochaskas exhort the importance of being adequately prepared with some stress management strategies to help deal with this and prevent relapse. They have found an especially helpful willpower strengthening tip to apply here. Instead of having only one way to deal with stress have two to three healthy choices. When we're cut off from one strategy (i.e., talking with friends, walking, practicing a relaxation technique) we can draw upon another. They have also found that more than about three choices starts to have a reverse effect by ushering in a feeling of being overwhelmed with too many choices.

Selecting the Actions to Take

Your client has no doubt been told by others (treatment team, friends, loved ones, etc.) what changes they should make to improve their wellness. Chances are great that they have heard it all before. The coach approach is different because we are not adding to that chorus for change. We are keeping the client in charge of choosing how they want to proceed with their own lifestyle improvement. We honor client autonomy. While it may be very tempting to prescribe a course of action, and our clients may actually plead for us to do so, helping our clients come to their own conclusion usually pays off much better.

What we can do, however, is help them to thoroughly explore their alternatives and base their choice in congruence with their values and their interests. There is much more potential for intrinsic motivation when a client is doing something they enjoy. Not everyone is a runner, cyclist, or the so-called gym rat. Perhaps your client would rather start with a walking group, or a dance class. Taking the time to explore a variety of ideas and discover where real interest lies is important.

Your client may also have preconceived notions about what will work best in terms of nutrition or exercise, for example. This is where we can help our clients to determine if they are operating on assumptions, misinformation, or evidence-based information.

The Maintenance Stage

Many of our clients have already been successful at lifestyle improvement. They may have even had multiple experiences of success at weight loss, smoking cessation, stress management, and more. However, success at maintaining those changes has usually been fleeting. Sometimes life events such as increased job or family stress triggered a return to their old lifestyle habits. Helping our clients to maintain their new lifestyle behaviors is where coaches can play, perhaps, their most vital role.

Having the support of a coach during the maintenance stage provides advantages our client may have never had before. Now the client is proceeding with a well-designed action plan, a true Wellness Plan. Now they have a system of accountability than ensures follow-through and consistency. Now they have their coach as an ally who can help them to strategize through the inevitable barriers that get in the way of change. At this time the coach has also been coaching for connectedness, helping the client to garner support in the rest of their life as well.

Lifestyle habits are often rooted in years and years of development and expression. Engaging in new behaviors to break old habits and to establish new ones requires a commitment to patiently persevere. TTM is quick to point out that the "21 days to change a habit" notion is a myth. The TTM uses six months as a criterion for staying in action, based on the amount of time it takes to arrive at decreased difficulty maintaining the behavior change, and therefore less risk of relapse. "The relapse curve does not level off until around six months. These findings convince us that those seeking change should be prepared for six months of concerted action" (Prochaska, J. 0. & Prochaska, J. M., 2016).

A significant challenge to maintaining such change efforts may be the practicality, financial and otherwise, of continuing the coaching relationship during this long period of time. Coaching with an independent coach may become increasingly unaffordable. An employee benefit of coaching may have a limit on the number of sessions. There are a couple of strategies that may be helpful in such cases. As the coaching has reached the maintenance stage, it may be possible to keep the client actively engaged in the maintenance process with less frequent appointments. Spacing out appointments from a weekly to bi-weekly to monthly basis may allow the client to have the benefit of coaching over a longer period of time as the new behaviors are taking hold.

When it is known that the coaching will have to cease before the maintenance stage is complete, the coach and client will be wise to work on how the client can acknowledge their need for vigilant work on this stage and concrete strategies for how to do so. Equipping your client with methods for effective tracking of the new behavior(s), such as a phone app, will be very helpful. Helping the client to develop more social connections to enhance accountability and support will be quite useful. Walking groups, even the social support option on tracking apps, can be resources for your client.

The 8th Principle of Progress: Counterconditioning to Use Substitutes for Unhealthy Habits to Move from Action to Maintenance

TTM makes use of a concept from behavioral therapy known as *counter conditioning*. We can't really unlearn a well-established habit. The old, and in this case unhealthy, habit is already hardwired in our brains along very well-worn neural pathways. However, our efforts at establishing new healthier behavioral habits can inhibit or block an old habit. Over time, these new behaviors become more powerful substitutes for the old neural pathways. The wellness field has long embraced the idea of positive addictions such as running and other healthy behaviors. These healthier behaviors also provide more intrinsic motivation for the client to continue them. Clients can often get very self-critical and impatient when they witness the re-emergence of old behaviors they are trying to eliminate. An understanding of how normal this re-wiring process is can provide reassurance and encourage self-compassion.

The 9th Principle of Progress: Reinforce Your Progress by Using Rewards to Move from Action to Maintenance

The Prochaskas were intrigued by how people attempting to make changes in their lives applied two basic principles of behavioral change: reinforcement and punishment. Studying 1,000 *self-changers* for two years they discovered that people used reinforcement the most in the Action Stage, and rarely relied on punishment. What may be most interesting for coaches is that they also found that subjects in the study "relied much more on self-reinforcement rather than social reinforcement from others" (Prochaska, J. 0. & Prochaska, J. M., 2016). They observed how subjects would report that while they often got lots of admonition and attention from family and friends for the need to change unhealthy behaviors (e.g., smoking), the same people would reinforce the client's efforts at change, but only a few times. It was like they would soon take the person's efforts at change for granted. When we think about it, it seems understandable. The process of change is lengthy and quite a project for the person making the change. It's not really something that others keep on their mind. "You need to be prepared to rely mostly on self-reinforcement or you may be disappointed by how little reinforcement you receive from others" (Prochaska, J. 0. & Prochaska, J. M., 2016).

The wellness coach may be able to add to the positive reinforcement for their client's efforts at change but may be wise to teach the client more about the need for self-reinforcement and how to do it.

Tips for Client Self-Reinforcement

- Learn to immediately use positive self-statements when healthy behaviors are performed. "Way to go! You remembered to check the calories before blindly ordering from that menu." "Super! You got out and walked even though it was raining!"

- Learn to notice (perhaps by tracking) and praise yourself for a reduction over time in the frequency, duration, and intensity of any unhealthy behaviors.

- Use a self-acknowledgment process such as writing down three acknowledgments per day. (See

Encouraging Self-Acknowledgment—Coaching
Experiment in Chapter Seven)

The 10th Principle of Progress: Foster Helping Relationships to Find Someone You Can Count on for Support to Move from Action to Maintenance

Helping relationships are vital to effective change and in recognizing this, TTM honors the foundational importance of the coaching alliance. The *Client-Centered* approach of Carl Rogers is embraced, and the facilitative conditions that we have featured in all of our coaching work are what make the coach a true ally in the change process. Unconditional positive regard, empathic understanding, and warmth and genuineness, from the coach, help make the coaching relationship work.

People who are successful at change also seek out formal and informal social support. Maintaining behavioral change long after coaching terminates is greatly dependent upon the kind of positive support people receive from others. Finding at least one other individual our client can confide in and feel true and lasting support from may be vital. This is where coaching for connectedness may solidify the support the client will need on their own for lasting lifestyle change.

The 11th Principle of Progress: Increase Personal Freedom Through Social Liberation by Noticing Social Trends to Move to Maintenance

"Social liberation is the process by which changes in society increase the options and opportunities for individuals to live healthier and happier lives" (Prochaska, J. 0. & Prochaska, J. M., 2016). There is no doubt that social and environmental factors form formidable social determinants of health. "Social determinants of health include factors like socioeconomic status, education, neighborhood and physical environment, employment, and social support networks, as well as access to health care" (Artiga, 2018). The environment in which our client lives, works, and plays can either make it easier or more difficult to change lifestyle behavior in a positive way. At times, coaches may need to help their clients learn how to be better equipped as self-advocates for their own wellness.

We can help our clients:

- Explore more options for better healthcare services.
- Find a way to be more appropriately assertive about their working conditions.
- Discover ways they can work with others in their community to make it a healthier place.

TTM also recognizes the power of positive social networks. The Prochaskas recommend helping clients to assess the positive or negative aspects of their social networks. How are they working for, or against their wellness? How can our client surround themselves with peer health norms that enhance their efforts at change? Making more positive social networks a conscious part of the client's Wellness Plan may be what catapults the client to not just initiating change, but more critically, to maintaining it.

The 12th Principle of Progress: Practice Stimulus Control to Manage Your Environment to Make Healthy Habits Automatic and Move to Maintenance and Beyond

TTM recognizes how "…unhealthy habits fall under the category of stimulus control when the presence or absence of something causes an action or behavior" (Prochaska, J. O. & Prochaska, J. M., 2016). In wellness coaching we can help clients realize how these connections show up in their lives by effective exploration that leads to insights. A client may explore their typical pattern of behavior in the evening when they return home from work and discover that they are triggered by certain environmental cues. Our overweight client may be stimulated to do unhealthy snacking right after watching a particular commercial on television, for example. Once identified, these automatic responses can be noticed, and a healthier response substituted.

Coach and client can work together to both identify these triggers and to strategize ways to break the cycle of stimulus and response. A common strategy might be to remove the unhealthy snacks from the house. I confess that I truly cannot allow organic corn chips into my home! This is just like the smoker or tobacco user who rids their home of such temptation. Instead, placing positive cues in more accessible places, such as moving fresh fruit onto the kitchen counter where it can be seen more easily, may stimulate a healthier behavior to take place.

The Termination Stage

How can our client realize that they are finally beyond the work of maintenance and can enjoy having arrived at their destination? At this point our client is no longer needing to work on changing; they can embrace the fact that these new behaviors are part of them now. It is no longer "What I'm working on;" it's "Who I am."

Coaching around the termination stage centers around two primary tasks:

1. Determining if we are indeed at the stage of termination.

2. Accepting the spiral (rather than linear) nature of change and preventing relapse as much as possible.

One of the key ways that I have found to help clients realize that they are in this final stage of change is to experiment with their tracking of behavior and see how consistent they can still be with their new healthy habits. Do they have to count every calorie now, or are they so good at meal planning, preparation, and choice that they continue to get the healthy results they want without laborious calorie counting? Can they let go of their close tracking or do they find that they still have to maintain it to be successful?

Are they finding that their old habits have lost much of their appeal, and their new positive health habits have much more intrinsic desire? Doughnuts taste too sweet now. Certain foods just seem too greasy. Being sedentary for too long feels very unpleasant.

The TTM's three criteria for termination of the old behavior and adoption of the new behavior are:

1. There is zero temptation to return to the previous behavior habit.

2. The individual has full confidence or self-efficacy that they won't return to the old behavior.

3. The individual is so comfortable with the change that they no longer have to make any effort to keep from relapsing.

Just as with the maintenance stage, we often don't get to continue coaching our clients all the way to the termination stage or do so for only some of the changes they want to make. Here it is important when preparing for the termination of coaching to equip our clients with some knowledge about how they can recognize their arrival in the termination stage. It is also important to help them be self-compassionate and realize that it is entirely normal to slip on that spiral staircase of change and have to climb back up again. Doing so with some understanding of the importance of each stage in the transtheoretical model of behavior change may prove very helpful to them.

Enhancing Goal Setting and Planning with TTM and WM360° ™

The Wellness Mapping 360° Methodology™, which I describe in my earlier book (*Wellness Coaching for Lasting Lifestyle Change*), goes beyond simple goal setting and emphasizes a fully integrated Wellness Plan completely co-created by the client and the coach. Areas of focus are identified and selected, then goals that will help attain the desired changes in each area are determined. Action steps are strategized and agreed upon with a system of accountability for each. Thus, we are not confusing goals with the action steps that help us to accomplish those goals.

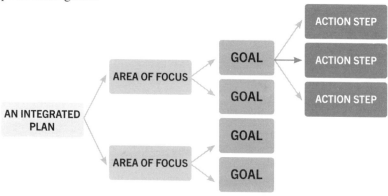

FIGURE 17—THE WELLNESS MAPPING PROCESS

Implementing all that we know about the transtheoretical model of behavior change in the selection of areas of focus and goals is crucial to the success of the Wellness Plan. Greater success can be attained initially by selecting areas of focus where the client is in the stages of preparation, action, or maintenance. As we know from studying the work of James Prochaska, a client can be in a different stage of change for each behavior. The client who is ready to begin modifying their diet today (action stage) may be only in contemplation about exercising and need further coaching to explore this. For areas of the person's life where they are still in precontemplation or contemplation, coaching may still address these areas, as we have seen, but they would not be included (yet) in the actual Wellness Plan. The coach could still work with their client to help them move from precontemplation to contemplation, or from contemplation to preparation, by setting small steps (goals and action steps) to move to the next stage. They could do this by helping their client to increase their knowledge of the pros, set aside their defenses, reduce the cons, or by recognizing the impact their risky behavior is having on others.

Starting out with small steps that have the highest probability of success helps to bolster self-efficacy. "Nothing succeeds like success!" is the oft-quoted coaching maxim. As the client experiences Bandura's mastery experiences, regardless of how small they may be, self-efficacy grows. As both Prochaska and Bandura have noted, success in one healthy behavior reinforces others. Clients gain confidence in themselves and their capacity for change. They also gain confidence in the coaching process and in the coaching relationship with their coach.

Having achieved success in a particular activity domain can create a more general sense of efficacy to learn in other life situations. To the extent that people consider their self-regulatory capabilities and learning efficacy in their self-appraisals, they will exhibit at least some generality in their sense of personal efficacy across different activities (Bandura, 2001).

A Wellness Coaching Example

Vivian began coaching with me in order to lose weight and get healthier after suffering a mild stroke at middle age. Her physician was vehement about her quitting smoking, as this would give her the strongest medical advantage post-stroke. Vivian's fear was that stopping smoking would drive her to eat more and gain weight instead of losing it. She considered herself in the precontemplation stage of change regarding this.

In co-creating her Wellness Plan we acknowledged the importance of smoking cessation but did not include it as an initial area of focus. To do so would have been, at that point, an exercise in futility. Instead we identified attaining and maintaining a healthy weight and managing stress more effectively as areas to work on. Though Vivian's level of self-efficacy at weight loss was marginal—she had struggled with a roller-coaster history of weight gains and losses—she was bolstered by the idea of having a coaching ally to help her this time. Her medical compliance/adherence was good so that was not an area of focus. We felt we could make progress in these areas first and build from there.

Within her weight loss area of focus we selected improved nutrition and eating habits, and increased exercise/movement as goals to work on. Throughout the coaching process we set specific action steps she would work on and follow up on at our appointments. She also tracked her food intake and her exercise frequency.

As we explored Vivian's life it became clear that managing stress was perhaps the lynchpin to the whole process. Her ups and downs with her eating and exercising all seemed to either be supported or destroyed by the stress she experienced at work. Her weight fluctuated greatly until we finally had a couple of breakthrough coaching sessions in which she gained tremendous insight about how she was adding to her own stress by operating on assumptions about work that were no longer true. She believed she had to work harder than everyone else just to be on the team. I challenged her to seek more support from her superiors who were more than willing to provide it. Her immediate boss even admonished her, "Quit working too hard!" Now the consistency in her efforts to eat better, exercise, and move more increased and the pounds began to drop as did her blood pressure readings.

The winter holidays caused a two-month hiatus in our coaching contact. When Vivian returned to our coaching during a phone appointment her voice almost shook with pride. "You know, I haven't had a cigarette since the day of our last appointment!" We celebrated and acknowledged this great accomplishment that we hadn't even worked on! Vivian's success in finally getting stress under control and losing weight gave her the courage and, yes, the efficacious belief that she could succeed at smoking cessation. She had initiated quitting on her own and continues to be tobacco-free.

Readiness for Lifestyle Change: Integrating Prochaska and Bandura

Several years ago, Deborah Arloski, M.S.W., and I combined our knowledge of the transtheoretical model of change and Albert Bandura's social cognitive theory so that wellness coaches could have a coaching conversation with their clients about lifestyle improvement guided by the best qualities of these two theories. We looked at Prochaska's stages of change and his process of decisional balance (weighing the benefits vs. risks of change) and considered all of this through the more social psychology lens of Bandura. We combined this with our knowledge of coach training and health and wellness promotion gained over the last forty years. The result was the development of a tool for guiding such a conversation—The Readiness For Lifestyle Change Tool©™.

We concluded that these theorists were pointing to seven key factors affecting the ease or difficulty of changing behavior.

To facilitate progress to action, adults need to:

1. Be ready.
2. See that the benefits outweigh risks.
3. Have adequate resources and opportunity.
4. Have enough time and energy.
5. Have sufficient support of others.

6. Believe in their own capacity.

7. Have adequate self-esteem.

We developed 10 statements for clients to respond to on a scale ranging 1-5.

THE READINESS FOR LIFESTYLE CHANGE TOOL™

1= Not True   2 = Rarely True   3 = True at Times   4 = Mostly True   5 = Very True

1. I am ready to make the changes needed in this area of my life.

2. I am capable of making the changes needed in this area of my life.

3. I believe making these changes will improve my life.

4. I have the resources and opportunities that will make these changes possible.

5. Making the changes in this area of my life is worth the time and effort.

6. I have the time to invest in making the changes needed in this area of my life.

7. I am excited to make the changes in this area of my life.

8. I am fearful of what might happen if I do not make the changes in this area of my life.

9. My environment supports me in making the changes in this area of my life.

10. I am choosing to make the changes to this area of my life.

© REAL BALANCE GLOBAL WELLNESS SERVICES, INC. 2020

Although a total score could indicate levels of readiness from low to high, we sought instead to create a tool that would elicit exploration by the client and processing with the coach. As our coaching students applied this tool to their work with clients, we found that the tool is best used in the actual coaching session, rather than it being an instrument suitable for self-completion, i.e., homework. As the coach and client explored each item in the context of a coaching conversation, clients would sometimes resolve ambivalence, and most importantly identify where the strengths were supporting change and where the barriers were located. We discovered the most valuable benefit of using this tool was to help coach and client identify areas upon which the coaching could focus and strengthen.

Pinpointing factors to draw upon as resources of strength supported a positive psychology approach to change. Upon taking stock of all the factors they had going for them and in support of change, clients were able to reduce their fear of moving forward and more willing to commit to change.

Targeting specific internal and external barriers (e.g., not enough time or resources; low environmental support, etc.) could then allow the client and coach to co-create strategies for best dealing with these barriers, addressing them head-on. I would encourage coaches to present each item to their client verbally and explore them together (very easy to do over the phone). Then, together have a coaching conversation around each item to the degree that it seems productive. What often results is a realization that willingness to commit to change in any area is really a combination of degree of self-efficacy (self-beliefs about confidence, capacity), motivation (excitement/fear), decisional balance (pros and cons, worth the effort), and both internal (cognitive/affective) and environmental barriers. With such identification accomplished, the coach and client can co-create stage-appropriate tailored action steps forward as identified earlier in this chapter.

The readiness tool has become one of our students' favorite instruments. Generally, the use of this tool would be reserved for clients who were feeling stuck or ambivalent about making changes in a specific area of their life, rather than being used with all new clients.

The Kaizen Approach to Wellness Coaching

Kaizen is not a theory of human motivation, but rather a strategic methodology to help people be successful at change. Developed as a management style during World War II in the U.S. manufacturing sector as a way to increase efficiency and productivity, the method was largely abandoned after the war. W. Edwards Deming brought the method to post-war Japan to help with rebuilding efforts. There, a little automaker named Toyota embraced the method and...the rest is history. Much of the success of the Toyota Corporation is attributed to "The Kaizen Way."

The word kaizen often translates as improvement or continuous improvement for the better. It is based upon the idea of continuous improvement through small, manageable steps. Neuroscientists tell us that our brains still interpret most all forms of change as threatening and triggering the midbrain's amygdala, which operates our stress response (aka fight or flight). Hence any change seen as sizable is seen as a threat and we react rather than respond. As we do so, our access to our higher brain, our cerebral cortex, is impaired. The kaizen strategy is to keep the change small enough that it is seen as easy, irrefutably doable, and therefore not an amygdala-triggering threat.

Psychologist Robert Maurer, author of *One Small Step Can Change Your Life: The Kaizen Way* (Maurer, 2014), presents this approach to change in a way that coaches can work with. Lifestyle change, as the kaizen approach would contend, often carries the implication of a whole new way of living, or at least revisiting some area of life where there have been emotionally upsetting failure experiences (diets that didn't work, smoking cessation failures, etc.). Clients, as we have said, often make the case for why they cannot change their behavior. The level of change that our client's treatment team is often seeking can be very intimidating, and sometimes very impractical given the barriers a person may face.

Maurer gives the example of a middle-aged woman who is over-weight and showing borderline symptoms pointing towards the development of some lifestyle diseases. Her M.D. wants her to immediately start exercising at the level recommended by the American Council on Exercise. Maurer is consulting with the M.D. and realizes that this woman is a single mother working full time and that attempting to meet such standards immediately is not only completely impractical, but also likely to be very frightening to the woman. Instead he urges the woman to simply begin by walking in place during commercials as she watches television in the evening. This allows the client to begin to do something, at least, and she comes to her next appointment asking to do more.

For the coach, starting our client out at a baby step level may be a very effective strategy. A client who has not exercised at all for years and needs to lose weight may begin by walking. Walking for twenty minutes three times a week will probably not make any significant difference in their weight loss efforts. However, merely initiating a new behavior may be the way to start. Once established, the level of exercise output can slowly be increased to a level where weight loss is experienced.

Breaking through a mindset of helplessness may be one of the biggest benefits of this kaizen approach. Here is an example from a coaching process I used during a training in China with one of our students.

> **Client:** Jenna—approximately 40-year-old high level
> executive and M.D., with a very demanding and
> stressful job. Married and caretaker of an older mother
> who is in failing health.

> **Concerns:** Jenna's health is currently good overall. She
> is slim and healthy but is experiencing the effects of
> too much stress. Difficulty sleeping. Feeling tense and
> anxious. She is worried about her own health since she
> has completely quit exercising or taking any time for
> herself. She would like to take more time to cook for
> herself and family and eat better. Feeling overwhelmed
> by work stress and caretaker stress.

Previous coaching attempts by other coaches in training had tried to help her find ways to return to exercising, get back to working out at a gym, improve her eating, etc. Jenna found nothing that seemed possible given her demanding schedule and obligations.

> **Coaching:** I explored the client's situation and responded
> with empathy and understanding. Together we looked
> at her work and home environments and together
> created a kaizen strategy. "Could you take five minutes
> to go out on your office balcony and simply breathe
> deeply and be quiet?" The client believed this was
> quite possible. Accountability was set around this. This

simple step caused her to break through her "I can't do anything!" thinking.

A six-month follow-up showed that she had begun taking more and more time for her own self-care. She had begun increasing exercise a small amount at a time. She also began using an app on her phone to track water intake and got her husband involved in her lifestyle improvement efforts.

People are experience-rich and theory-poor... people who are busy doing things don't have opportunities to collect and organize their experiences and make sense of them.

—**Malcolm Gladwell**, *The Tipping Point and Blink*,
New York Times interview

Masterful Moment

How competent do I feel about behavioral change theory?

Am I at a point where theory allows me to think on my feet without tripping over the theories themselves?

This chapter was about creating forward momentum, going beyond great listening and helping the client to understand their current reality well enough to make progress on change. We began by helping our client to adequately explore and take stock of their wellness. We made the distinction between merely reporting on current behavior and delving into it in a way that could yield insight and understanding. To help with this process we focused on how the coach can share observations that they have for their client's benefit.

The time and way to go forward is mediated by a sound understanding of the concept of readiness for change. Thus, we took an extensive dive into the transtheoretical model of behavior change. We demonstrated how to apply this to your wellness coaching and introduced the readiness for lifestyle change scale to help you and your client to identify how they can move forward on improving a particular aspect of their lifestyle. Lastly, we looked at how making small changes can be an effective strategy for initiating change by implementing the principles of the kaizen approach.

In Chapter Nine we will learn more about how to coach through the internal barriers to change. Internal barriers are about our attitudes, beliefs, and fears. Addressing the emotional aspects of change are critical to success and we will provide guidelines for how to effectively do process coaching. Beliefs and emotions are often mixed about change so we will delve into the relevance of motivational interviewing and how to apply it in our coaching.

REFERENCES

Arloski, M. (2014). *Wellness coaching for lasting lifestyle change.* (2nd Ed.). Whole Person Associates.

Artiga, S. (2018, May 10). Beyond health care: The role of social determinants in promoting health and health equity. *Kaiser Family Foundation.* https://www.kff.org/disparities-role-of-social-determinants-in-promoting-health-and-health-equity

Bandura, A. C. (2001). Sociocognitive self-regulatory mechanisms governing transgressive behavior. *Journal of personality and social psychology*, 125-135.

Gannes, L. (2014, May 1). Recode: Social sharing makes losing weight contagious. *MyFitnessPal.* https://www.vox.com/2014/5/1/11626338/social-sharing-makes-losing-weight-contagious-finds-myfitnesspal

Maurer, R. (2014). *One small step can change your life: The Kaizen way.* Workman Publishing.

Prochaska, J. O., & Prochaska, J. M., (2016). *Changing to thrive: Using the stages of change to overcome the top threats to your health and happiness.* Hazelden Publishing.

Prochaska, J. O., Norcross, J. C., DiClimente, C. C. (1994). *Changing for good.* Quill/Harper Collins Publishing.

PART THREE
What to Do

Chapter 9—Coaching Through the Internal Barriers to Change

CHAPTER NINE

Coaching Through
the Internal Barriers to Change

How can we walk with our clients through the landscape of emotion and stay on solid and fertile ground? How can we avoid the mud, or even the quicksand of faux counseling/psychotherapy? We want our clients to harvest the insights and benefit from the emotional release that comes from telling their story while feeling heard, understood, and even affirmed. We want them to know that we are true allies who won't abandon them the first time they reach for a tissue.

Coaches, at times, treat the world of feelings like they are all stored in a Pandora's Box. Open the lid and we may be headed straight for disaster. Better to keep it closed tight. I've been alarmed to hear reports of health and wellness coaches who work in systems where they say, "We don't do emotions."

Probably the most challenging territory for coaches who do not have a mental health background is how to perform what the life coaching profession calls process coaching (Kimsey-House, 2018). Sure, it's easy to hear a client say they want to lose 30 lbs. and quickly construct a Wellness Plan that has them increasing activity and improving their diet. Goals and action steps are set up and a system of tracking behavior may be implemented. Sounds great…until your client comes in talking about how they only walked one time last week. They feel embarrassed. They say they are sorry they let you down. And now they are almost crying as they relate how frustrating and painful it has been to be overweight most of their life. Like it or not, you've got to stay with them as they explore these feelings. Shut them down by either changing the subject or non-verbally communicating your discomfort, and you will likely damage the coaching relationship and the client will lose the opportunity to integrate their emotions around this important subject. The client needs to process their feelings.

Exploring both the external barriers to change and the internal barriers is an essential part of most effective coaching. Clients benefit greatly by looking at their own self-defeating behavior patterns and do not always do so dispassionately. It may be essential for a client to ask for support in their life with their lifestyle improvement efforts. Yet, their reluctance to ask for help may be an emotional issue. Its roots most likely do not reach Freudian depths. Your client may simply need to get in contact with their feelings, realize how tender this subject is for them, then, with the unwavering support of their coach, take the risk of reaching out to others.

Process Coaching

More masterful coaching recognizes that it is about the client's experiences of their life as it intersects with this world. Continually there is much to integrate. There is also a great deal of growth that is possible. Laura Whitworth, Henry Kimsey-House, Karen Kimsey-House, and Phil Sandahl, the authors of *Co-Active Coaching* (Kimsey-House, 2018) share this guidance:

These authors urge us to look at feelings as information rather than symptoms. What are they teaching us? Our inescapable humanness demands that we accept the fact that we are emotional beings. Coaches will sometimes avoid delving into feelings as though they were distractions from the real business of coaching. Just as Whitworth, et al. remind us, unless we help our clients work their way through the emotional (internal) level, and perhaps do this first, we may not see real change in actual behavior.

Resolution vs. Relevance

Coaches often cautiously retreat from the affective level for fear of crossing the line into therapy. A client may speak of any manner of unresolved conflicts, a history of trauma, even abuse that they have experienced. It may be about family of origin issues, or any sort of unfinished emotional business. This does not immediately indicate the need for a referral. The reality is that many, if not most, people carry around their unfinished business and function quite well. The challenge for the coach is not to take the bait of problem solving and seeking to resolve these old issues.

The key here is to discover how the emotions of the client are relevant to the progress they are attempting to achieve in coaching. Perhaps a coach and client create action steps in their Wellness Plan, various self-care activities, and yet the client repeatedly holds themselves back from engaging in these. As this is discussed in coaching, an internal barrier may be identified that traces back to their family of origin. Perhaps a critical parent harshly enforced that all work must be done before one does anything for one's self. Doing process coaching around this, the savvy coach seeks not the resolution of all of the feelings and unfinished business with that parent (be they dead or alive). Instead, they coach to help their client gain insight regarding how things learned in the past are holding them back today. If the client is able to gain such insight and translate it into action (moving ahead with self-care) then the process coaching is achieving its goal. If the client continues to only process feelings and does not gain insight or does not succeed in shifting their behavior, then we have probably identified an issue that is significant enough to warrant the encouragement of referral to a counselor or therapist.

Putting It into Words

> **Client:** *You know, I love this idea of taking time for myself to do just what I enjoy, but every time I do, I just feel really guilty.*

> **Coach:** *Tell me more about how this guilt shows up.*

In this example our coach begins by requesting clarification in a very neutral way. This allows the client to go further without having to go in the direction a question would have taken them.

> **Client:** *Well, like last week when I said I would connect with one of my good friends on the weekend and go do something fun. The whole time we were hanging out together I kept thinking about all of the things on my to-do list at home, and how I probably should be doing things for my family instead.*

The coach then responds empathically and reflects feeling. This gives the client permission to go further into the feeling level. The coach is attempting to help the client identify a pattern.

> **Coach:** *That must have really taken some of the pleasure out of being with your friends and trying to have fun. You sound really disappointed.*

> **Client:** *Yeah. I am. We were just trying to relax and enjoy the day and I was only about half into it.*

The coach inquires about past experiences with the same thing.

> **Coach:** *Has that happened before, when you've been unable to fully enjoy the moment like that?*

> **Client:** *Definitely! It seems to happen all the time. I keep thinking of what I didn't get done around the house, and about what is still hanging incomplete at work. It's almost like I can hear my parents, years ago, always pushing me hard to get all of my work done before I could do anything I wanted to do. They were really strict and on top of that they would forbid me to do most of the things I wanted to do anyway.*

The coach again expresses empathy and reflects feeling. The coach is conveying to the client that the coach can handle talking about feelings. This enhances the coaching alliance and builds trust. The coach is also not jumping into problem solving and thereby dampening down the emotions.

> **Coach:** *It must be extremely frustrating having thoughts like that get in the way today.*

> **Client:** *Frustrating indeed. When I think about them, and the hard time they gave my siblings and me, I really can get upset.*

Here the coach validates the client's reality and empathizes. The coach then requests clarification but does so in a directive way that nudges the client back to relevance to their Wellness Plan.

> **Coach:** *Your tough upbringing was very real. It sounds painful to remember those experiences. Tell me more about how it gets in the way of you giving yourself permission to practice more self-care.*

> **Client:** *I guess it keeps me from either planning something good for myself, like how I cancelled getting a massage again last week. Or, when I'm finally out there doing something I want to do to relax and unwind, I distract myself thinking of what I should be doing.*

The coach follows the client's examples by not asking for details, but instead by sharing an observation in a gentle confrontation with the client.

> **Coach:** *Are you hearing how you are allowing all of that history to get in your way today, in the present?*

> **Client:** *Yeah. That's exactly what I'm doing.*

Finally the coach empowers the client to own their decision-making power and enquires how they can provide support. More coaching would then follow.

> **Coach:** *How can I support you in making your own decisions about what's good for you?*

Reflection of Feeling

Through my training experience, I've observed that the coaching skill that shows up the least is reflection of feeling. While coaching can often focus on problem solving, two huge oversights seem to frequently appear: 1) forgetting to express empathic understanding, and 2) reflecting feeling. By not doing these two things coaches can miss tremendous opportunities to enhance the coaching process. When we express empathy and reflect feeling we open the coaching conversation to the emotional realm. This provides a number of important advantages.

1. Acknowledging the emotional side of coaching builds trust and builds the coaching alliance. The client knows that they have a true and courageous ally who is not afraid to deal with what they are feeling. The client doesn't have to hide; they can be true to themselves. When the feelings of the client are honored and met with unconditional positive regard, instead of judgment, the coaching alliance deepens.

2. Acknowledging the emotional side of coaching validates what is figural for the client. In the Gestalt sense of awareness, the emotional component, when strong, is often figural (in front, most aware, occupying more of one's consciousness). If this is avoided, coach and client struggle and tend to focus on the background. Acknowledging the affective is acknowledging what is real for the client.

3. Acknowledging the emotional side of coaching taps into energy! Emotion is often described as energy in motion — E-motion. When the client makes more contact with their emotions, more energy is accessed and can be utilized in the coaching process.

4. Acknowledging the emotional side of coaching connects with motivation! We move on what we are passionate about. We also can address the fear that often results in lack of movement. Clients are not going to progress towards action when they are frozen with fear. Emotion provides the fuel that allows values and priorities to be expressed.

5. As we know, self-efficacy, the degree to which one believes that they can affect change in their life, is pivotal to success in lifestyle improvement. One of Bandura's four ways to build self-efficacy is termed Physiological States. Emotions, moods, physical reactions, and stress levels influence our levels of confidence and our own personal evaluations of our abilities. Anxiety can foster self-doubt, thereby lowering self-efficacy. As we help our clients to safely contact feelings and explore their life-relevance, they learn that they have more control over emotions, and how to interpret and evaluate their emotional states. All of this can have a positive effect on their self-efficacy.

6. Acknowledging the emotional side of coaching builds progress in readiness for change. In the *Transtheoretical Model of Behavioral Change*, the Prochaskas list dramatic relief as the third principle that allows a client to move emotionally out of recontemplation (See Chapter Eight.) (Prochaska, 2016).

Ten Guidelines for Process Coaching

1. The vast majority of your clients are functioning at a level where they can handle emotions well. They can gain insight from talking about their feelings.

2. In your initial discussions with your client about coaching you make it clear in your coaching agreement that coaching is not a

substitute for any form of treatment. (This should be in writing in your coaching agreement form.)

3. Be incredibly clear about the distinction between coaching and counseling/therapy.

4. Get yourself out of the way! But stay with your client. Realize when the difficulty you are having exploring emotions with your client (or your reluctance to) is really about your own feelings. You may have some emotional work to do yourself. You may have come across an area so tender for you that you have to ask the client's permission to not explore this topic and help them find other resources to do so.

5. Use the basic active listening skill — reflection of feeling. Don't just paraphrase what the person says. Offer your observation about the feeling that is apparent in your client as they speak. Helping your client to name what they are feeling leads to clarity and progress. This also opens the invitation to explore the emotional level. It gives them permission to go further into their awareness of their feelings.

6. When your client begins to dive deeper into their history of an emotional issue, presentify it. That is, ask the client to tell you how that experience/history relates to today. *"So, I understand how critical your parent must have been, but how does that affect your taking time for self-care today?"* Remember, relevance over resolution.

7. Ask permission. Don't assume that it's okay with your client to go forth into a new area that is likely filled with emotion. The necessary trust may not be there yet.

8. FAVE: First Acknowledge, Validate, and Empathize. (See Chapter Four.)

9. Allow your client to feel what they feel. Check your temptation to rescue your client when they are still in the shallow end of the pool. Convey your supportive presence as they contact their sadness, grief, joy, or anger. Allow for the expression of emotion before you make any attempt to have them think in a more adaptive or productive way. Reminding a client that they have choice about

their feelings before they emote will usually bring out an angry or resentful response from your client. They will believe that you are trying to shut down their right to express their feelings or that you are judging that their feelings are somehow wrong. If you go toward the cognitive prematurely it may end badly.

Allow your client to go beyond an intellectual conversation about feelings. Connection with feelings often is what allows a shift to take place within your client and through the resultant insight the path to action opens up. Don't ask why the person feels the way they do. Explore it and acknowledge it. Let the client work with their own emotions, with your support and non-judgmental trust. Again, your job is to facilitate their work.

10. Forward the action. Real progress occurs when clients can take their new awareness and translate it into action. Coaches can get stuck on a carousel of feeling exploration that can go on infinitely. Develop your coaching skills for forwarding the action. Ask powerful questions that explore what the client is ready to do about their new awareness. How can they take what they are now aware of and apply it to what they want in their life? How can what they now realize help them make progress towards their goals? Co-create experiments for the client to try out and support them by helping them with ways to be accountable to themselves for carrying it out. Do so while applying readiness for change theory. Do they need to contemplate further and process it with you more? Is it best now to take preparatory steps? What action steps are they ready to move on?

When clients stay stuck in a labyrinth of emotion—when they seem unable to translate their new awareness into action—it is most likely that you are looking at the need for a referral to a counselor/therapist. This, in fact, is one of the best indicators of the client's ability to handle emotion and make great use of coaching…or not.

Staying with your client is critical when they are wading into the deeper waters of feeling. Reassure them that you are right there with them. This alone has a calming effect. Remain as centered as possible and focus on the here and now. Your coaching presence carries the day. If you retreat, the trust with your client can be damaged. Be courageous and stay with them by exhibiting excellent body language and by conveying your presence through active listening skills such as paraphrasing, acknowledgment, and the use of empathic statements.

Emotions and Making Lifestyle Choices

Research in the science of emotion "…reveals that emotions constitute potent, pervasive, predictable, sometimes harmful and sometimes beneficial drivers of decision making" (Lerner, 2015). Part of the coaching journey is to assist our clients in sorting out their feelings so they can make the best decisions possible. That may mean acknowledging the validity and importance of certain emotions.

Think of a client who decides to live according to their values of closeness with their family and turns down the well-paying job offer that would keep them on the road most of every month. Emotional decisions can be just as valid and functional as logical ones. We sometimes call these heartfelt decisions.

So, if our lifestyle choices are a primary determinant of our health and well-being, then how do our emotions affect how we make these decisions? It seems straightforward that making the *right* or *healthy* choice should be a rational process based upon having the best information. Yet anyone in the healthcare or wellness field is keenly aware that clients don't always opt for the best or healthiest lifestyle choices. They often observe clients changing these choices for no apparent reason. One day our client is convinced to start working towards a mostly plant-based diet, and on another day, they show little if any desire to do so. We can explore ambivalence, of course, but what is really going on in our client's decision-making process?

A wellness coach may think that it is their job to get their client to make the *right* lifestyle choices, the evidence-based healthy living standards of information with which we are quite familiar. Making lifestyle choices are like any other decision-making process—they are more complicated than it seems at first. Understanding how our emotional bias fits into this process may help coaches to be less perplexed by some of the self-defeating lifestyle choices we see our clients make.

Emotions are a heavily researched area of psychology, and it is easy to get lost in its vast literature. In a very succinct article, executive coach Svetlana Whitener synthesizes the work of several key researchers and conveys a useful paradigm to coaches to learn from (Whitener, 2018).

Emotions emerge as a response to external stimuli, or the recollection of it, or the imagining of it.

> That stimulus generates an unfelt emotion in the brain, which causes the body to produce responsive hormones. These hormones enter the bloodstream and create feelings, sometimes negative and sometimes positive... So, to review, it's stimuli, then emotions, then hormones and, finally, feelings. In other words, your emotions impact your decision-making process by creating certain feelings (Whitener, 2018).

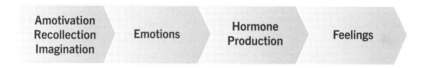

FIGURE 18— GENERATION OF EMOTIONS AND FEELINGS

How we interpret or frame those feelings and how we respond to them results in our choices executed in our behavior.

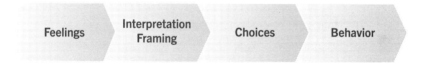

FIGURE 19— FEELINGS TO CHOICES TO BEHAVIOR

In this model it is not the emotions that we are aware of, it is the resultant feelings that we feel. When our clients contemplate making lifestyle changes, they often experience a variety of feelings. They may experience positive anticipation or dread. The memory of past failures may bring up fear resulting in feeling embarrassment, regret, shame, or guilt. Likewise, a history of more pleasant experiences may lead to positive anticipation. What stage of change the client is in may be heavily influenced by the feelings they are experiencing.

Understanding this model can allow the coach to be more patient with the client's decision-making process. It can help the coach to accept the validity of our client's emotions amid their lifestyle decision-making. The coach can also work with the client on exploring different ways to reframe or interpret their feelings. We can then help our clients to attain clarity about their lifestyle choices and help them to follow through with improved lifestyle behavior.

How the Coach Can Help:
Coaching with Emotions and Feelings

Coaching Presence – Your coaching presence sends an ongoing message that either gives permission to explore feelings or denies it.

Notice – Be keenly observant of the emergence of feelings on the part of your client. Be continually scanning not just their words, but how they say them. Hear the changes in tone of voice, volume, rapidity, etc. Notice all of the nonverbal information you can gather.

Contact – Help your client to connect with their feelings. Use the active listening skill of reflection of feelings. Share observations of patterns you see. "I'm noticing that each time you talk about taking time for self-care you begin speaking about your partner."

Name It – Help your client to name their feelings. As we saw above, emotions can generate a wide variety of feelings. Expand your own emotional vocabulary and help your client to drill down to what they are truly experiencing. "Well, it's not really just sadness, it's more like regret."

F.A.V.E. – First **A**cknowledge the client's experience and what they have been through. Then **V**alidate their feelings. It's okay for them to feel the way they feel about it (regardless of how irrational or inappropriate their feelings may seem). You absolutely must not judge their feelings. Most importantly **E**mpathize. Show real empathy and compassion and put it into words.

Process – Help your client to explore and process their feelings. Allow them to expand and talk about them. Once the initial release has taken place, they will usually start to analyze what is going on for them, looking to make sense of (and find meaning from) their feelings. What are they learning from the information these feelings are providing? How does it relate to their situation and their lifestyle choices? This is referred to in TTM as dramatic relief.

Insight – Is your client able now to gain some insight from what they have learned in this process?

Application/Integration – Are they able now to take their insights and turn them into action? Now you can coach your client on ways they can modify their behavior or create experiments in their lives to improve their lifestyle.

Note – If you find that you are answering the questions in the last two items with the negative, your client may benefit more from counseling instead of (or in addition to) coaching.

Relevant Theory—Motivational Interviewing

Improving one's lifestyle is seldom a singular decision arrived at through a simple, logical process. To move forward with an attempt at change often means encountering conflicting thoughts, pulling the client in opposing directions. I would have to say that most of the clients I have worked with have not been terribly ambivalent about improving their lifestyle, and their lives. They have usually been at a point of appreciating the assistance of an ally to help them clarify what they want and to work towards getting it. They have often had to overcome low self-efficacy, all kinds of internal and external barriers, etc. They have not always had the kind of support that they need to succeed, and when this was the case, we could work on building that support. Ambivalence does not always enter into the picture, but when it does, the more masterful coach needs tools, techniques, and an understanding of the change process that can help their client to resolve that ambivalence and move forward. That is where motivational interviewing shines.

William Miller and Stephen Rollick's work with motivational interviewing first emerged in the 1980s with a focus on helping individuals with addiction. Since then it has evolved into an evidenced-based counseling method for facilitating the course of change across a broad range of behaviors. It is supported by many years of corresponding research and randomized clinical trials. As in any methodology, to become truly skillful in the application of motivational interviewing requires training and experience. MI and health and wellness coaching share many concepts, skills, and methods. Here we will provide a theoretical overview and thoughts about its application in wellness coaching and show its many commonalities.

For Health and Wellness Coaches, learning about motivational interviewing can greatly enhance understanding of how to work with ambivalence and resistance to change. Miller and Rollnick emphasize the critical importance of:

- Recognizing ambivalence as a normal human experience.
- Engaging in deep appreciation and respect for everyone.
- Working with ambivalence rather than against it.
- Not trying to rush the process.

In what is probably the single best MI reference, *Motivational Interviewing: Helping People Change, Third Edition*, Miller and Rollnick define MI as "a collaborative conversation style to strengthen a person's motivation and commitment to change" (Miller, 2013) and a form of counseling to effect lifestyle behavior change. Health and wellness coaching is not counseling. However, MI and health and wellness coaching share two critical points of convergence: being client-centered and tapping into the individual's motivation to change. In both, the process is collaborative and honors client autonomy.

Miller and Rollnick describe MI as both client-centered and directive. Its principles are firmly rooted in the client-centered therapy of Carl Rogers and, as such, share a mutual foundation with the coaching field. They seek to help their client to come to their own conclusions about changing rather than trying to convince or persuade their client about what they should do.

Common Ground—Motivational Interviewing and Coaching

My own exposure to MI came long after I had been thoroughly trained in life coaching, and, of course, subsequent to my education and work as a psychologist. The more I learned about MI, the more I was impressed with how similar it was to all the principles of life coaching as defined by the ICF core competencies and the co-active coaching work of Whitworth, Kimsey-House, et al. (Kimsey-House, 2018). I imagined the evolution of coaching and MI as a vision of two people walking down *Carl Rogers Avenue* on opposite sides of the street. After years of walking along the same foundational path they suddenly became aware of each other and were shocked at how much commonality there was in what they both had learned about how to effectively help people change and grow.

If you are already grounded in coaching and delve into learning more about MI you will recognize many of the mutual acquaintances on that same avenue. MI has different terms for many of the same principles, methods, and techniques. This is especially obvious when Miller and Rollnick speak of the Spirit of motivational interviewing, which is very similar to what we call the coaching mindset.

The Spirit of Motivational Interviewing

1. Collaboration (vs. Confrontation)

The MI approach is collaborative and contrasts greatly with other approaches that impose a more hierarchical relationship. MI entered the world of addiction treatment with a radically different way of relating to their clients. The Rogerian Client-Centered foundation put the client in charge of their own life, and the MI counselor in the role of ally, not expert, just as in coaching. Building trust and forming a true alliance with their client enhances the therapeutic process. At the same time the MI counselor and the client may not see the nature of the client's problems or ways of improving them the same way, but what pervades the relationship is the Rogerian concept of unconditional positive regard. MI uses the term absolute worth for this.

2. Evocation (Drawing Out, Rather Than Imposing Ideas)

As we discussed in Chapter One, the coach's job is to evoke, to bring forth from within the client their own wisdom and their own motivation. The MI approach understands that external pressure for change is usually resisted, even when a person may agree that such change would be beneficial. So, rather than imposing the motivation, the commitment to change from the outside, MI seeks to draw out from within the individual their own reasons for change.

Again, we really can't convince or persuade someone to be well. Change from within is recognized as far more enduring. As directive as MI may be in terms of methodology and techniques, it never takes the stance of telling people what to do. MI is directive in that the MI therapist knows where they want the client to go (toward health and wellbeing).

3. Autonomy (vs. Authority)

Coaching always speaks of supporting client autonomy, and, just as we saw in Chapter Six, self-determination theory recognizes autonomy as one of the three basic needs of human beings. Likewise, MI keeps the client "in the driver's seat," encouraging them to make their own choices. MI helps the client to develop a menu of options and then encourages the client to do what works best for them and their lives. The MI counselor, may, however, actually provide the client with a menu of options based upon past success they have had with similar clients. MI is, simultaneously, a client-centered and directive approach.

4. Compassion

There is no better description of this than Miller and Rollnick's.

> To be compassionate is to actively promote the other's welfare, to give priority to the other's needs. Our services are, after all, for our clients' benefit and not primarily for our own. Virtually every major world religion advocates the cultivation and practice of this virtue, to benevolently seek and value the well-being of others. Compassion is a deliberate commitment to pursue the welfare and best interests of the other (Miller and Rollnick, 2013).

Ambivalence

The intent of MI is to help clients move out of ambivalence by choosing one path and then facilitating movement along that direction. Just like our clients, we all know the experience of feeling trapped between two conflicting perspectives. Furthermore, when the story on both sides of the ambivalence remains equally compelling and it feels impossible to choose a direction, often the only relief comes from dropping the topic altogether and focusing elsewhere. As Prochaska would say, "When in doubt, delay."

Not knowing how to effectively help clients navigate that stuck place can decidedly be one of the most challenging and frustrating experiences for health and wellness coaches. Despite all good intentions, ineffective strategies often lead to one or both of two unfortunate outcomes:

- On the client side: a reinforced sense of being stuck or even strengthening the negative side of the ambivalence because they feel demeaned, judged, or criticized.

- On the coach side: exasperation that leads to blaming the client, labeling them as resistant or oppositional and walking away.

Identifying the Language of Ambivalence

MI explores the self-talk that promotes continued resistance to change and inertia. It refers to this as *sustain talk*. Essentially this kind of self-talk sustains the status quo. Change talk "is any self-expressed language that is an argument for change" (Miller, 2013).

The whole MI approach is to be aware of and acknowledge our client's inner and outer dialogue about the pros and cons of change. The coach will be acknowledging the sustain talk that the client is using and supporting the use of change talk that they are hearing.

MI breaks *change talk/sustain talk* down using two acronyms—DARN and CAT. As the client is working through the pre-contemplation and contemplation stages of change, we hear examples of:

Preparatory Sustain Talk:

- **Desire:** characterized by, "I don't want to."

- Ability: characterized by lack of self-efficacy. "I've tried, and I don't think I can." Worries about being able to change.
- Reasons: characterized by client identifying barriers and a lack of perceived benefit. "I don't have time." Counter arguments.
- Need: characterized by client's perception of need for the current habit. "I have to smoke. I can't go without it."

We hear these arguments from our clients as they make the case for why they cannot change. Ironically the same DARN acronym shows up again on the change talk side of ambivalence representing the client's desire, ability, reasons, and needs for change to take place.

Preparatory Change Talk

- Desire: characterized by "I really want to." Expressing a wish to succeed.
- Ability: characterized by greater feelings of self-efficacy. "I've had some success before. I think I can do it this time."
- Reasons: characterized by client minimizing barriers and recognizing perceived benefit. "I believe I can find the time, and it will help me be healthier."
- Need: characterized by client's perception of their need for overcoming the current habit. "I really want to be smokeless around my grandchildren." May overlap with Reasons, but feels more imperative, more of the emotional argument for change.

So, our ambivalent client is teetering back and forth between the DARN aspects of sustain talk and change talk.

As the coach hears their client give voice to this internal debate, they respond without judgment, reflecting back to the client what they are hearing. All the while the coach is guiding the client away from sustain talk and towards change talk.

D.A.R.N.	CHANGE TALK	SUSTAIN TALK
DESIRE	It would be great to be able to get down on the floor and play with my grandchildren and then get up easily. I would love to do that.	I just can't do what I used to be able to do. I'm just getting old. Everyone gets out of shape as they age.
ABILITY	Sure, I'm not as flexible as I used to be, but I can still touch my toes, walk easily, and can even dance! I guess I could start looking into yoga and such.	I'm really stiff in the morning, and, well, most of the day. I have to sit a lot on my job and then I ache when I start moving.
REASONS	My grandchildren are so much fun to play with and they won't be young forever. I don't want to lose my ability to move well and become a burden for others. I might have less headaches and backaches too.	I have to get to work early so there's no time to stretch or exercise in the morning, then when I get home, I've got to make dinner and then I'm just exhausted. Watching TV is about all I've got the energy for.
NEED	I've really got to start doing something to help with flexibility. I'm not getting any younger. I can't keep on doing less and less.	I've got to just accept that it's all part of growing old. I get along just fine in daily life. I don't need to take classes to learn how to move my own body.

Despite the emergence of more change talk, there is still no real indication that change is going to take place. Saying one *wants* to lose weight is not the same as stating that one *will*. As they say, talk is cheap, but it is a critical start. Taking the MI process further is all about *mobilizing change talk*. This kind of commitment language involves Commitment, Activation, and Taking Steps, CAT.

If our client is not ready to change and is still resistant to efforts at change, we will hear the sustain talk side of CAT.

- Commitment: An assertion that the client is going to remain the same. "Forget exercise. I hate it and I'm not doing it." "No more stupid diets! That's final."

- Activation: Expressing an unwillingness, a lack of readiness. Willing to accept the consequences of no change.

- Taking Steps: Action in the opposite direction of healthy change. "I canceled my enrollment in that dance class." "I returned the bicycle I bought last week."

Mobilizing Change Talk

- Commitment: Signals likelihood of change taking place. "I will…." "I intend to…." Shows a decision to proceed with change, even if there is still some doubt.

- Activation: Movement towards action. "I'm ready to...." "I'm okay with…." "I'm willing to…." Not a complete promise, but an implied commitment.

- Taking Steps: Client is speaking of taking some kind of steps towards actual change. They are reporting what they have already done. "I enrolled in that tai chi class yesterday!" "I checked out membership at three different fitness centers."

The MI Hill

Don't be unnecessarily concerned with classifying the change talk you hear. The important thing is to recognize it. Just by virtue of being social animals people already have an intuitive sense of how this works. We can suggest that change talk is a bit like walking up one side of a hill and down the other. The uphill side represents preparatory change talk (like DARN), and the downhill side is mobilizing change talk (like CATs). One thing to ask yourself during a session is where you are on the hill (Miller, 2013).

Miller and Rollnick see the preparatory change talk up the hill as part of the pre-contemplation and contemplation process. Then, hopefully at some point, you and your client crest the hill and begin to hear more and more mobilizing change talk. This shows that your client has moved into the preparation and action stages of change on the downhill side.

I appreciate it when Miller and Rollnick urge us, "Don't be unnecessarily concerned with classifying the change talk you hear" (Miller, 2013). MI has a plethora of classifications of terms and concepts, skills, and methods. For the beginner it is easy to get lost in them. With practice, the process becomes more natural, especially as you realize how much it has in common with the coaching process with which you are already familiar. There is an applicable quote here, usually attributed to George Bernard Shaw or Oscar Wilde:

"Britain and America are two nations divided by a common language."

One place where MI and coaching use disparate terminology to say essentially the same thing is in the area of skills. Again, keen on acronyms, MI speaks of using OARS skills to row the communication boat. OARS skills are adapted from the client-centered model.

OARS—Open-ended Questions: Affirmation, Reflection, and Summarize

OARS—Open-ended Questions: Just as in coaching, open-ended questions are used to help the client explore and elaborate. Closed questions are avoided as much as possible.

OARS—Affirmation: In coaching terminology this is the active listening skill of acknowledgment. Here we are recognizing and acknowledging the client and their experience. The coach will be seen to support and encourage the client without resorting to praise, per se. The relationship needs to be maintained as that of equals, with the coach not holding a one-up position handing out praise or withholding it. "In general, avoid affirmations that begin with the word 'I,' because these focus more on you than on the client. 'I am proud of you,' for example, may be well intentioned and even well received, but clearly has parental overtones. Like good reflecting, good affirming usually centers on the word 'you'" (Miller, 2013).

OARS—Reflection: A primary MI skill, reflection includes the active listening skills of paraphrase and restatement, and reflection of feeling. "The essence of a reflective listening response is that it makes a guess about what the person means" (Miller, 2013). That seems about as simple as it gets, but they make an excellent follow-up point. "But why not just ask people what they mean? Pressing people with questions to explain themselves and their meaning actually seems to distance them from what they are experiencing. They step back to analyze and begin to ask whether they really do or should feel what they have expressed" (Miller, 2013). I would add that doing so may also weaken the coaching alliance causing the client to assume implied criticism, or by bringing out a defensive need to justify what they have expressed.

There are five varieties of reflection in the MI lexicon.

1. **Simple Reflection:** a rephrasing of what the client has said.
   Example:
   Client: *I'm feeling kind of anxious today.*
   Coach: *You're feeling sort of tense.*
   This can be the use of the active listening skills of paraphrase, restatement, or reflection of feeling. You are keeping the reflection quite simple and if relied upon too much the coaching doesn't seem to gain any forward momentum.

2. **Complex Reflection:** This is a reflection inferring a meaning and/or emphasis to what the person has said. You could be making a guess about the unspoken content of the client's communication. This could be an example of the active listening skills of reflection of feeling or using intuition.
   Example:
   Client: *I know I should get my bloodwork done and get in to see my doctor. I guess I'm better off staying ignorant about what's going on.*
   Coach: *Sounds like it reminds you of how your father found out about his diabetes, and that's very scary.*

3. **Amplified Reflection:** Reflecting this way when the client is offering sustain talk is intended to evoke a shift to change talk (and such thinking). The coach amps up the intensity of the client's statement when

they essentially paraphrase what the client has said. The coach will tend to use absolutes such as any, none, impossible, couldn't possibly be better, etc. This way of taking the client's statement to an extreme gets the client to essentially challenge their own perspective. Example:

Client: *I don't have time to exercise at all. Every minute of my day is booked!*

Coach: *I hear you saying that it's impossible for you to fit any extra movement into your schedule.*

4. **Double-Sided Reflection:** In this kind of reflection the coach has an opportunity to both acknowledge the sustain talk of their client, validating how real it is for them, and then to offer a different perspective by drawing upon the client's previous change talk. Example:

Client: *Doing these rehabilitation exercises hurts so much! I don't think my knees can take it anymore.*

Coach: *The rehab stretches are really painful, that's for sure, and I know how important you've said getting your full range of motion back is to you.*

5. **Shifted Focus Reflection:** When it seems that coach and client have reached an impasse on a particular topic, the coach might decide to strategically shift to a topic where there is less resistance. Example:

Client: *Eating more fruits and vegetables is going nowhere. My family just doesn't want to change, and I guess neither do I.*

Coach: *So, changing diet is not working out right now. Let's move on to talking about the walking group you started participating in.*

Summarize: To summarize is, of course, to use the active listening skill of summarization. MI goes on to break summarization down into three types and shows the value of each. An important point that Miller and Rollnick make is that we can never summarize everything a client says. So, we have to make a judgment (in their context they would call it a clinical judgment) about what to summarize and what not to.

1. **A collecting summary** recalls a series of interrelated items as they accumulate.

2. **A linking summary** reflects what someone has said and links it to something else you remember from the prior conversation.

3. **A transitional summary** wraps up a task or session by pulling together what seems to be important.

All summarizations can be combined with affirmations that might, for example, link it to someone's strengths or assets they have that will help them to succeed at change. When we summarize, we are helping our clients stay focused and we are, as we said in our section on active listening skills, showing evidence that we are listening well. In the MI book for health professionals (Rollnick, 2007) the example of a bouquet is used. The MI coach collects all the little DARN change talk statements (flowers) and pulls together a bouquet of flowers presenting them back to the client. Hearing their own arguments for change in this way helps further the client's movement towards change.

When change talk begins to shift towards preparation for taking action it is time to do more than just continue to elicit change talk. This is very much like what coaching terms forwarding the action. Now we are shifting from evoking change to planning.

The Foundational Principles of Motivational Interviewing

These principles move clients towards action. "When the client entertains that change is possible and change talk starts, motivation is tapped into, and this can lead to developing action steps for change. The small wins towards change create a spiral towards sustaining goals that can lead to new goals, new relationships, and new insights about what is possible" (Miller, 2013).

1. Express Empathy

Perhaps nothing helps develop rapport and shows acceptance of our client like the expression of empathy. Empathetic understanding is one of the facilitative conditions of therapy that Rogers spoke of and that we have adapted (Chapter Four) as one of the primary facilitative conditions of coaching. Miller and Rollnick define empathy as "the extent to which the clinician understands or makes an effort to grasp the client's perspective and feelings: literally, how much the clinician attempts to 'try on' what the client feels or thinks" (Miller, 2013).

2. Develop Discrepancy

Work with clients so they discover how their current behaviors may not match their values. Help them see how they want their life to evolve. So, I hear you saying that you really want to set a healthy example for your children, yet would you say that the way you relate to food is doing that?

MI sees developing a perception of discrepancy as a key motivator of change. Miller and Rollnick originally saw this as the psychological concept of cognitive dissonance. They found that a simpler way was to think of it "…as a discrepancy between present and desired states; the distance between a personal goal and the status quo. Goal-status discrepancy is one of the most fundamental drivers of motivation for change" (Miller, 2013)(Ford, 1992).

Miller and Rollnick point out that many of our clients show up aware of these kinds of discrepancies in their lives, especially when it comes to health behavior. Smokers know it is bad for them. Overweight and obese people are usually very aware of how their weight does not line up with the kind of healthy life they want to live. So, Miller and Rollnick ask, why doesn't this awareness of discrepancy lead to change? They convey a point that is very important for health and wellness coaches to grasp. The degree of discrepancy needs to be just right to encourage change. "If the discrepancy is too small, it may not appear important enough to prompt action. If it is too large, the needed change may seem beyond reach" (Miller, 2013). Low self-efficacy can be a huge factor as well in preventing movement towards change despite a perception of discrepancy.

Awareness of such discrepancy may actually be how the client recognizes their ambivalence about change. Change talk often initiates discrepancy awareness. A trusting client-centered relationship of acceptance, non-judgment, and empathic understanding helps the client open up to discrepancy with less defensiveness.

3. Roll with Resistance

When we think of resistance, we often think of it as defiant or oppositional. It's easy to demonize it.

> There is nothing inherently pathological or oppositional about sustain talk. It is simply one side of ambivalence. Listen to an ambivalent person and you are likely to hear both change talk and sustain talk intermingled. When ambivalent, people naturally voice sustain talk in response to their own or others' arguments for change. To call this "resistance" is to pathologize what is a perfectly natural part of the process of change (Miller, 2013).

Miller and Rollnick found that the exhibition of much of what we call resistance depends upon what the counselor (coach) is doing. When we try to counter our client's sustain talk with arguments about why the person should change, when we are correcting them, or interrogating them, clients will dig in their heels and become defensive. They will resist even more. When a client starts to express sustain talk again, the coach knows they are pushing too hard and need to be more patient and roll with it.

So, what MI discovered long ago is what I've termed a coaching Aikido move. They roll with resistance. Rolling with it means turning alongside your client, so to speak, as opposed to butting heads with them. You turn and look at what they are saying from their point of view. You acknowledge what they are saying, validating their feelings.

> **Client:** *I know I'm not getting nearly enough sleep, but I really enjoy finding late night shows to watch. I've learned some very interesting things. It takes me forever to wind down anyway.*

> **Coach:** *So, even though you're up late, you're finding some real value in how you spend that time.*

> **Client:** *Yeah, I don't think people need as much sleep as doctors say. I'm a night owl. I like how quiet and peaceful it is late at night.*

Coach: *There's a lot you enjoy about staying up late. Tell me what you know about what doctors say about getting enough sleep.*

Rolling with resistance is not the same thing as collusion. We're not agreeing with our client that their unhealthy habits are okay. What we are doing is allowing them to process the pros and cons of change, to go back and forth with their ambivalent process of sustain talk versus change talk. If we don't allow the sustain talk to be fully expressed, and that includes on the emotional level, then resistance is likely to heighten. When we roll with it, communication keeps rolling and the client feels freer to explore their thinking. Eventually, we can support the change talk as it emerges. We can ask questions that help the client consider new perspectives without imposing them on the client.

Coaches speak about this process when they talk about dancing in the moment. It means going with your client in a dance-like fashion rather than wrestling with them. "It is said that people do not resist change, but resist being changed" (Miller and Rollnick, 2013).

4. Support Self-Efficacy

MI recognizes the crucial role that self-efficacy plays in determining the likelihood of change occurring. As we saw in Chapter Six, the work of Albert Bandura showed us that our client's belief in their own capabilities to effect change has a profound effect upon their motivation to improve their lifestyle. Supporting the growth of the confidence that their wellness efforts will pay off and that they can succeed at executing them becomes a major focus of the MI approach as our clients move forward.

The practice of MI also has four more guiding principles that coaches will find helpful. Loving acronyms, MI refers to these as **RULE**.

R: Resist the Righting Reflex with Clients

Imagine you are in a session with your wellness coaching client and they mention how a particular dietary habit is perfectly fine for them to do as they struggle to manage their diabetes. As a well-informed wellness coach who is aware of solid, evidence-based healthy living guidelines, you immediately rush to correct your client's faulty eating practice. While you may be absolutely correct, how did your need to set your client right affect the coaching conversation, and perhaps the coaching alliance? People don't like to feel corrected and usually resist what sounds like persuasion, especially when they may be ambivalent anyway. It may have felt quite authoritarian to your client. Will they shut down and pull back? Will they get defensive and argue with you about your point? Will the interruption caused by you exercising your righting reflex cause the flow of the conversation to be completely disrupted?

It is much about timing. If you can catch yourself in time, note what your client is saying and return to it later, at a more neutral time when your client may be more receptive to exploring alternative information.

For the coach, the righting reflex is a holdover of the educating or consulting mindset. Our default setting causes that reflex to fire just as surely as a physician tapping someone's knee with a rubber hammer makes the leg kick. Catching ourselves and staying in our coaching mindset saves the day.

U: Understand the Client's Motivations

Staying true to client-centered principles, MI recognizes that it is the client's own motivations that trigger change, not the urgings of the person in the helper role. The MI counselor, or the wellness coach using this MI guiding principle, will work to evoke from within the client the values, concerns, and perceptions that drive motivation. Again, there is recognition that we are not there to motivate our client, but to help them discover their own motivations.

L: Listen to the Clients

Clients often expect the professional to have all the answers and direct them in ways that will result in successful change. As directive as MI is, it remains dedicated to listening to the client as much, or even more than informing them. The real answers are there within the client to be evoked and discovered. There is a real emphasis on coaching active listening skills, and operating, once again, from a coaching mindset.

E: Empower the Client

MI recognizes that the client is the ultimate authority on their own life. They know how best to implement the kinds of changes that will improve their lives. The coach's challenge is to help them discover strategies to do so with the client in the lead. We coach supporting client autonomy. We coach supporting self-advocacy. As clients find their own answers and get validation and support from their coach, behavior change starts to take root.

Integrating MI and Wellness Coaching

Motivational interviewing is a separate methodology from coaching with its own research and language. At the same time, most health and wellness coach training programs integrate at least some of it as a core method. MI is most often recognized by coaches as a useful tool for helping our clients to resolve ambivalence. The more masterful coach, with a lifelong dedication to continuous improvement in their knowledge and skills, will find a great deal in Miller and Rollnick's book *Motivational Interviewing: Helping People Change, 3rd ed*. Within all of the ways that the authors break down MI into principles, acronyms, and the like, and weave profoundly astute pearls of wisdom about how any helping professional can do their work better and hone their craft.

Masterful Moment

How can you blend aspects of MI into your own coaching style? What elements do you find real value in? You may discover that you already coach using all of the types of reflection, for example, without consciously categorizing them in MI terminology. There may be other times when you very consciously reach for the utility of an MI method. Think of coaching and MI as not an either-or, but rather as a "yes-and" inclusive approach.

Coaching Caution —The Limits of Coaching

While coaches often shy away from the affective domain, there are also coaches who are more than willing to jump into the territory of emotion. I was alarmed when I discovered a group of coaches who, on their website, promised "deep emotional healing." It did not appear that any of them were licensed mental health professionals, yet they were inviting clients to come to them to deal with their trauma. As a psychologist who has dealt with the full range of mental health problems and crises, I believe it is far beyond the scope of practice for coaches to enter this realm. It is dangerous and unethical for coaches who fancy themselves as "healers" to offer such misleading services.

Increasingly, licensed mental health professionals are adapting coaching methodology to their work, and are able to do so within their scope of practice. It does not work the other way around for coaches without such professional education and licensure to attempt to practice in the realm of counseling and psychotherapy. Coaches who have familiarized themselves with any of the numerous psychological self-help books on the market should not think that this prepares them to engage in coaching using such methods. These self-help books are often of great value to individuals and can be grounded in excellent theory and research. A coach, however, should not think that once they have read such books, or even attended a workshop on such topics, that they are in any way qualified to delve into these methods in coaching. Even the authors of these books would be the first to advise that the coach leave work on family of origin issues, deep shame, trauma and abuse, etc., to the qualified professional. An article in *Psychology Today*, entitled "Life Coaches and Mental Illness," looks more deeply at how coaching is being applied in this area and underscores some of the cautions that coaches should be mindful of (Ley, 2014). The author goes on to state that "By and large, I think this is a positive trend, emerging in response to need. However, there are important issues to consider, as coaching intersects more explicitly with mental illness" (Ley, 2014). He enumerates serious concerns about

- Ethics and boundaries
- Client abandonment
- Confidentiality

- Liability
- Medical and medication issues
- Suicide
- Self-care, and
- When coaches are in over their heads—knowing when they are in need of consultation.

Coaches can often coach effectively with mental health patients, if they limit their work to coaching and leave the counseling to the mental health pros. In fact, mental health patients, as a whole, have health statistics that indicate a much greater struggle to be healthy and well. Rates of obesity, smoking, and chronic illness among these populations are higher than the average. Access to wellness coaching could potentially be of great benefit to people with mental health challenges. A wellness coach can be part of the support team that helps a mental health patient work on improving their lifestyle, their organizational skills, finding needed resources, and more.

It is very common for coach and client to discover that additional services are needed. These may include seeking the help of:

- A dietician, nutritional therapist
- Fitness trainer
- Couples counselor
- Career counselor
- A qualified mental health professional

The key is for the coach to support these additional services and draw a distinction about whom and what to seek guidance about.

Coaching a Client Through to a Mental Health Referral Using the Stages of Change

Times arise when it becomes apparent to a wellness coach that their client would benefit from working with a mental health professional. In 2018 the International Coach Federation created a whitepaper (available as a PDF) entitled "Referring a Client to Therapy: A Set of Guidelines" that provides a useful definition.

Making a referral means inviting a client to discuss referral, co-creating options, and empowering the client to take action by identifying resources or making an appointment. A referral to another helping professional is warranted when a client delves into an issue that goes beyond a coach's competency level (The International Coach Federation, 2018).

I am particularly pleased with how this ICF project committee chose their words in their definition. The referral process is not a sudden abandonment of our client. It begins with an invitation to discuss the topic—together. It shows us that as coaches we work with our client to co-create options. We empower our client to take action with concrete steps that we help the client to follow. We can see that making a referral is also a process, not an event.

The need for referral may be urgent and involve client safety as when there is a threat of harm to self or others. That rare situation is more clearly recognized, referral is made, and coaching is usually terminated. Standard reading for every coach should be the "Top Ten Indicators to Refer a Client to a Mental Health Professional," also an ICF resource available as a pdf (Meinke, 2017). This article provides excellent guidance for recognizing the signs of serious depression, harm to self or others, etc. While coaches who are not licensed mental health professionals should never be placed in a position where they are responsible for any kind of mental health screening, a familiarity with these indicators is a must.

More common is the situation where the client raises issues presenting no immediate danger or threat, but indicates either a history of unfinished emotional issues, or current circumstances that are creating barriers for the client's effectiveness at succeeding at lifestyle improvement. In such situations, having a thorough working knowledge of the difference between coaching and therapy is essential for a professional coach.

When the issues are beyond the scope of coaching and are interfering with client progress, then extending that invitation to discuss a referral needs to be made. How to make this referral work successfully is not as simple as explaining the benefits of therapy and providing resource information. Often clients are ambivalent, or even outright resistant to a mental health professional referral. The thought of reconnecting with all of the unpleasant emotion involved in working directly on their issues in therapy brings up fear. Unfortunately, coaches sometimes drop such a client quickly when they are not ready to jump into action and seek out the therapy from which they would benefit. Such a client would benefit from a coach who implements a stages of change approach.

As we mentioned in the last chapter, James and Janice Prochaska make the point that most of the people we all work with are not in the action stage of change on any particular behavior. They estimate that only about 20% are actually ready to jump into action. Why would this be any different when it comes to engaging in counseling or psychotherapy? Yet, sometimes, when the client balks at following through on a psychological referral, coaching is abandoned. Instead, think of it as our job to help the person to weigh the pros and cons of engaging in counseling as they sit in the contemplation stage of change. We are helping them with decisional balance. Taking a page from motivational interviewing, we coach as they work through their ambivalence. We want to roll with resistance instead of accepting it as a rejection of our referral recommendation.

Coach Through to Referral

Coach: *So, I hear your hesitancey when I suggest that counseling might be the best way forward with this.*

Client: *Well, yes. I've been in counseling before and I don't know if I want to open up that whole issue again.*

Coach: *Sounds like you possibly have some fear about talking about such uncomfortable subjects again.*

Client: *Yeah. Growing up in my home was not a pleasant thing!*

Coach: *I know it holds a lot of negative memories for you. You've shared some stories about how bad it was. Yet, I also hear you saying that it's frustrating to have these things hold you back from doing what you want to do today to be healthy and well.*

Client: *Right! It's really frustrating! I know I need to get more active and take more time to eat right, but then I feel so guilty when I take time for myself.*

Coach: *So, on the one hand you really want to make these improvements to your lifestyle, but when you attempt to do so, these barriers, these thoughts get in the way.*

Client: *Exactly! I appreciate your help, but it seems like whenever we set up action steps, I never follow through on them, even though I know I need to.*

Coach: *Yes, we've explored how it's all related, but we still seem stuck. What do you think would be the benefits if you did get back into counseling about this?*

Client: *Well, I guess I could really open up about it and try to unload some of this frustration. I'm just so tired of having the past hold me prisoner!*

Coach: *So, a counselor could actually help you explore that and really make some progress in this area, perhaps result in some relief.*

Client: *Yeah. Okay. So, what's next?*

Coach: *Let's work together on reconnecting you with some counseling. Let's see what steps you can take to find the resources you need.*

In this example the coach meets the client where they are. They help their client to contemplate the idea of returning to counseling. Acknowledging the client's fears and validating their feelings, the coach helps the client to begin to weigh the reasons to return to counseling and the reasons to avoid it. The family of origin stories are referenced, but not delved into deeply. Instead, the emphasis is on relevance. How the past is getting in the way of the present is the essence of the contemplation. Then, at the end of the example we begin to move into the next stage of change: preparation.

Coaching works because we are the client's ally through the whole behavioral change process. When referral comes up, we remain their ally. Then to help them actually follow through and make it to the referral resource, we help them with the process of identifying such resources, making the appointment, and attending the appointment. We offer support and accountability with all of the action steps required to achieve this preparation. We acknowledge the courage, the valuing of one's self that is required for each step along the way.

The excellent article by Meg Jordan and John Livingstone (Jordan, 2013) "Coaching versus Psychotherapy in Health and Wellness: Overlap, Dissimilarities and Potential for Collaboration" is an essential resource for all coaches. The authors outline how coaching and therapy draw from the same research and some of the same approaches such as positive psychology and mindfulness. Both disciplines focus on client strengths and abide by professional conduct and ethics. However, they note the vast differences in training and client expectations. They point out that while coaches seek to evoke from their clients a way forward, "This evocative inquiry is an essential difference between coaching and psychotherapy or coaching and health education. Psychotherapists and health educators may be quicker to provide the client with information or interventions in the moment, since they are socially conditioned and educated to be expert resources and provide essential knowledge…"(Jordan, 2013).

Masterful Moment

Trusting in the Coaching Process

Coach someone well and long enough and you will enter with them into the realm of emotions. As you do so it is a time to stay centered and trust the coaching process. If you have been honoring your client's feelings all along, reflecting back to them your observation of their feelings as they arise, the entrance to a more profound level of feelings won't feel like such a big jump.

When my client contacts powerful feelings I can feel myself sitting up straighter, feet flat on the floor, shoulders relaxed, my breath a bit deeper. That physical centering helps to center me mentally and emotionally. I feel ready to respond quickly and easily in any direction.

What allows me to enter this realm with my client more easily are a couple of things. First, I have done a lot of my own work. Over the years, I've sought to grow personally and to heal from my emotional issues. That causes me to rarely be triggered by the emotions of others. It permits me to keep my own stuff out of the way. Secondly, I practice the ultimate Aikido move of the empath—I realize that when a person is emoting and unloading their pain, their anger, their fears, their sorrow—they are not dumping it on me. Instead I see me standing side-by-side with my client and helping them dump it, getting it out, but not dropping it on me.

Knowing that my client's baggage is their own, and that when they express it, it does not become my burden, allows me to stay right there with them as they feel what they feel. I don't have to tamp it down, minimize, or discourage my client from expressing their feelings. I hold the space with my client from a stance of compassionate detachment.

Because I am operating as a coach, I am not striving to delve deeper into my client's feelings. Instead we are seeking insight together. The emotional expression is relieving anxiety. Reflecting my client's feelings back to them is giving it a name, a handle my client can grasp and work with. As my client strikes upon an insight there is a relief that is experienced by both of us. Then we seek to make use of that insight and see how it applies to the client's life. Having seen this sequence come full circle helps me to trust the coaching process more every time I participate in it.

This chapter explored the way in which coaches can effectively work with their client's emotions without crossing the line into therapy. We looked at the necessity of addressing the affective side of things and how to do process coaching. We also explored the great role that emotions and their resultant feelings play in lifestyle decision making. We reviewed all the major aspects of motivational interviewing and how this can be integrated into the repertoire of a more masterful coach. Lastly, we demonstrated how to facilitate referral to mental health services when they are required.

In our next chapter we will take what we have learned and apply it to working with clients who either have or may want to prevent major health challenges. We will look at the continued importance of coaching presence as we delve into the more medical world without shifting into a treatment-oriented mindset. We'll explore the role of identification with one's illness and how coaches can empower their clients to take charge of their own health.

REFERENCES

Ford, M. (1992). *Motivating humans: Goals, emotions and personal agency beliefs.* Sage.

International Coach Federation. (2018, April). *Referring a client to therapy: A set of guidelines.* https://coachfederation.org/app/uploads/2018/06/Whitepaper-Client-Referral-June-2018.pdf

Jordan, M. L. (2013). Coaching versus psychotherapy in health and wellness: Overlap, dissimilarities and potential for collaboration. *Global advances in health and medicine,* 44-51.

Kimsey-House, K. K., Kimsey-House, L., Sandhal, P., & Whitworth, L. (2018). *Co-Active Coaching: The proven framework for transformative conversations at work and in life.* (4th ed.). Nicholas Brealey.

Lerner, J. S. (2015). Emotion and decision making. *Annual review of psychology,* 799-823.

Ley, D. J. (2014, February 24). Life coaches and mental illness. *Psychology today.* https://www.psychologytoday.com/us/blog/women-who-stray/201402/lifecoaches-and-mental-illness

Meinke, L. F. (2017, December). Top ten indicators to refer a client to a mental health professional. *International Coach Federation.* Coachfederation.org: https://coachfederation.org/app/uploads/2017/12/WhentoRefer.pdf

Miller, W. R. (2013). *Motivational interviewing: Helping people change (*3rd Ed.*).* Guilford Press.

Rollnick, S. M. (2007). *Motivational interviewing in health care: Helping patients change behavior.* Guilford Press.

Whitener, S. (2018, May 9). How your emotions influence your decisions. *Forbes coaches council.*

PART THREE

What to Do

Chapter 10—Covering the Whole Continuum

Covering the Whole Continuum
—Coaching Clients With Health Challenges

Wellness coaches work with clients who stretch across the whole continuum of health, from the healthy person who needs a plan to maintain their high level of wellness to the person challenged by a life-threatening disease. In fact, for most wellness coaches, the majority of their clients are already dealing with some kind of health challenge. It might be in the warning category, like a client with elevated blood lipid levels, or something as daunting as a recent diagnosis of heart disease, diabetes, COPD, or cancer.

Coaches may feel intimidated when faced with clients struggling with serious illnesses and health conditions. That is very understandable. The key is to realize that the coach does not need to have a treatment level of knowledge about an illness or condition to be effective at helping that person succeed at the lifestyle behavioral changes that will improve the course of that illness or condition.

Once coach and client are well grounded in the reality of the client's health challenge, the coaching process will be essentially the same regardless of the specific health challenge. You will proceed as a coach, not a treatment expert.

The evidence of the effectiveness of wellness coaching in working with health challenged clients is robust and accumulating fast. The best research guide at this time is the Compendium of the Health and Wellness Coaching Literature (Sforzo, 2017) and the Compendium of Health and Wellness Coaching: 2019 Addendum (Sforzo G. A., 2019).

The National Board for Health and Wellness Coaching was established to create standards and credentialing for our young profession. Here is the guidance of their Scope of Practice statement (National Board for Health and Wellness Coaching, 2020).

Scope of Practice for the Wellness Coach

While health and wellness coaches per se do not diagnose conditions, prescribe treatments, or provide psychological therapeutic interventions, they may provide expert guidance in areas in which they hold active, nationally recognized credentials, and may offer resources from nationally recognized authorities such as those referenced in NBHWC's healthy lifestyle curriculum. As partners and facilitators, health and wellness coaches support their clients in achieving health goals and behavioral change based on their clients' own goals and consistent with treatment plans as prescribed by individual clients' professional health care providers.

Simply put, the role of the wellness coach is to be the behavioral change expert, the client's ally, and not the treatment provider. Coaches may combine education about healthy lifestyles from evidence-based authenticated sources. Coaches must be careful to avoid providing direct advice in areas where they are not qualified as described above. Recently wellness coaches have found themselves in legal trouble in some states by offering nutritional guidance when they were not qualified to do so. It is important that wellness coaches are never placed in a position to do any kind of medical or psychological screening when they are not professionally qualified to do so.

The Coaching Mindset

When faced with a client who is challenged by lifestyle related illnesses and medical problems our challenge is to maintain our coaching mindset. The medical nature of our client's challenges seems to bring forth the need for diagnostic thinking. Stay client-centered and integrate the coaching with the work of the client's treatment team.

The client with a health challenge needs to be somebody's patient. Realizing that our client already has a treatment professional and/or a treatment team, we are free to be their coach. We can concentrate on building the coaching alliance and helping the client to fill the lifestyle prescription of lifestyle improvements that their treatment team has written for them. We can remain in our coaching mindset.

Getting on the Same Page—Your Client's Story

Connecting with your client begins with information and progresses into your client's story. It incorporates both how to be and what to do with your client. Much of a client's health and wellness information may be ascertained from the information they share in their welcome packet. Other information will have to be obtained through an effective coaching conversation. This is an opportunity to build the coaching alliance and help the client to see you as an ally, not just another health professional filling out forms.

Getting on the same page with your client in terms of the health challenges they are dealing with allows the coach to gain insight and understanding of their client's needs and experience. Convey your interest in your client as a person first, and as a medical patient second. You can use this as a way to build trust and establish your relationship with them as a caring ally.

Here are some important questions to explore with your new health-challenged client to build an understanding of who they are, what challenges they are facing, and how you can assist them.

- What are my client's known medical challenges?
  - Discover what your client's current health status is.
  - Do they know when their last medical evaluation was?
- When was the onset of their challenge(s)?
  - There are huge differences between the person with recent onset and someone with a long-term chronic condition.
  - Ask if there are multiple health challenges, and when and how they appeared.

- What treatments, medications, and self-testing or monitoring are they engaged in?
  - If you are not familiar with some of these factors, what more do you (the coach) need to know?
  - You may have to spend some time looking up information.
  - You don't need treatment-level knowledge about your client's health challenges, but the client/coach relationship will benefit from the experience of you both speaking the same language. For example, know what their A1C score means.

- What is your client's level of knowledge about their challenge(s) and treatments?
  - Medical patients who know more about their illnesses and treatments improve both medical compliance and outcomes (The Wellness Network, 2016).
  - How well informed are they about their illnesses and how to manage them?
  - Note that helping your client find the health education that they need may be part of the coaching you do in your upcoming sessions.

- What, specifically, have they been told by their medical treatment team that they need to change about their lifestyle (the lifestyle prescription)?

- What is their level of medical compliance?
  - Take note of this and see if improving this will become part of the co-created Wellness Plan.

- How fear-based is their motivation?
  - Is fear of increasingly poor health or premature death their sole motivator?
  - What other sources of motivation do they already have? You may be able to help them discover more.

- Are they participating in the coaching for themselves, or for others?
  - How volitional is their presence in coaching?
  - Are they coaching at the behest of their physician, their partner, or others?
  - This answer gives you an idea of how external their motivation is.
- To what do they attribute the cause of their health challenge?
  - Do they see the cause of their challenge as external or internal?
  - Is there anger towards themselves, their family, their culture, etc.?
  - This may be something important to work through later in coaching.
- How strongly do they believe that improving their lifestyle will help? (Self-efficacy.)
  - How confident are they that all of this wellness effort will be effective and helpful?
  - How confident are they that they are capable of being successful at lifestyle improvement?

During the Foundation Session encourage your client to educate you about their health challenge. Convey your curiosity in a helpful way that allows the client to feel empowered by sharing what they know with you. Inquire. This may also expose how little your client may actually know about their health challenge, its treatment, etc.

After the foundation session, ask yourself, "What else do I need to know?" You may need to take time to do some research to become better informed about your client's health challenge. You may be surprised to learn how lifestyle improvement may be quite relevant to their particular illness. Taking the time to look up a medication, a particular treatment, or a self-care protocol may allow you to connect much better with your client. Again, you don't have to have a treatment level of knowledge, but you do need to be able to relate to your client's experience.

How To Be—Connecting with Your Health Challenged Client

In both the foundation session and every subsequent session, it is important to check in with your client and get a feel for their current level of functioning. You are not doing a clinical assessment (unless you are a clinician and that's part of your role with this client). Knowing more about your client's immediate status may be vital to the success of your coaching session.

Explore with your client, through both questions and your observation, their immediate status regarding:

- Energy level. Energy levels are affected by many things, but for your health challenged client this may be a critical factor in the success of the session. To what degree is your client able to concentrate and stay focused? Have they been getting adequate rest? Ask them to rate their energy on a 1-10 scale if it seems helpful.

- Medications and treatment effects. Your client's energy and ability to concentrate, stay focused, and be insightful may be interfered with by their medication. Meds can also interfere with your client's ability to get adequate rest.

- Pain. Clients often minimize how severe their pain is. Yet, it can interfere tremendously with the coaching you are trying to accomplish if it is too intense. If your client is still in recovery from any kind of surgery, or has had some kind of medical treatment recently, inquire directly, with great compassion, about their immediate pain level. Pain can interfere with a client's perception of what has gone on in a session. It can cause them to miss what is being said, to not realize how empathic the coach is being, or to have a distorted recollection of what actually happened. Again, use a 1-10 scale for a rating.

- Reschedule the coaching session if any of these factors will be enough to make the experience unproductive or negative for your client.

Connecting with Your Health Challenged Client—Empathy

Usually when a coach expresses empathic understanding their client welcomes it. Trust is fostered and all is good. With the health-challenged client that is most often the case, but it may also be met with suspicion, resentment, or other surprising feelings. Empathy can be a touchy subject.

To deeply understand empathy, imagine that it is you who has experienced what your client has experienced. What would it be like for you to receive a diagnosis of a life-threatening illness? Your client is in a position where receiving genuine empathy can benefit them tremendously, but if they suspect that it is in any way disingenuous, the coaching relationship may be irreparably harmed.

Your client may also be in a place where they are so engulfed by their identification with their illness that the attempts by others at empathizing elicits, "How can you know what I'm going through?"

When you can relate to your client's experience through your own you can certainly empathize. You may also find a degree of self-disclosure to be valuable.

The caution, again, is to avoid expecting your client's experience to be just like yours. You may find that your illness/wellness journey with the same condition is very different from theirs.

Client Identification with Their Illness

We like to say that a coach listens to a person's story and helps them to realize that they are *not* their story. For the health-challenged client, their illness, conditions, or health experience is a huge part of their story. "Although most patients succeed in adjusting to their illness, some patients experience substantial difficulties which can negatively affect their physical and psychosocial functioning" (Morea, 2008). Much of that difficulty comes when a client has over-identified with their health challenge. "I am a diabetic." While this is true, how strongly does the person now see themselves through this lens? What effect could it have on someone's self-efficacy? How different it might be if they could say, "I'm a person challenged by diabetes."

In 2016 an international team of scientists sought to understand the concept of illness identity more deeply. They were inspired by the work of Erik Erikson on lifespan ego development (Erikson, 1968) and viewed identity "as the degree to which an individual integrates different self-assets into a coherent sense of self, and such a coherent sense of self translates itself into daily life and guides choices and values" (Oris, 2018). When we think about a sense of self-guiding choices and values and apply this to making lifestyle choices, illness identity could play a huge role.

Their work with adolescents dealing with Type One diabetes led this team to develop the Illness Identity Questionnaire and identify four illness identity dimensions or states: engulfment, rejection, acceptance, and enrichment (Oris, 2016).

> Rejection was related to worse treatment adherence and higher HbA1c values. Engulfment was related to less adaptive psychological functioning and more diabetes-related problems. Acceptance was related to more adaptive psychological functioning, fewer diabetes-related problems, and better treatment adherence. Enrichment was related to more adaptive psychological functioning (Oris, 2016).

Think of the term engulfment. Your client may be completely engulfed by their illness. This is "the degree to which chronic illness dominates a person's identity and daily life. Individuals completely define themselves in terms of their illness, which invades all domains of life, at the expense of other important self-assets" (Morea, 2008). If your client feels in the grip of such an illness, how hopeful are they? How disempowered do they feel that they cannot do anything about it?

For other clients, or perhaps for the same client as they move into a different illness identity dimension, their story becomes one of rejection. "…rejection refers to the degree to which the chronic illness is rejected as part of one's identity and is viewed as a threat or as being unacceptable to the self." The rejecting client avoids thinking or talking about their illness and they tend to neglect it, which results in poor treatment adherence. In TTM terms, we would say that this is a client in the pre-contemplation stage of change, far from the action stage.

The acceptance dimension of illness identity shows a client who is not overwhelmed by their chronic illness, does not deny it, but rather accepts that this is their reality. "Chronic illness plays a peripheral role in one's identity, besides other personal, relational, and social self-assets, and does not pervade all life domains" (Morea, 2008).

The fourth illness identity dimension, enrichment, provides the coach with a unique situation. Here the client has developed to where they frame their illness as an opportunity for growth. They see positive changes in themselves having taken place as a result of these negative developments in their health. "Such positive changes manifest themselves in different ways, including an increased appreciation for life, changed life priorities, increased personal strength, and more positive interpersonal relationships" (Tedeschi, 2004). Coaching a client who has reached this state of identity with their illness is a delight. Here the focus might be more upon maintaining good self-care and treatment adherence, and possibly upon continued improvement in health. Such a client might be motivated to work on disease reversal through lifestyle improvement such as we see with programs like that of Dean Ornish (Ornish, 2020).

Identity, Grief, and Loss—Astonishing Noncompliance

"My presumptive world was shattered." Those were the words one of our students uttered as she relayed what she had experienced when she received a diagnosis of a life-threatening disease. What happens to that coherent sense of self that Erickson spoke of when a sudden diagnosis or health event turns a person's world upside down? Much of our identity is our sense of who we are and where our life is headed. It is connected to our state of health. Seeing one's self as a strong, robust person with a bright future suddenly can be lost and replaced with a void easily filled by numbness, fear, and confusion. I would contend that one is impacted not only with the sense of engulfment that we spoke of above, but a profound sense of loss.

The sudden loss of our good health can initiate:

> ...a cascade of other forfeitures.... Depending on the nature of the illness, these losses may include comfort, sexual function, career, income, self-efficacy, freedom, cognitive function, intimacy, pride, joy, self-esteem, self-control, independence, mental health, hope, dignity, and certainty. In the most extreme cases, one illness may bring about all of these losses, sometimes over and over again in many ways (Jackson, 2014).

A loss of health is a loss, and losses have to be grieved. Grieving, however, is an incredibly individual process.

Elizabeth Kübler-Ross' often-used guide *On Death and Dying* (Elizabeth Kübler Ross Foundation, 2013) acquainted us with the five stages of grief (denial, anger, bargaining, depression, and acceptance). The Kübler-Ross' model, which I spoke of in my previous book, has come under considerable criticism (Konigsberg, 2011) that we should note. The model was not based upon empirical research, but on interviews that Kübler-Ross did with terminally ill patients. I have never viewed the model as one of stages that a bereaved person goes through in order. Grief is a very messy thing, not a series of steps that one progresses through to a final sense of completion and acceptance. While Kübler-Ross meant for her work to be descriptive, it has too often become prescriptive with people being admonished that these are stages that they need to go through.

We can, however, look at the so-called stages as a list of potential experiences, feelings, and emotions that a person in loss may feel. A very common observation by healthcare providers and wellness coaches is a person who has just experienced a loss of health (as we described above) express these emotional processes. The relevance is how their experience of loss affects their efforts (or lack thereof) at lifestyle improvement.

Frequently, the patient who experiences a health crisis receives instructions from their treatment team to make immediate lifestyle changes. They are directed to quit smoking, lose weight, adopt the Mediterranean Diet, reduce salt intake, manage stress, and more. They have every reason in the world to make these changes in order to improve their chances of returning to better health, or even of survival itself. What we often see is something I refer to as *astonishing noncompliance*.

The astonishingly noncompliant (or non-adherent) client, may be experiencing denial. They minimize the importance of their health event, downplay its seriousness, and do all they can to return to business as usual. Talking about the event or diagnosis becomes a forbidden subject, and the person may become quite defensive. They may be angry that this tragedy has befallen them, and understandably depressed about what has happened, and the state they are in. The idea of change has very little appeal. They seek the comfort of the familiar — including self-soothing habits such as smoking, overeating, etc. All of this happens in no particular order and becomes that person's unique way of coping. We might even theorize that their health crisis has been such a shock to their own identity that integrating it into that coherent sense of self is not yet possible.

For the healthcare provider, the coach, and for the client's loved ones, there is true astonishment at the client's lack of response to this call-to-arms for change. They need to follow their lifestyle prescription. There is greatly perceived medical urgency!

Coaching with clients around medical compliance and adherence to the lifestyle prescription is the place where Prochaska's *Readiness for Change*, Elizabeth Kübler-Ross' *Stages of Grief*, and Maslow's *Hierarchy of Needs* all intersect. A depressed client, in denial of the seriousness of their health crisis, may be much more likely to now be in precontemplation or contemplation at best, when it comes to making certain lifestyle improvements. They are in the midst of dealing with the effects of their health crisis, motivated primarily by Survival when we look at Maslow's Hierarchy of Needs (Maslow, 1998).

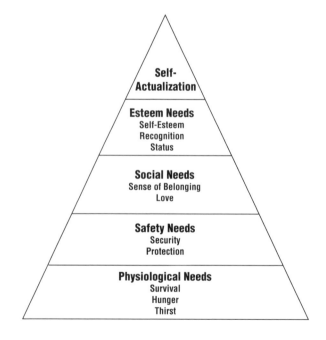

FIGURE 20—MASLOW'S HEIRARCHY OF NEEDS

Survival Level

Maslow's theory of motivation contends that as people get their needs met at the lower levels of the Hierarchy of Needs pyramid they naturally move on up to the higher levels (their being needs). When we encounter a client who fits the picture we are talking about here, do we acknowledge where they are in this hierarchy and do we help them get their needs met at that level? Or, do we demand immediate behavioral change just because the value and urgency of it is so great?

A brush with death, or even the news that such a threat is imminent, can automatically push us into survival mode. No matter at what level we were in getting our needs met on Abraham Maslow's hierarchy of needs, such an experience necessarily drives us down to the survival level. We feel profound threat to our physiological needs and safety needs. Our very physical existence is threatened. Life becomes about the real basics of survival: the next breath, food, water, shelter. It becomes about the basics of safety, feeling secure, going back to the familiar, whatever reassures us that we will be okay. It is no wonder that people going through such a thing may embrace the status quo, resist change, and psychologically minimize the threat that they perceive.

Such an experience may make it difficult for your client to meet their physiological and safety needs when they are encumbered by the initial experience of grief. Rising up through both the stages of readiness for change and the lower levels of the needs on Maslow's model may be delayed considerably if they are experiencing grief in the way Kübler-Ross describes.

Our first job is to help our client to feel like they have an ally, someone who supports them and has their best interests at heart. This helps meet their safety needs and even some of their social needs. We then need to check in with the client and see how they are doing at the survival level. Are they receiving the medical care they need? Is their living situation allowing them to cover the basics of shelter, food, and safety? Much of this comes down to how their health challenge affects their job security. It is their perception of their situation that counts. How do they perceive their health challenge as a threat to their livelihood? Do they fear losing their job, falling behind in production, having their business falter or fail? To what extent are they engaged in catastrophic thinking about all of this?

What is more frightening than to believe we are powerless? The threat to our very survival is there. If our client feels powerless to affect the course of their illness, then they wonder why should they make all the effort required to achieve lifestyle improvements. For our client to let go and trust in the change process their physiological and safety needs must be met. If they doubt this, they may give the appearance of compliance, but their probability of follow-through is questionable.

Beyond Survival

Beyond the very basics of survival, we can help our client get their needs met in the next two levels of Maslow's Hierarchy: social needs (sense of belonging, love) and self-esteem needs (self-esteem, self-worth, recognition, status). This is where coaching for connectedness plays a priceless role. We know that isolation is a real health risk and at this crucial time the presence and engagement of an extended support system can provide many benefits. Our client will need the help of others in many practical ways, but they will fare far better if they are getting the emotional support that comes with getting their needs for belongingness, acceptance, and compassion met. We, the helper, can only provide a very small part of the support needed.

Some of our best efforts may be to help the person we are working with find, develop, and expand sources of support in their lives. This person needs understanding, empathy, and support, not criticism and pressure to make lots of changes immediately. We need to encourage our client to ask for the support they need in the ways that they need to receive it. It might be beneficial for the client to connect with some people experiencing a similar illness who are further down the path of lifestyle improvement that they are beginning to contemplate.

Coaching to improve self-esteem allows the client to move through Maslow's pyramid to the next level. We all need to feel good about ourselves, to receive recognition and praise. When one is hit with a health challenge it may threaten how one views themselves. Helping the person to regain a sense of power and control in their life can also reclaim self-esteem. When we feel powerless to control events and circumstances in our lives, we can feel weak, vulnerable, and impotent. When we discover what we can actually do through our own lifestyle choices to affect the course of our illness for the better, we feel empowered and regain confidence and strength.

Ten Ways to Effectively Coach Clients Faced with a Loss of Health

When we encounter the person who has had a heart attack or other health challenge, we must remain coach-like. In each step consider that their readiness for change will be determined in part by their grief and where they fall in Maslow's hierarchy of needs. How quickly they move through the change process will be in part determined by past experiences and in part by the support they have in the present for change.

1. **Meet Your Client with Compassion, Not Judgment.**
   Pause and look at your client with a mind of compassion. Connect with what their experience is. Inquire and listen with the intent to understand their experience and take it in without judgement. Convey to them your empathic understanding of what they are going through.

2. **Acknowledge and Explore Your Client's Experience.**
   Ask them what it was like when they found out about their health challenge, diagnosis, or what is was like when they experienced this health event. Don't jump to solutions or start problem solving. Just listen, really listen. Reflect their feelings. Acknowledge what was and is real for them. Explore it with them and see if there isn't some fear that needs to be talked about in this session. You may be the first person that they feel they can truly open up with. Many people in this situation seek to protect their loved ones by downplaying the seriousness of their health challenge or minimizing their story about how frightening it was for them to experience.

3. **Don't Push, Stay Neutral in Your Own Agenda, and Explore More.**
   While it may feel like this person needs to take swift action and/ or feels tremendous urgency, be patient. Readiness for change grows at a different rate for each step of the journey.

4. Be Their Ally.

Help your client feel like they are not facing this alone. This helps meet their need for safety and some of their social needs. Does the client understand their health challenge? To what degree does the client understand and buy into the lifestyle changes recommended?

5. Address Survival First.

Do what you can to make sure your client is getting all the medical help and information they need. Explore their fears about maintaining income, job, career, business, and how it all will be impacted by their health challenge. Help them gain a sense of control and feel more safe and secure in all ways. Help them to see that they are not completely helpless and vulnerable, but that there are ways they can affect their situation.

6. Help Them Process the Loss.

Talking through the grief is very powerful. The loss of health is felt to the level that it is perceived. That perception will be part reality and part fear. Help your client to process their feelings, to give a voice to the part of them that is afraid. Accept their initial tendency to minimize but slowly help them feel safe enough to move through the other expressions of grief.

7. Help Them Form a Plan.

Even if it is very basic, help your client develop a plan for becoming healthy and well again and how to face their health challenge. Meet them where they are currently, remembering that preparing to take action is a vital readiness for change stage. What do they need to know? Having a plan will give them both hope and a sense of purpose and direction, a map to find their way out of their current situation. It is something to hold on to and builds a sense of esteem.

8. Coach for Connectedness.

If basic survival needs feel met the person can reach out to others and will benefit from a sense of belonging. Family and friends need to be inclusive and not critical. Support from co-workers is also extremely helpful. Coach your client through their own reluctance to asking for support. More formal support groups that allow your client to connect with others faced with a similar health challenge may be most valuable.

9. Build Self-esteem.
Recognize, acknowledge, and reinforce all progress. Help your client to exhibit greater self-efficacy because as they take charge of their health and their life, their self-esteem grows.

10. Nothing Succeeds Like Success.
Help the health-challenged person to take small steps to prepare for change and then experiment with actions where they are most ready. Build on these easier successes and leave the tougher challenges for later after confidence has been built.

Maslow reminds us that "growth forward customarily takes place in little steps, and each step forward is made possible by the feeling of being safe, of operating out into the unknown from a safe home port, of daring because retreat is possible" (Maslow, 1998). To emerge from that home port, our client needs to be in the process of working through their grief, they need to be moving up the spiraling stages of change, and what better way to set sail towards the unknown lands of change than with a good ally?

Coaching for Medical Compliance, Adherence, and Growth

Most clients who struggle with medical adherence to the lifestyle improvements recommended by their treatment team benefit from the structure that wellness coaching provides as well as the power of the coaching alliance. Clients are attempting to adopt new behaviors, shift from old unhealthy behaviors, and often reorganize their lives radically to do so. They benefit from partnering with their coach to co-create a well-designed plan that addresses their overall wellness and makes medical adherence a part of it. It becomes one area of focus in a fully integrated Wellness Plan.

Health and wellness coaches who work with clients challenged by chronic illness, and even more acute medical challenges are counted on to help with medical compliance and adherence. The clients themselves count on their coach as they may struggle with medical self-testing, taking medication properly, following up with appointments, exercising, and fulfilling the recommendations of their lifestyle change prescription. Coaches are also counted on by those providing healthcare services, insurance services, employee benefits, and more, to help manage costs through better overall patient compliance/adherence. This often becomes a large part of a wellness coach's job.

The job is valued because the need is great. First of all, when clients fail to take their medication properly, or don't manage their blood sugar levels well by doing their self-testing regularly, etc., they suffer. There are more hospitalizations, trips to the emergency room, more chance of complications, and more disease progression.

The Network for Excellence in Health Innovation calls improving patient medical adherence a $290 Billion Opportunity (Network for Excellence in Health Innovation, 2019). That is what is lost in U.S. healthcare spending each year due to poor medication adherence alone. The same source goes on to say that "when patients with severe or chronic conditions do not take their medications, the consequences can be extreme. Health outcomes are affected by non-adherence. For example, those with 80-100 percent adherence rates are significantly less likely to be hospitalized than their counterparts."

Lack of follow-through on medications, and other types of medical directives can be due to many different reasons, some of which are not the fault of the patient. Cost of prescriptions and supplies in the United States are often a huge factor. Inadequate instructions from the healthcare provider, a lack of self-care education, access to treatment and/or education, etc. accounts for about 31% of the reasons for poor adherence. The other "69% of the problem is behavioral, such as perceived benefits, poor doctor-patient relationship, medication concerns, or low self-efficacy" (Rhodes, 2017).

A note on terms:

Noncompliance—More of a refusal, a decision. Can be medical or lifestyle prescriptions. May be due to external causes (like cost). Not complying with medical directives, prescriptions, etc. Medical providers may take on a more judgmental way of viewing this.

Example: A patient decides that their physician is basing a prescription on inadequate information and decides not to take prescribed statins.

Non-adherence—not following through consistently with the treatment plan including the lifestyle prescription. Not adhering to the plan. More likely due to inabilities, difficulties executing the plan, etc.

These terms are sometimes interchangeable in the professional literature.

Research on health and wellness coaching has shown significant effectiveness in improving adherence and compliance (Thom, 2015). Unfortunately, most of the research narrowly focuses on one research variable, one aspect of medical compliance/adherence—medication adherence. In a study of the impact of health coaching with patients with poorly controlled diabetes, hypertension, and/or hyperlipidemia, "Health coaching by medical assistants significantly increases medication concordance and adherence." Ruth Wolever and Mark Dreusicke found that integrative health coaching led to an increase in medication adherence and that better adherence correlated with a greater decrease in HbA1c (Wolever, 2016).

Many of the studies appear to be concluding that it is the coaching methods that make a real difference in effectiveness. Wolever and Dreuskicke concluded that "Medication adherence requires underlying behavior skills and a supporting mindset that may not be addressed with education or reminders." So, though helpful, clients often need more than just text messages sent on their smartphones. Amanda Rhodes, in a 2017 article takes on a more corporate perspective in showing how coaching is beneficial to both patients and the pharmaceutical and healthcare companies that serve them. What her company's research emphasized was how client-centered the whole approach needs to be.

Patient-centered behavioral coaching is designed to help patients determine the way in which THEY believe they need to change their behaviors to achieve their goals. Patients who feel listened to are more comfortable with the care they receive and are more likely to adhere. (Rhodes, 2017).

Alliance Fosters Compliance

For the wellness coach and the clients they serve, the heart of the matter is the coaching alliance. As seen in the articles we've spotlighted here, adherence comes not from only medical directives. It comes from a client developing self-determined goals that they are motivated to pursue. It comes from having an ally to help them navigate through the barriers they face to achieving the high level of health and wellness that all people want. The coach may be well aware of the medical urgency for a client to quit smoking or take their medication properly. But as we've learned from all forms of behavioral change efforts the process, ultimately, must be self-directed. That is, the client has to see the value in making the change, be ready to make it, and have both a concrete plan of action and the support they need to achieve it. Tempting as it may be for the coach to become extremely directive and take over the action planning, they must remain in a true coaching mindset and be the ally the client needs in their own process. This requires patience, but as is often the case, patience pays off.

A Fully Integrated Wellness Plan

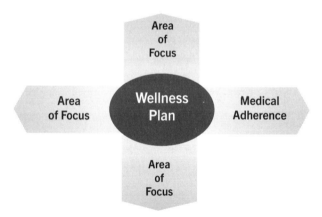

FIGURE 21—INTEGRATED WELLNESS PLAN

Co-creating a fully integrated Wellness Plan may well include medical adherence/compliance as an essential part of it. The client and coach work together to determine what the other areas of focus will be, based upon readiness for change theory, the directives of the lifestyle prescription, the values and interests of the client, and all of the exploration and assessment that the coach and client have done together. Other areas of focus could include such things as: attaining and maintaining a healthy weight, smoking cessation, achieving greater social support, and the like.

Areas of focus break down into goals and the specific action steps that the client will engage in to achieve those goals. All of this is co-created, not dictated.

In the focus on medical adherence, coach and client co-create a way to identify the specific behaviors that are needed to either develop or change. They then strategize the best action steps that will be an optimal starting point for success. They develop tracking strategies, so the client will know when they are taking medications on time, staying organized enough to follow through on medical appointments, etc. The key to tracking, whether done on phone apps, or good old pencil and paper is following up with accountability. Sending the coach information from an app, or text message, or simply reporting in at the next coaching appointment will help the client feel accountable to themselves to achieve what they want to get done.

Coach your client to determine what the components of medical adherence are for them. Don't just focus on medication. Help them see that their best strategy is to live the healthiest life possible in all dimensions of their wellness.

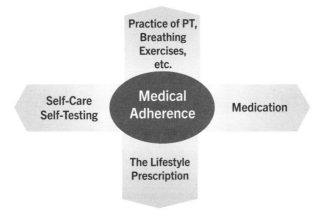

FIGURE 22—MEDICAL ADHERENCE PLAN

The coaching alliance also takes on a myriad of barriers, both internal and external, that get in the way of reliable medical adherence. Strategizing through barriers such as a lack of family or workplace support, checking out fearful assumptions (especially about side-effects), all increase the likelihood of success.

The Three R's of Medical Adherence/Compliance

Remember
Alarms/Reminders
Clients can use smart phones, etc. to set reminder alarms. Counting on other people for reminders is unreliable. Coaches should avoid supplying clients with reminders.

Associative Reminders—Combine the new behavior with an already established habit, such as taking medications when you brush teeth.

Record
Tracking methods. What works is the system your client will use. Calendars, notebooks, smartphone apps, etc.

Report
Coaching Accountability Agreements. Set up solid accountability agreements that your client will appreciate. Most often this is reporting in at the next coaching appointment but can also be sharing app information with the coach or sending emails or texts at agreed upon times.

Wellness Coaching and Lifestyle Medicine

The primary reason that health and wellness coaches are working with people with chronic illness, and many types of medical concerns is because there is overwhelming evidence that lifestyle affects the course of illness and health (American College of Lifestyle Medicine, 2019). More and more healthcare providers are shifting to a lifestyle-based view of practicing medicine. Lifestyle medicine practitioners prioritize, whenever possible, the use of "lifestyle interventions" as the first line of treatment. Lifestyle improvement is viewed not just as preventative, but also as curative and even preferential mode of treatment.

I often begin a presentation on lifestyle medicine by talking about two people whom we imagine to be identical demographically.

A Tale of Two People

Let's say our two people both experience being diagnosed with Type Two Diabetes at the same time. During the next two years Person A is the model patient, working diligently on losing weight, stopping smoking, following their recommended diabetic diet, getting better rest, and managing their stress better. They succeed in achieving very positive results in all of these areas in addition to being fantastic at their adherence to their medical treatment program. At the end of two years Person A will be moving toward thriving. Their disease will be managed well. They may even have made progress at diabetes reversal.

Then we look at Person B. They do not follow their diabetic diet well. They don't succeed at losing weight, stopping smoking, or any of the other lifestyle improvements that Person A accomplished. Their medical adherence was very poor throughout the subsequent two years. Now their health is failing. Their progressive disease has worsened and they may have developed serious co-morbidities. What was the difference between Person A and Person B? One word. Behavior.

Lifestyle medicine is showing us what *behavioral* health really is. As the field developed, there has been an increasing awareness that simply prescribing orders for their patients to get more exercise, improve their nutrition, manage their stress, etc., does not result often enough in actual behavioral change. Physicians, nurses, and other healthcare providers are studying wellness coaching in order to foster success in their patient's journey to wellness. Nurses, in fact, have developed a whole professional coaching association and body of literature (Dossey, 2013). Many experiments are also underway to integrate health and wellness coaches into the treatment teams of more and more healthcare delivery venues, including primary care. The wellness coach is a unique part of the treatment team in that they do not provide treatment. They do, however, help integrate the treatment plan with the Wellness Plan.

How the Wellness Plan Supports the Treatment Plan

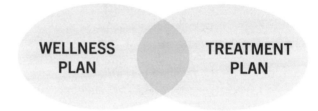

FIGURE 23—WELLNESS/TREATMENT PLAN

Any person under active medical care should have a treatment plan that was devised by their treatment team to enhance their health and wellbeing. The advent of patient-centered care and shared decision making (Barry, 2012), has helped open the gate for health and wellness coaching to enter into the medical world in a more congruent way. The inclusion of the patient in the treatment-planning process requires healthcare providers to integrate the attitudes, values, and behavior of their patient. Now, wellness coaching is being seen as the delivery mechanism for the behavioral change the treatment team desires to see.

The wellness coach can play an interconnecting role between the client and the treatment team. The nature and function of that role will vary depending upon the model being used. Since most healthcare providers do not have the time for actual coaching sessions, relying upon a coach to have greater contact time with their patient fills an important gap. Providing coaching can be an affordable option for a medical organization when the person doing the coaching does not have to be a high-level medical professional. The wellness coach is fully qualified to deliver these services.

Regardless of the model or the situation where an independent coach is working with a client and coordinating with the treatment team, communication is key. Whenever possible it is ideal for the coach's client to be the one communicating directly with the treatment team. Coaches need to check with their client about such communication and urge their client to do so consistently.

Integrating the Treatment Plan and the Wellness Plan

- Client provides the coach with all relevant medical information.
  - Current health challenges.
  - Current treatments, medication, etc.
  - Current lifestyle prescription.
- Coach and client explore client's level of:
  - Knowledge about their health challenges, treatments, medication, self-care, etc.
  - Medical compliance.
  - Medical adherence.
  - Together they explore the dynamics of:

    Success, failures, barriers.

    Work together for improvement.
- Coach and client co-create a Wellness Plan that includes:
  - Supporting the treatment plan.
  - Succeeding at filling the lifestyle prescription.
  - Creating areas of focus, goals, and action steps based upon the client's stage of behavioral change for each behavior.
  - Helping the client receive any health education they need about medical self-care, disease management, etc. This may include consulting with professionals such as diabetes educators, registered dieticians, physical therapists, and so on.
  - Creating a life of optimal health and well-being.

- Coach communicates with the treatment team primarily through their client, encouraging the client to communicate directly with their treatment team regarding:

  — Any changes in health.

  — The fact that they are participating in wellness coaching.

  — Any lifestyle practices that might affect treatment, such as relaxation training, diet, and exercise.

- Any direct communication between the coach and the treatment team needs to have written permission given by the client.

- The coach helps their client with organization, accountability, etc., improving attendance for medical appointments and management of medications, self-testing/self-care.

- The coach helps their client make best use of medical appointments (self-advocacy).

- Coaching can help the client report more accurately to the treatment team about changes in lifestyle (frequency of exercise, improvement in diet, sleep, etc.)

- Coaching can help the client bring better questions to their treatment team that will help them receive the care they need and learn more of what they need to know to be more effective in their own health improvement.

Coaching Through the Three Rs
of the Comeback Trail

Most of the work that the wellness coach will be doing with health-challenged clients pertains to chronic illnesses or conditions. At times, however, the coach may be working with a client whose life has been impacted by an acute health event. Heart attack, surgery, a tragic accident, or other sudden circumstances may set the client on a journey through a process of recovery, rehabilitation, and reclaiming their life. Even though it might seem that such health events would be dealt with in an entirely medical manner, there is still a lifestyle component, a behavioral aspect that affects a person's recovery.

Coaching Recovery from a Health Event

One might think that if there was excellent medical treatment little else would be needed for successful recovery. Yet, we see many cases where sterling treatment was followed by unsuccessful recovery. The difference is often in the way in which the patient goes about their recovery process. There is a surprising amount of behavioral change that the patient has to make for successful recovery.

- To what degree is the patient medically compliant/adherent?

  —Medication usage.

  --Medical self-care—wound care, self-testing, etc.

  —Follow-up appointments and treatments.

  —Practicing post-surgical breathing exercises.

  —Practicing range of motion exercises.

- What kinds of lifestyle changes have already been recommended and how well is the patient adhering to those recommendations?

  —Dietary changes—low salt, heart-healthy, etc.

  —Smoking (or other tobacco use) cessation.

  —Exercise recommendations.

- How successful is the client at getting adequate sleep and rest?

Each of these questions can, in an empathetic and compassionate coach-like way, be explored. Coaches can co-create with their clients' strategies to accomplish these behavioral tasks using the coaching methodology we have expounded upon earlier.

There is more to coaching someone through the process of recovery than just focusing on accomplishing behavioral change. There is also a role to play helping our client to process what has happened to them on a more emotional level. You may be the first person that the client trusts enough and believes is removed enough from the situation that they can open up and process their experience. Surgeries, even when anticipated, accidents, and other health events can be quite traumatic. Your client may need to share how terribly frightened they were, something they feel they can't really share with others. Talking through the experience allows your client to find relief from some of this anxiety. Processing it may help them understand the experience better and to integrate the change more completely.

There can also be a connector type of role for a coach to play as the client is going through recovery. Remember, most of the recovery process takes place at home, not in a hospital. Coaches can help clients to gather the support they need from others. Not all clients are surrounded by caring family and friends. Coaches can help clients to work through their reluctance to ask for the help they need. We can help our clients with very practical and logistical tasks such as finding and making use of available resources such as free rides to medical appointments, home nursing, and support services.

Coaching Your Client Through the Rehabilitation Process

To return to good health and prevent relapse, to restore adequate physical functioning, your client may require benefit from a course of rehabilitative therapy. Depending on your client's health challenge, this could be cardiac rehabilitation, pulmonary rehabilitation, physical therapy following joint surgeries, and a myriad of others.

The American Heart Association makes a convincing case for cardiac rehab, but sadly acknowledges how underutilized it is.

"Each year, roughly 915,000 Americans will have a heart attack and more than 30% will have a second and potentially fatal event."

1. Cardiac rehabilitation (CR) reduces the risk of a future cardiac event by stabilizing, slowing, or reversing the progression of cardiovascular disease (CVD).

2. Patients with other cardiovascular diseases such as valve repair and heart failure also benefit from a CR program, such as exercise rehabilitation.

Yet despite its clear benefits, CR remains underutilized, particularly among women and minorities. Only 14% to 35% of eligible heart attack survivors and 31% of patients after coronary bypass surgery participate in a CR program. The utilization rate for eligible Medicare beneficiaries is even lower; 12%. However, evidence clearly shows that the more sessions patients attend, the better their outcomes and the lower their risk for heart attack and mortality compared with those who do not participate (American Heart Association, 2011).

If our client sees the benefit of cardiac rehab but has not had it prescribed (a surprisingly common case), we can coach for self-advocacy to help our client get it ordered by their physician. If it has been prescribed but our client has not followed through, we can help them to weigh the pros and cons and help them move from contemplation to preparation and finally take the action of attending. This would be another application of our knowledge of TTM. We could use a motivational interviewing approach if our client shows ambivalence about this decision. We can help them process internal and external barriers to participation.

Once our client is participating in whatever type of rehabilitation they need, the coach can be of value in two more ways. They can help their client to attend rehab consistently by making it part of the client's Wellness Plan and setting up support and accountability. They can help their client to reframe their rehab experience as a new way of life (exercising regularly, etc.) instead of a temporary remedy.

Coaching for Reclaiming the Best of Your Client's Life

There is life before a health event and life after where we can see a list of abilities and activities that have been lost. Perhaps a process the client will truly value is to have a wellness coach help with sorting out, realistically, what is temporarily lost and what is permanently lost.

When we look at the temporary losses, we start to hear our client categorizing what they are ready, willing, and able to actively pursue reclaiming, and what they are not so sure about. When these activities are not fully pursued, they might never be reclaimed. A person may be left with avoidable incomplete range of motion, inadequate lung capacity, or other hardships.

Active Pursuit of Reclaiming Activities—Milestones

When your client is ready to pursue reclaiming activities that are important to them, they need a plan for how to accomplish this. With the coaching process and the support of an effective coach their chances of success are much greater.

Have your client make a list of all the activities that they have not been able to do since their health event. Have them list activities that they have only started to reclaim, such as walking. Go through the list together and explore what activities they feel are important to them, a real part of who they are, and discuss their motivation for reclaiming those activities.

Now, coach your client to help them prioritize what activities are most important and the most doable (cleared medically, and most likely to be successful) for them. Co-create a plan for reclaiming those activities using coaching methodology. Start small and set a series of milestones…short-term goals to shoot for that are, with concerted effort, achievable.

- Reclaiming goal—hiking in the mountains again.
  - —Milestone #1—walking around the block.
  - —Milestone #2—walking a mile on flat ground.
  - —Milestone #3—hiking to the top of a very small hill.
  - —Milestone #4—hiking to the top of a challenging hill.

Coach through the barriers, both internal and external, to achieve these milestones. To reach each milestone there will be many action steps along the way. Co-create these with your client, helping them see a motivational link between what they are doing and the goal they want to achieve. Encourage them to carefully track their behavior as they work on each action step. Set up helpful accountability to support their follow-through. Help them find additional support in their family and community of friends, co-workers, etc. In other words, use the well-established coaching process and celebrate every bit of success. (Refer to Appendix C: The Milestones Reclaiming Tool.)

Exploring Your Client's Reclaiming Reluctance

It's not unusual for a client to show reluctance about reclaiming activities that have been set aside by a health event, or to have mixed feelings about doing so. There are definitely realistic fears but there are also fears based upon inadequate information, misleading information, and assumption. There is an old saying that **FEAR** is an acronym for False Evidence Appearing Real. We all tend to fill-in-the-blank with either assumptions or whatever information we have. Discover with your client where their information came from. Was it from a valid source? Would looking into a second medical opinion be advisable? What does your client know about their prognosis? Have they asked their treatment team the specific questions that they need answered? Sometimes treatment professionals are reluctant to give much of a prognosis or may be unable to, for that particular case. This leaves the client less confident about how to proceed with reclaiming certain activities. They may be told only ten percent of patients can do this activity again. Why not be part of that ten percent?

You can also help your client to process their fears on a more emotional level. Perhaps the coaching experience is their best opportunity to safely name and explore what their fears are. Empathically explore the nature of their fears. What are they afraid would happen if they tried to reclaim these activities? Just processing their concerns with a coach may help the person to release some of their anxiety and worries.

Self-Efficacy and Support During Reclaiming

It would be only natural for a significant health event to have a strong effect on a person's self-efficacy. Explore with your client how confident they are that making the effort to reclaim these activities will be worth the effort, and how confident they are that they can succeed at it. Help them build on small successes (mastery experiences) while receiving acknowledgement from you, their coach. Help them find inspirational examples of people with whom they identify being success at reclaiming (modeling). Use what you know about building self-efficacy to help your client reclaim the best of their life. (Chapter Six)

Reclaiming the activities that make life healthy and enjoyable is much more difficult when one receives a lack of support to do so, or worse yet, discouragement. Again, coaching for connectedness is vital to your client's success. You may want to co-create with your client ways they can get the support they need. This may involve helping them to work through their own reluctance around asking for the help they need.

Thrive Don't Just Survive

Don't assume that your client with a serious health challenge is not thriving, or capable of thriving. Tremendous medical progress has been made allowing people with illnesses to not only manage their disease or condition well, but to thrive in most areas of their lives. Cancer treatments have come a long way and we see people going into remission and becoming cancer free. Lifestyle change may play a key role in prevention of reoccurrence. People with heart disease, diabetes, and many other health challenges are finding that they can affect the course of those illnesses in a positive way through lifestyle improvement and proper disease management.

We are even seeing success at disease reversal for heart disease and diabetes. These programs have substantial evidence backing them up (Ornish, 2020) (Esselstyn, 2016) (Hallberg, 2019). When patients commit to a disease reversal program, they launch on a journey that affects all aspects of their lifestyle. Coaches are beginning to be utilized to help people succeed with the behavioral changes and the concerted effort these programs require. At Tufts Medical Center, their coaching program has achieved impressive results. For people with Type Two Diabetes "one in three have achieved remission, with blood sugar levels at or near normal without medication" (Dansinger, 2020).

The well-respected program for heart disease reversal developed by cardiologist Dean Ornish, focuses on four important areas of one's life:

- What you eat.
- How you manage stress.
- How much you move.
- How much love and support you have.

Achieving success with this lifestyle medicine approach might be enhanced by participants having the support of a coach. If your client is interested in enrolling in a program like this, your work with them could be most helpful.

Whole Person Wellness Approach

There has been a seismic shift in the world of healthcare. I'm not referring to the application of the business model, but rather to the combined awareness that we must work with, care for, and treat the whole person.

We see this in the shift toward:

- Patient-centered care.
- Shared decision making.
- Integrative medicine.
- Lifestyle medicine.
- Population health.
- Social and environmental determinants of health.
- Wellness coaching, to help people accomplish the lifestyle improvements that will help them attain and maintain optimal health and wellbeing.

Health and wellness coaching is beginning to be applied in a wide variety of clinical settings, and this will only grow. The models being used and the experiments underway are too numerous and fluid to illustrate here. As coaches integrate their work into these settings it is key that they remember their role as professionals is to assist their clients in lifestyle behavioral change. Your job as a coach is to help people to grow. You are not staging an intervention upon your client's life. You are not treating them. You may be working side-by-side with treatment professionals, but remember, you are the behavioral change expert. Keep returning to the foundations of coaching. The client's agenda is the agenda. That you are there to evoke their inner wisdom. Even as you become a masterful coach, keep your own self-vigilance alive and your ego out of the way. Realize the valuable role you have to contribute and coach on!

Backing Away from the Cliff: A Wellness Coaching Case Study

Imagine that you are a 47-year-old man named "Jim" who works in the shipping department of a food manufacturing company. Though you were diagnosed with diabetes 14 years ago you have received virtually no education on how to manage your disease.

Though your job isn't particularly stressful, you're stuck on the 4 p.m. to midnight shift. Other than the movement on the job, you get very little exercise. Snack foods and sodas from the vending machine at work tempt you. When you come home late at night, before bedding down at two in the morning, you eat.

Weighing in at just over 240 lbs. (+108 kg.), you have become hypertensive (blood pressure = 170/90). As your disease has progressed it has precipitated other conditions such as hyperlipidemia and diabetic neuropathy. Recently you were diagnosed with gout. You're now using an insulin pump, frequently depleting your daily maximum dosage of 130 units. You are frustrated that the pump would not let you administer any more even though you have tried. Your doctor recently informed you that you are going into renal failure. Fortunately, your wife is very supportive of you improving your health.

Imagine what you, as Jim, are feeling right now. You've had no education about how to manage your illness or what to eat. What do you need to learn? What do you need to change? This was the situation when this real-life client was referred to a registered dietician who was trained as a health and wellness coach. This description of Jim and his sessions with the coach whom we will call "Laverne" comes from her case study.

Coaching With Laverne

Laverne is a registered dietician and wellness coach working for a disease management company that contracts with Jim's workplace. In her first session with Jim, Laverne clearly communicated that she would be primarily doing two things. The first was working as a dietitian to provide him with the information that he would need to improve his health conditions. The second was working as a coach to help him incorporate that information into his lifestyle, focusing on lasting eating behavior change.

> *I explained that this was a nutrition program that would be customized according to the rate at which he learned and adopted new habits. I told him that the helping relationship/ alliance we were creating, including the fact that I was there to help him accomplish what he wanted...not what I wanted him to accomplish. I shared the fact that we would not be making overnight changes but changing just two or three things every time we spoke. I reassured him that this ap-*

proach was designed not to overwhelm but to help him move towards eating healthier without feeling tortured or stressed out about it.

My client expressed his appreciation that I was working with him. I communicated that there was hope as long as he had the desire to do this. I expressed that I sensed his strong motivation to change and that it was very possible to achieve his targets for improving his diet.

After setting the foundation for their coaching—becoming clear about what coaching is, how it works, going over ethical and professional guidelines, and how the coach would be integrating her role as a dietician with that of a coach—Laverne began exploring Jim's current situation and the way that he had been eating.

Our initial appointment revealed his diet was very high in sugar, fat, sodium, and caffeine. These came from highly processed and refined foods like potato chips, corn chips, regular sodas, white bread, hot dogs, bologna, bacon and sausages, ice cream. He consumed quite a bit of meat/animal protein and fruit juices and reported that he ate out often. He did not drink nearly enough water (currently just about 8-16 oz. per day).

Co-Creating the Relationship

Fortunately, Jim was at a point where he was very open to coaching. He was already motivated to make changes to his eating behavior so co-creating a relationship was not difficult.

This client was very open and transparent, and I was totally myself: open and sincere. I showed genuine concern for his current health situation. I also showed empathy that he never received a formal nutrition education.

I could tell that his mindset was where he knew he needed to do something to change his current picture. I shared with him that I was there to work with him as an ally. I communicated that he was not going to have to figure things out on his own. I did not have a judgmental or condescending tone. Even though his diet was very unhealthy, I did not make him feel terrible about it. I focused on the future and the how we could, as we work together, make a difference not in just the way he ate but also in his lab values.

I listened to the client's agenda. He told me that even though he has been a diabetic for many years he never took it seriously. He said he was ready to make changes to the way he ate. I listened to his concerns. One of his main concerns was that he did not want to go into renal failure and end up on dialysis. His doctor told him he had protein and blood in his urine, and they wanted to draw labs to check his kidney function. I mirrored and reinforced his feelings and concerns and also his belief that he could do something now that could make a difference. I asked open-ended questions that allowed the client to express himself.

Wearing Two Hats

Laverne very skillfully integrated her consultative role as a registered dietician with that of a coach. We often refer to this in coaching as wearing two hats, and Laverne wore them both well.

> *The client was open and motivated to make changes even before we spoke. He was also very teachable. I provided insight regarding the foods that he was eating and described exactly how they were causing the very symptoms he wanted to avoid. We made a powerful connection because Jim was able to see how foods he was eating were affecting various aspects of his health. For example, how high sodium and caffeine intake and an absence of produce affected his blood pressure; large amounts of orange juice, enriched grains and regular sodas and their effect on his blood sugar. I was able to clearly break down the relationship between the foods he chose and his health.*

> *I told him the things that were happening to him were real. But I emphasized that just as they were real, so would be the results we could achieve in working together on changing the current picture. When he heard these things and how powerful they were, he was even more ready to make changes. We talked about how his behavior became a pattern and explored the idea that we can create new patterns through repetition and reprogramming. We discussed how his desire for change would literally fuel our efforts in getting change to occur.*

One of the most rewarding things about wellness coaching is when we see our clients succeed at making concrete behavioral change. Through a combination of consultation and education that showed Jim what he needed to change, and a coach approach that helped him discover how to make those needed changes happen, great progress was made in very measurable terms. In Laverne's case, her licensure as a registered dietician allowed nutritional consultation to be included in her scope of practice. A coach without this qualification would need to refer their client to a qualified nutritional consultant and then work with their client about how to implement the nutritional recommendations.

Specific Changes that Occurred (Mental, Behavioral, Lifestyle)

By our third session my client had lost 8 lbs. He was no longer drinking 18 oz. of orange juice in the morning. He actually stopped drinking juice and was drinking water and eating fresh fruit instead.

He became aware that there was a very direct relationship between what he was eating and the numbers he was getting from his blood pressure monitor and blood glucose meter. He also became aware that changing the things he ate, even though he ate that way all his life, was not as hard as he previously thought, especially when you look at it in smaller chunks.

He was eating a high fiber breakfast and had not had sausages, cheese, etc., at breakfast since out first session. He increased his water intake to 48 oz. per day and had 2 healthy snacks throughout the day. Our goal for water intake is still 64 oz. per day. We are still slowly building up to that amount.

We had a challenge when he was hungry when he came home after work late at night. In reviewing his food recall we found that he was going too long without eating in the evening. We included an additional snack during that time so he wouldn't be famished when he got home.

As a result of the changes he made, he reported that his blood pressure was down, (he checked it every day) and he was no longer maxing out on his daily insulin dosage. We will be evaluating his labs to determine if, over time, any improvement to his renal function occurs.

In the short amount of time that Laverne spent coaching Jim, a real shift took place. Jim was able to reverse years of self-defeating health behaviors and, we might say, pull himself back from the medical cliff he was heading towards. This coach helped her client avert a real health crisis.

As Laverne concluded her case study she reflected upon where she and her client needed to go from this point forward. She especially considered how to make these *improvem*ents in lifestyle last.

I realize that there is some fear-based motivation (fear of renal failure for example). I am aware that this will not help with lasting change. My future sessions with him will include helping him to be aware of this and the fact that this will wear off. To help deal with this, I plan to help him stay connected with what he truly wants for his health and connect fundamentally with the foods that can help give him what he wants as opposed to focusing on what he doesn't want. I will communicate the fact that change doesn't occur overnight but is a process that we work towards every day.

I will continue the coaching process, troubleshooting and addressing challenges and helping him work on the important principles of eating behavior change that will set him up for success. I will also watch for signs of spiraling back to earlier stages of change, help him realize what is happening and coach him towards going forward.

What the Coach Learned

I learned that many times people want to make changes but feel as though, for one reason or another, they cannot. It seemed like before we spoke, healthy eating was a mystery to him. A mystery he never bothered to find out about or solve. As I broke down the mystery into terms he could understand, you could actually feel his self-efficacy rising. It was almost tangible. I also learned that he didn't want to be sick. He didn't want to go in the direction of kidney failure. He needed some help in finding the right path to better health that would work for him. I found it really sad that after all these years he never received any information as to how to manage his condition.

Not all clients are going to be as motivated and engaged in the Action Stage of Change as our client Jim was. Coaches often must draw upon all that they know about coaching and behavioral change theory (e.g., The Transtheoretical Model of Behavioral Change) to coach each client effectively. What Laverne was able to do so well was to combine her nutritional expertise with her high level of competency as a wellness coach to help her client make such dramatic changes in lifestyle and health. Case studies, being only in the form of the written word, do not easily convey all that took place that allowed for success. The coach's own style and presence, her ability to empathize and show unconditional positive regard, even when presented with a client engaged in an almost self-destructive pattern of eating, was a real key to unlock the door of change. It was not just the nutritional knowledge she conveyed to her client; it was the way that she was doing so that allowed him to be open to it, absorb it, and apply it. We can also speculate that the supportive role of the client's wife was essential, as well as the support of friends and co-workers. The coach was able to offer the client vital information, a relationship of support and a coaching methodology to carry it out.

Masterful Moment

How confident do I feel about coaching people with health challenges?

How does my own history or family history around health challenges affect my coaching?

Am I attracted to developing a specialization in coaching people with a specific health challenge?

Coaching for a Lifetime of Wellness

Long-term success at lifestyle improvement, keeps coming back to the concept of sustainability. Diets are inherently unsustainable, as are crash exercise programs. When our client finds a new way of living that they can maintain for the rest of their life they have greater health, joy and wellbeing. As we support client autonomy throughout the coaching process, we enable our client's independence and equip them to remain successful long after coaching is complete.

The question of making health behavior change endure is a puzzling one. What little we know comes down to essentially a shift in self-concept and community support. A lifetime of wellness may very well require helping our client to think of themselves in a new way. Helping them employ or develop the support they need to make their lifestyle changes last is a process that the coach will be engaged in with their client from the first coaching session to the last. To do so well will require you to know who you are, how you need to be, and what you need to do to be a true ally for your client's wellness.

Masterful Moment

The masterful coach is continually seeking out new knowledge. What do you see as your way forward in developing your own craft as a wellness coach? Where is your own growing edge? What self-awareness have you gained and what has it taught you about yourself as a coach? How dedicated are you to your own personal growth, actualizing your own potential as a human being?

We cannot of course save the world, because we do not have authority over its parts. We can serve the world though. This is everyone's calling; to lead a life that helps.

—**Barry Lopez**

REFERENCES

American College of Lifestyle Medicine. (2019). Evidence Overwhelmingly Support Efficacy of Lifestyle Medicine. Retrieved from American College of Lifestyle Medicine: https://www.lifestylemedicine.org/Scientific-Evidence

American Heart Association. (2011, May). Retrieved from Cardiac Rehabilitation Putting More Patients on the Road to Recovery: https://www.heart.org/idc/groups/heart-public/@wcm/@adv/documents/downloadable/ucm_449722.pdf

Arloski, M. (2014). Wellness Coaching for Lasting Lifestyle Change, 2nd Ed. Duluth, MN: Whole Person Associates.

Barry, M. J. & Edgman-Levitan, P. A. (2012). Shared decision making—pinnacle of patient-centered care. New England journal of medicine , 780-781.

Dansinger, M. (2020). Lifestyle Coaching Program for Diabetes and Weight Loss. Retrieved from Tufts Medical Center Endocrinology, Diabetes and Metabolism: https://www.tuftsmedicalcenter.org/patient-care-services/departments-and-services/endocrinology/clinical-care-services/lifestyle-coaching-program-for-diabetes-reversal

Dossey, B. H. (2013). The Art and Science of Nurse Coaching: The Provider's Guide to Coaching Scope and Competencies. American Nurses Association.

Elizabeth Kübler Ross Foundation. (2013, August 16). On Death and Dying. Retrieved from Elizabeth Kübler Ross Foundation: https://www.ekrfoundation.org/5-stages-of-grief/on-death-and-dying/

Erikson, E. (1968). Identity: Youth and crisis. W.W. Norton & Company.

Esselstyn, C. (2016). Homepage. Retrieved from Dr. Esselstyn's Prevent & Reverse Heart Disease Program: http://www.dresselstyn.com/site/

Hallberg, V. M. (2019). Reversing type 2 diabetes: A narrative review of the evidence. Nutrients, 766.

Jackson, K. (2014, July/August). Grieving chronic illness and injury—Infinite losses. Retrieved from Social Work Today: https://www.socialworktoday.com/archive/070714p18.shtml

Konigsberg, R. (2011, January 29). New Ways to Think About Grief. Retrieved from Time Magazine: http://content.time.com/time/magazine/article/0,9171,2042372,00.html

Maslow, A. (1998). Toward a Psychology of Being, 3rd Ed. Wiley.

May, M. G. (2005). Am I Hungry: What to Do When Diets Don't Work. Nourish Publishing.

Morea, J. M. (2008). Conceptualizing and measuring illness self-concept: 571 a comparison with self-esteem and optimism in predicting fibromyalgia adjustment. Research in Nursing and Health, 563-575.

National Board for Health and Wellness Coaching. (2020). NBHWC Scope of Practice. Retrieved from NBHWC National Board for Health and Wellness Coaching: https://nbhwc.org/wp-content/uploads/2019/04/FINAL-NBHWC-Health-Wellness-Coach-Scope-of-Practice-4_15_19.pdf

Network for Excellence in Health Innovation. (2019). Improving Patient Medication Adherence: A $290 Billion Opportunity. Retrieved from NEHI Network for Excellence in Health Innovation: https://www.nehi.net/bendthecurve/sup/documents/Medication_Adherence_Brief.pdf

Oris, J. S., Luyckx K., Rassart J., Gourbert L., Goossens E., Aters S., Art S. , Vandenberghe J., Westhovens R. & Moons P. (2016). Illness Identity in Adolescents and Emerging Adults With Type 1 Diabetes: Introducing the Illness Identity Questionnaire. Diabetes Care, 757-763. Oris, L. L. (2018). Illness Identity in Adults with a Chronic Illness. Journal of Clinical Psychology Medical Settings, 429-440.

Ornish, D. (2020). *Ornish Lifestyle Medicine*. Retrieved from https://www.ornish.com

Ornish, D. (2020). *Undoit With Ornish*. Retrieved from Ornish Lifestyle Medicine: https://www.ornish.com/undo-it/

Ory, M. L. (2010). The Science of Sustaining Health Behavior Change: The Health Maintenance Consortium. The American journal of health behavior, 647-659.

Rhodes, A. (2017, June 29). The Impact of Behavioral Coaching on Adherence. Retrieved from DTC Perspectives: http://www.dtcperspectives.com/impact-behavioral-coaching-adherence/#_edn3

Sforzo, G. A. (2019). Compendium of health and wellness coaching: 2019 addendum. Amercian journal of lifestyle medicine.

Sforzo, G. A. (2017). Compendium of the health and wellness coaching literature. American journal of lifestyle medicine.

Tedeschi, R. G. (2004). Posttraumatic growth: conceptual foundations and empirical 604 evidence. Psychological inquiry, 1-18.

The Wellness Network. (2016, October 4). The impact of knowledge: Patient education improves compliance and outcomes. Retrieved from The Wellness Network: https://www.thewellnessnetwork.net/health-news-and-insights/blog/the-impact-of-knowledge-patient-education-improves-compliance-and-outcomes/

Thom, D. W. (2015). The impact of health coaching on medication adherence in patients with poorly controlled diabetes, hypertension, and/or hyperlipidemia: a randomized controlled trial. Journal American board family medicine, 38-45.

Wolever, R. A. (2016). Integrative health coaching: a behavior skills approach that improves HbA1c and pharmacy claims-derived medication adherence. BMJ open diabetes reserach & care.

NBHWC
Health and Wellness Coach
Scope of Practice

Health and wellness coaches work with individuals and groups in a client-centered process to facilitate and empower the client to develop and achieve self-determined goals related to health and wellness. Coaches support clients in mobilizing internal strengths and external resources, and in developing self-management strategies for making sustainable, healthy lifestyle, behavior changes. While health and wellness coaches per se do not diagnose conditions, prescribe treatments, or provide psychological therapeutic interventions, they may provide expert guidance in areas in which they hold active, nationally recognized credentials, and may offer resources from nationally recognized authorities such as those referenced in NBHWC's Content Outline with Resources. As partners and facilitators, health and wellness coaches support their clients in achieving health goals and behavioral change based on their clients' own goals and consistent with treatment plans as prescribed by individual clients' professional health care providers. Coaches assist clients to use their insight, personal strengths and resources, goal setting, action steps, and accountability toward healthy lifestyle change.

How to Coach with the Readiness for Lifestyle Change Tool

The Readiness for Lifestyle Change Tool integrates the concepts of behavior change developed by James Prochaska and associates—Transtheoretical Model of Behavior Change—with the research of Albert Bandura and his Social Cognitive Theory. This tool is designed to help a coaching client to become more aware of how ready they are to begin working on lifestyle improvement and to identify critical factors that will influence those efforts.

The best use of this tool takes place when it is used during a coaching session as a way to facilitate a conversation about change. It is not designed to be used as a homework tool that a client would fill out on their own. Explaining the tool to your client and then working with them in a coach-like way will allow them to explore the factors in their life that support and inhibit change taking place.

The score that the total yields is, frankly, not as important as the process that takes place in the coaching conversation. The total score is intended to give a rough estimate of readiness but is by no means precise. It can be used to help the client realize how ready they are for making changes or not.

Perhaps the greatest value of the tool is identifying areas to focus on for continued coaching. For example, if the client rates statement #9 as a 2—Rarely True—then you can explore what aspects of their environment do not support them in their life, and you can co-create strategies for garnering more support.

The best application of this tool is when a client has an area of their life that they want to improve but are feeling ambivalence or conflict about moving forward. The tool is excellent for helping them to weigh the pros and cons of change.

Here are some guidelines and tips for using this tool:

- Use the Readiness for Lifestyle Change Tool in a live coaching session, not as homework.

- Use the tool to facilitate a coaching conversation.
- You will not want to use this tool with every client for every area of their life that they want to improve. Save it for the areas where there is more ambivalence or conflict. Use it strategically.
- Take your time. Allow for greater exploration and coaching as you move through each item.
- When you have completed the 10 items with your client and totaled the score, explore what they learned or realized by completing it.
- Then review the highest rated items first. Acknowledge how these items support change.
- Then go on to explore the lower rated items. These will help you and your client to identify areas for growth and focus for coaching.

Readiness for Lifestyle Change Tool ©

Use this tool after you have created your well life vision and have decided the areas of your life you want to focus on. Explore each statement and rate how true each statement is for you at this time in your life and then talk about them with your coach. Once you rate yourself for each statement add your numbers together to gain your total readiness score.

Please respond to each question answering:

1= Not True   2 = Rarely True   3 = True at Times   4 = Mostly True   5 = Very True

1. I am ready to make the changes needed in this area of my life.

    1   2   3   4   5

2. I am capable of making the changes needed in this area of my life.

    1   2   3   4   5

3. I believe making these changes will improve my life.

    1   2   3   4   5

4. I have the resources and opportunities that will make this change possible.

    1   2   3   4   5

5. Making the changes in this area of my life is worth the time and effort.

    1   2   3   4   5

6. I have the time to invest in making the changes needed in this area of my life.

    1   2   3   4   5

7. I am excited to make the changes in this area of my life.

    1   2   3   4   5

8. I am fearful of what might happen if I do not make the changes in this area of my life.

    1   2   3   4   5

9. My environment supports me in making the changes in this area of my life.

    1   2   3   4   5

10. I am choosing to make the changes to this area of my life.

    1   2   3   4   5

Please total your score for this section _____

Readiness—What does your score mean?

40–50 pts.   **High level of readiness**

Congratulate yourself. You are ready to make the changes you have selected!

30–39 pts.   **Moderate level of readiness**

What would help you be more ready to make the changes you have selected?

20–29 pts.   **Low level of readiness**

Explore your answers with your coach. What is holding you back?

Below 20 pts.   **Very low level of readiness—**

Explore your answers with your coach. Consider choosing another focus area.

Based on the behavior change theories of James Prochaska and Albert Bandura.

Wellness Mapping 360°© Tools for Living Well Copyright 2021 Real Balance Global Wellness Services, Inc.

Milestones Reclaiming Tool

(2021 Real Balance Global Wellness Services, Inc.©)

Historically milestones have been used to "mark the way" to one's destination, often letting you know how far you have come, or how far you have to go. Use this tool to help you understand where you are at on your own reclaiming journey. Let the tool help you to be successful at getting to your destination.

List (in no particular order) personally meaningful/fun/rewarding activities that you used to do, but have not done since your health challenge appeared. (Examples: dancing, bicycling, having sex, visiting friends, air travel)

1. _____

2. _____

3. _____

4. _____

5. _____

6. _____

7. _____

Choose 5 activities from the list above and rate them using the following scale.

Activity 1. _____

Doing this activity again is:

MEDICALLY NOT POSSIBLE   A BIG CHALLENGE   POSSIBLE   DOABLE   LIKELY

How important is reclaiming this activity as part of your life?

NOT IMPORTANT	SOMEWHAT IMPORTANT	IMPORTANT	VERY IMPORTANT	EXTREMELY IMPORTANT

Notes: _____

_____

Activity 2. _____

Doing this activity again is:

MEDICALLY NOT POSSIBLE   A BIG CHALLENGE   POSSIBLE   DOABLE   LIKELY

How important is reclaiming this activity as part of your life?

| NOT IMPORTANT | SOMEWHAT IMPORTANT | IMPORTANT | VERY IMPORTANT | EXTREMELY IMPORTANT |

Notes: _____

_____

Activity 2. _____

Doing this activity again is:

MEDICALLY NOT POSSIBLE   A BIG CHALLENGE   POSSIBLE   DOABLE   LIKELY

How important is reclaiming this activity as part of your life?

| NOT IMPORTANT | SOMEWHAT IMPORTANT | IMPORTANT | VERY IMPORTANT | EXTREMELY IMPORTANT |

Notes: _____

_____

Activity 3. _____

Doing this activity again is:

MEDICALLY NOT POSSIBLE   A BIG CHALLENGE   POSSIBLE   DOABLE   LIKELY

How important is reclaiming this activity as part of your life?

| NOT IMPORTANT | SOMEWHAT IMPORTANT | IMPORTANT | VERY IMPORTANT | EXTREMELY IMPORTANT |

Notes: _____

_____

Activity 4. _____

Doing this activity again is:

MEDICALLY NOT POSSIBLE   A BIG CHALLENGE   POSSIBLE   DOABLE   LIKELY

How important is reclaiming this activity as part of your life?

NOT IMPORTANT	**SOMEWHAT IMPORTANT**	**IMPORTANT**	**VERY IMPORTANT**	**EXTREMELY IMPORTANT**

Notes: _____

_____

Activity 5. _____

Doing this activity again is:

MEDICALLY NOT POSSIBLE   A BIG CHALLENGE   POSSIBLE   DOABLE   LIKELY

How important is reclaiming this activity as part of your life?

NOT IMPORTANT	**SOMEWHAT IMPORTANT**	**IMPORTANT**	**VERY IMPORTANT**	**EXTREMELY IMPORTANT**

Notes: _____

_____

Now, identify your **three most important and doable activities**.

1) _____

2) _____

3) _____

Next list the first activity that you want to reclaim and **identify three or four milestones** that will be "markers" or steps along the way towards completing the task of doing that activity again.

Example:

1. Activity = bicycling

Milestones along the path toward my goal:

    1. Get in good enough shape to receive my doctor's permission to bicycle

2. Finish at least half of my rehabilitation sessions
3. Find someone to bicycle with and set a date

Example:
2. Activity = hiking in mountains
Milestones along the path toward my goal:
    1. Walk around the block.
    2. Walk one mile on flat ground.
    3. Hike to top of a small hill.
    4. Hike to top of challenging hill.

My Milestones

Activity #1

Milestones along the path toward my goal: Date I reached it!

1. _____   _____

2. _____   _____

3. _____   _____

Notes: _____

_____

_____

Activity #2

Milestones along the path toward my goal: Date I reached it!

1. _____   _____

2. _____   _____

3. _____   _____

4. _____   _____

Notes: _____

_____

_____

Activity #3

Milestones along the path toward my goal: Date I reached it!

1. _____   _____

2. _____   _____

3. _____   _____

Notes: _____

_____

_____

Real Balance Coaching
Self-Observation Tool©

CLIENT:_____ DATE OF SESSION:_____

COACH:_____

Listen to a recording of a client session observing your coaching for:
- Consistency.
- What you did well.
- Where you missed opportunities to use your coaching skills.
- How you could coach better?
- Rate your coaching on a 1–3 scale or note N/A for what did not apply to this session.

1 = SATISFACTORY	2 = ADEQUATE – could be better	3 = MISSED OPPORTUNITY or needs to improve	N/A = Not applicable – did in session

The coach:

Creates and sustains rapport with client.	1	2	3	N/A
Demonstrates effective use of voice, e.g., tone and language.	1	2	3	N/A
Reflects or summarizes what the client communicates to ensure clarity and understanding, thereby demonstrating the ability to actively listen to the client.	1	2	3	N/A
Assists the client to create new awareness and assists the client to explore beyond current thinking.	1	2	3	N/A
Questions are consistently open-ended.	1	2	3	N/A
Demonstrates a balance between questions and active listening skills.				
Creates or allows space for silence, pauses, or reflection.	1	2	3	N/A
Partners with the client to manage the time and focus of the session.	1	2	3	N/A
Responds in a consistently non-directive manner.	1	2	3	N/A

Elicits and explores client's thoughts, what the client knows and wants to know before making suggestions or offering resources.	1	2	3	N/A
Asks permission to share resources, to make suggestions, or to switch hats.	1	2	3	N/A
Shares observations of client's behavior and speech in a neutral and helpful way.	1	2	3	N/A
Notices, acknowledges, and explores the client's emotions, energy shifts, nonverbal clues or other behaviors.	1	2	3	N/A
Invites the client to generate ideas about how they can move forward and what they are willing or able to do.	1	2	3	N/A
Partners with the client to design doable action steps and accountability measures that integrate and expand new learning.	1	2	3	N/A
Acknowledges and supports client autonomy in the design of goals, actions, and methods of accountability.	1	2	3	N/A
Explore session focus in sync with client's stage of readiness for change.	1	2	3	N/A

In this session what strengths of yours did you demonstrate? What do you believe you did well?

_____

_____

_____

_____

_____

_____

_____

Reviewing this session, what are some areas that you feel you need to work on? What are some areas that you recognize as needing growth?

_____

_____

_____

_____

_____

WholePerson

Whole Person Associates is the leading publisher
of training resources for professionals who empower people to
create and maintain healthy lifestyles by addressing
stress management, wellness promotion,
and mental health issues.

Proud member of IBPA — Independent Book Publishers Association